ATS-106 ADMISSION TEST SERIES

This is your PASSBOOK for...

Certified Dental Technician (CDT)

Test Preparation Study Guide Questions & Answers

NLC®

NATIONAL LEARNING CORPORATION®

COPYRIGHT NOTICE

National Learning Corporation

212 Michael Drive, Syosset, NY 11791
(516) 921-8888 • www.passbooks.com
E-mail: info@passbooks.com

PUBLISHED IN THE UNITED STATES OF AMERICA

PASSBOOK® SERIES

THE *PASSBOOK® SERIES* has been created to prepare applicants and candidates for the ultimate academic battlefield – the examination room.

At some time in our lives, each and every one of us may be required to take an examination – for validation, matriculation, admission, qualification, registration, certification, or licensure.

Based on the assumption that every applicant or candidate has met the basic formal educational standards, has taken the required number of courses, and read the necessary texts, the *PASSBOOK® SERIES* furnishes the one special preparation which may assure passing with confidence, instead of failing with insecurity. Examination questions – together with answers – are furnished as the basic vehicle for study so that the mysteries of the examination and its compounding difficulties may be eliminated or diminished by a sure method.

This book is meant to help you pass your examination provided that you qualify and are serious in your objective.

The entire field is reviewed through the huge store of content information which is succinctly presented through a provocative and challenging approach – the question-and-answer method.

A climate of success is established by furnishing the correct answers at the end of each test.

You soon learn to recognize types of questions, forms of questions, and patterns of questioning. You may even begin to anticipate expected outcomes.

You perceive that many questions are repeated or adapted so that you can gain acute insights, which may enable you to score many sure points.

You learn how to confront new questions, or types of questions, and to attack them confidently and work out the correct answers.

You note objectives and emphases, and recognize pitfalls and dangers, so that you may make positive educational adjustments.

Moreover, you are kept fully informed in relation to new concepts, methods, practices, and directions in the field.

You discover that you are actually taking the examination all the time: you are preparing for the examination by "taking" an examination, not by reading extraneous and/or supererogatory textbooks.

In short, this PASSBOOK®, used directedly, should be an important factor in helping you to pass your test.

Certified Dental Technician

INTRODUCTION

WHAT IS CERTIFICATION?

Certification is the professional standard in dental laboratory technology. It is the means for the dental profession, the dental laboratory industry and all others with an interest to identify dental technicians and dental laboratories that have demonstrated their technical qualifications and their commitment to maintaining high standards in dental technology.

The CDT Program is a national program. Since certification is voluntary, it represents not only compliance with documented standards, but also a special personal commitment to quality and professionalism. Each Certified Dental Technician (CDT) has met industry standards of required knowledge and applied skills through the successful completion of examinations and compliance with continuing technical education requirements.

The CDT is recognized and endorsed by the National Association of Dental Laboratories (NADL), the American Dental Association (ADA) and the American College of Prosthodontists (ACP). It also receives outstanding support and participation from U.S. military services. The CDT program is accredited by the American National Standards Institute (ANSI).

For those engaged in the practice of dental technology, certification offers:

- An incentive to achieve proficiency;
- Criteria for maintaining continuing education;
- Improved career opportunities;
- Peer recognition; and
- Enhanced professional visibility.

For the dentist-client, certification offers:

- Reinforced credibility through the use of credentialed support services;
- A means to encourage proficiency and advancement; and
- An enhanced source of specialized expertise.

Finally, for the dental patient, dental technology certification could establish:

- An enhanced perception of the value of dental services; and
- A positive perception of (and respect for) the career of dental technology.

WHAT ARE THE SKILL STANDARDS?

The goal of the CDT examination is to measure competence or the mastery of a predetermined body of knowledge and the skills deemed to represent the successful, professional-level practice of dental technology. To become a CDT, a technician must demonstrate their knowledge and applied skills, from start to finish in their chosen specialty, in the manufacturing procedures common in contemporary practice. There are five (5) specialties currently recognized by the NBC: Ceramics, Complete Dentures, Crown & Bridge, Orthodontics and Partial Dentures.

THE EXAMINATIONS

The examinations given by the NBC are the result of years of continuing development. Questions on the tests originate with technicians in the field. Special task forces (comprised of technicians, laboratory owners, educators and dentists) have been appointed by the NBC to conduct regular reviews, revisions and updates of the exams. All examination content is also subject to ongoing statistical analysis based on actual usage of exam questions, as well as peer review, to ensure relevance to current practices in dental technology.

From the official announcement for educational purposes

The following examinations must be passed successfully to become a Certified Dental Technician (CDT):

- The Comprehensive examination (or the Recognized Graduate examination, if eligible);
- The Written Specialty examination; and
- The Practical examination (in the same specialty area as the Written Specialty examination — Ceramics, Complete Dentures, Crown & Bridge, Orthodontics or Partial Dentures.)

Candidates may sit for the examinations in any order but all three (3) exams must be passed within four (4) years of the date that the first exam was passed.

About the CDT Examinations

TYPES OF EXAMINATIONS

The goal of the CDT examinations is to measure competence or the mastery of a predetermined body of knowledge and the skills deemed to represent the successful, professional-level practice of dental technology. To become a CDT, a technician must demonstrate their knowledge and applied skills, from start to finish in their chosen specialty, in the manufacturing procedures common in contemporary practice.

Each of the CDT examinations must be passed successfully within a four (4) year period to become a CDT. The candidate must test in the same specialty area for both the Written Specialty exam and the Practical exam. The examinations may be taken in any order that the candidate desires.

THE COMPREHENSIVE EXAM

Current Recognized Graduates may waive the Comprehensive exam requirement, but all other technicians must pass the Comprehensive exam before being recognized as a CDT. The Comprehensive examination is the measure for basic knowledge in history, ethics and the five specialties.

The Comprehensive examination is a written multiple-choice test. There are 160 questions on the exam, covering basic dental laboratory knowledge: oral anatomy, tooth morphology, materials science, health & safety, fundamental theory and terminology across the five specialties tested by the NBC (Ceramics, Complete Dentures, Crown & Bridge, Orthodontics & Partial Dentures).

Candidates have up to two and one-half (2 ½) hours to complete the examination; they may use as much or as little of this time as they require.

THE WRITTEN SPECIALTY EXAM

The Written Specialty examination is a requirement for all CDT candidates. This exam tests a candidates' knowledge in his or her chosen specialty area.

The Written Specialty examination consists of eighty (80) multiple-choice questions. Each test item will consist of a question and four (4) possible answers, or an incomplete statement and four (4) possible ways to complete the statement. Of the four possible responses, the candidate must select the best answer.

Candidates have up to seventy-five (75) minutes to complete the examination; they may use as much or as little of this time as they require.

THE PRACTICAL EXAM

The Practical examination is a requirement for all CDT candidates. This exam is a hands-on exam that requires candidates to demonstrate their competence over a range of procedures normally associated with their respective specialties. The Practical exam consists of preliminary procedures that must be performed in each candidates' own laboratory prior to the exam date, plus specific steps which must be completed under the observation of three (3) NBC Examiners at the exam site.

Approximately four (4) weeks prior to the exam date, the NBC Headquarters provides candidates with detailed instructions, molds from which the candidates must work and a Candidate Identification Number. At the same time, candidates also receive contact information for the host facility so that they may contact the host about any specific needs they may have, including site soldering capabilities, available air hand piece connections or borrowing equipment (like porcelain ovens). Whenever possible candidates should bring their own equipment and supplies to the exam site (including porcelain furnaces and pumps, if needed). If this is impossible, candidates must contact the host facility for permission to borrow the items needed. Neither the NBC nor the exam host site can guarantee borrowed equipment or materials. Every effort will be made to assist candidates, but there is no guarantee that the equipment will function correctly (or as candidates are accustomed to) nor that time-critical equipment will be available only to a specific candidate.

On the day of the exam, candidates usually arrive at about 7:00am for an exam that begins at 7:50am. Candidates must bring all preliminary work with them; verify their identity; locate the work station that displays their Candidate Identification Number; and set up their materials and equipment. The NBC Lead Examiner will give candidates specific information and instructions that must be followed. These instructions will be simple, but are extremely important. Candidates should be certain that they understand all instructions before proceeding with their examination.

Candidates have exactly five and one-quarter hours (5 1/4) to complete the examination; they may use as much or as little of this time as they require. During this period, the NBC Examiners will carry out specified security measures, monitor candidate work, and begin the evaluation of the work done in the preliminary portion of the examination.

EXAM PREPARATION & SAMPLE QUESTIONS

Preparation for all of the exams leading to certification begins at the technician's first introduction to the dental laboratory. Ideally, it is a process of training, education, experience and continuing education. In publishing this manual, the NBC is not attempting to teach the competencies measured by its examinations, but rather to give technicians an understanding of examination content, structure and procedures so that they may approach the CDT examinations with the confidence that comes from knowing what to expect.

It is to each candidate's advantage to plan, work and practice towards the completion of their examinations. Candidates are required to complete all parts of their examinations without aid or assistance. Exam Proctors and NBC Examiners may not define terms or answer questions relating to the exam content.

The Comprehensive examination is designed to measure the equivalent of a formal education in dental technology. Technicians who have on-the-job training or have learned their skills in other settings may find it useful to review certain parts of various publications to broaden and/or reinforce their understanding of dental technology. Technicians who have experience in narrowly defined specialty areas should use the preparation for this examination as an opportunity to broaden their theoretical knowledge to include fundamental concepts throughout the range of specialties offered in dental laboratories.

For the Comprehensive exam and the Written Specialty exams, candidates will be instructed to read the question carefully, select the best answer and then locate the question number on the answer sheet and mark the circle corresponding to the answer selected. The questions on the examinations will look something like this:

QUESTIONS:	ANSWERS:
1. The cutting edge of an anterior tooth is called: A. Buccal B. Incisal C. Distal D. Mesial	1. ○A ●B ○C ○D
2. What is measured by a Boley gauge? A. Inches B. Centimeters C. Millimeters D. Picas	2. ○A ○B ●C ○D

Practical exam candidates should bring their preliminary work and should be prepared to complete all other portions of their examination on-site. The Practical examinations are designed to enable candidates to display their abilities by performing representative procedures that are normally associated with practice in their respective specialties. Day-to-day, hands-on experience is the primary preparation for this portion of the examination. In addition, candidates may be able to improve their comfort and performance levels by studying, planning and practicing the required steps prior to the exam date. To help reduce the stresses on exam day, candidates should ensure their readiness by bringing or arranging for their equipment and materials and by having a plan. It may also help candidates to realize that time management is important.

Examination Content & Tasks

COMPREHENSIVE EXAM

The Comprehensive examination is the measure for basic knowledge in history, ethics and the five specialties. The following subjects may be included:

GENERAL

I. Anatomy & Terminology
- A. Occlusion
- B. Tooth morphology
- C. Basic anatomical landmarks
- D. Identification of muscles

II. Materials
- A. Gypsum products
- B. Waxes
- C. Resins
- D. Metals
- E. Acids

III. Fabrication & Technique
- A. Handling and interpretation of dental prescriptions or work authorizations
- B. Use and maintenance of laboratory equipment
- C. Weights, measures and chemical symbols used in the laboratory

IV. The Dental Profession & the Dental Laboratory Industry
- A. History
- B. Industry and professional organizations
- C. The CDT program
- D. Dental laws and ethics
- E. Infection control

CERAMICS

I. Impression Materials
- A. Types
- B. Handling
- C. Custom trays

II. Cast Fabrication
- A. Materials-physical properties
  - 1. Stone
  - 2. Epoxy and resins
  - 3. Refractory materials
- B. Techniques
- C. Dies
  - 1. Types of preparations
  - 2. Margins
  - 3. Undercuts
  - 4. Alternatives to die preparation
  - 5. Spacers-lubricant
  - 6. Die stability

III. Articulation
- A. Types
- B. Uses
- C. Occlusal registrations
- D. Mounting procedures (face bows, etc.)

IV. Materials- Types, Physical Properties & Handling Characteristics
- A. Gypsum
- B. Waxes
- C. Metals, alloys and solder
- D. Porcelain, composites and stains
- E. Separating materials
- F. Fluxes and anti-fluxes
- G. Alcohols
- H. Acids and pickling agents
- I. Wetting agents
- J. Wax solvents
- K. Abrasives and polishing agents
- L. Laboratory gases
- M. Investments/refractories

V. Pattern Design & Fabrication
- A. Abutments
- B. Pontics
- C. Connectors

VI. Spruing
- A. Sprue materials
- B. Techniques
  1. Venting
  2. Resevoirs
  3. Auxiliary sprues
  4. Direct and indirect
  5. Specific gravity

VII. Investing
- A. Technique
  1. Hygroscopic
  2. Thermal
  3. Vacuum pressure
- B. Handling

VIII. Wax Elimination (Burnout)

IX. Casting & Divesting
- A. Centrifugal
- B. Induction
- C. Vacuum
- D. Weights and measures
- E. Divesting

X. Finishing Procedures for Substructures

XI. Soldering — Pre- & Post-porcelain

XII. Tooth Morphology/Terminology
- A. Anatomy
- B. Occlusal function
- C. Contour

XIII. Metal Preparation
- A. Aluminum oxide blasting
- B. Cleaning (steam, ultrasonic)
- C. Oxidation

XIV. Opaque Technique
- A. Spraying
- B. Brush
- C. Instruments

XV. Porcelain Application
- A. Internal modifications
- B. Contouring
- C. Buildup and condensing

XVI. Firing Technique
- A. Opaque
- B. Body
- C. Add-on
- D. Stain and glazes

XVII. Finishing

COMPLETE DENTURES

I. Oral Anatomy & Physiology
- A. Muscles
- B. Anatomical landmarks
- C. Occlusion

II. Impressions — Materials & Handling
- A. Preliminary impressions
- B. Custom trays
- C. Final impressions

III. Casts — Materials & Fabrication

IV. Trial Denture Bases

V Occlusal Rims

VI. Articulators & Articulation of Casts

VII. Prosthetic Teeth
- A. Selection (types and materials)
- B. Arrangement

VIII. Denture Base Fabrication

IX. Flasking
- A. Gypsum materials
- B. Mold preparation

X. Packing & Processing Dentures
- A. Materials
- B. Casting methods
- C. Processing equipment and techniques
- D. Remount and corrections
- E. Removing cast from dentures

XI. Finish & Polish Denture Base
- A. Equipment (lathes, handpieces)
- B. Abrasives and polishing agents
- C. Techniques & procedures

XII. Post-delivery Laboratory Procedures
- A. Rebase
- B. Reline
- C. Repairs

CROWN AND BRIDGE

I. Impression Materials
- A. Types
- B. Handling
- C. Custom trays

II. Cast Fabrication
- A. Materials
- B. Techniques
- C. Dies

III. Articulation
   A. Types
   B. Uses
   C. Occlusal registrations
   D. Mounting procedures (face bows, etc.)

IV. Materials- Types, Physical Properties & Handling Characteristics
   A. Gypsum
   B. Waxes
   C. Metals, alloys and solder
   D. Composites and resins
   E. Separating materials
   F. Fluxes and anti-fluxes
   G. Alcohols
   H. Acids and pickling agents
   I. Wetting agents
   J. Wax solvents
   K. Abrasives and polishing agents
   L. Laboratory gases
   M. Investments/refractories

V. Pattern Design & Fabrication
   A. Abutments
   B. Pontics

VI. Spruing
   A. Sprue materials
   B. Techniques

VII. Investing

VIII. Wax Elimination (Burnout)

IX. Casting & Devesting

X. Finishing Procedures
   A. Full cast (finishing and polishing)
   B. Substructure (finishing)

XI. Soldering
   A. Technique
   B. Investing
   C. Devesting

XII. Tooth Morphology/Terminology
   A. Anatomy
   B. Occlusal function
   C. Contour

ORTHODONTICS

I. Orthodontic Appliances — Fixed
   A. Types
      1. Passive
      2. Active
      3. Functional
   B. Identification
   C. Function

II. Orthodontic Appliances — Removable
   A. Types
      1. Passive
      2. Active
      3. Functional
   B. Identification
   C. Function

III. Materials
   A. Wire
   B. Plastics
   C. Waxes

IV. Clasps
   A. Types
   B. Functions and uses

V. Auxiliaries
   A. Springs
   B. Screws
   C. Coil spring (open and closed)
   D. Labial bows
   E. Other (bands, etc.)

VI. Acrylics
   A. Vacuum formed
   B. Sprinkle technique
   C. Dough pack (cold cure)
   D. Light cured
   E. Heat cured
   F. Finishing and polishing

VII. Soldering/Welding
   A. Materials
   B. Equipment
   C. Finishing and polishing

VIII. Appliance Repair
   A. Replace auxiliaries
   B. Acrylic repair
   C. Metal repair
   D. Infection control

IX. Study Casts
  A. Pouring
  B. Triming
  C. Measurements
  D. Infection control
X. Equipment
  A. Hand instruments
  B. Bench equipment
  C. Maintenance and safety
XI. Splints

PARTIAL DENTURES

I. Components of Framework
  A. Major connectors (types and functions)
  B. Minor connectors (types and functions)
  C. Direct retainers
  D. Indirect retainers
  E. Rests
  F. Denture bases
  G. Vertical stress eliminators
II. Cast Fabrication
  A. Impression materials and handling
  B. Cast materials and handling
  C. Diagnostic casts
  D. Master cast preparation
III. Articulation of Casts
  A. Jaw relations records
  B. Hand articulation-plasterless articulators
IV. Survey & Design
  A. Surveyors (path of insertion)
  B. Technique for surveying
  C. Clasp selection
  D. Major connectors
  E. Beading outline
  F. Relief for acrylic retention
V. Refractory Cast Fabrication
  A. Refractory materials (qualities)
  B. Duplication
VI. Preparation of Refractory Cast - Transfer Design
VII. Fabrication of Partial Dentures
  A. Pattern application
  B. Spruing
  C. Investing
  D. Burnout
  E. Casting (types)
  F. Retrieval of casting
  G. Altered (split) cast technique
  H. Finishing and polishing of metal framework
  I. Selection and arrangement of artificial teeth
  J. Fabrication of resin saddles
VIII. Repairs & Additions
IX. Wrought Metals

WRITTEN SPECIALTY EXAM

The Written Specialty examination is the measure for specific knowledge in the specialty area selected by the candidate. The following breakdown outlines some of the subjects that may be included:

CERAMICS

This examination is similar to the Crown & Bridge examination with the addition of specific concentration on porcelain and porcelain-fused-to-metal restorations and materials.

COMPLETE DENTURES

Subject matter includes oral anatomy; occlusion; the physical properties and correct handling of materials; fabrication procedures and techniques; and the design and use of restorations and appliances normally associated with the Complete Denture specialty.

CROWN & BRIDGE

Subject matter includes tooth morphology; occlusion; the physical properties and correct handling of materials; fabrication procedures and techniques; and the design and use of restorations normally associated with the Crown & Bridge specialty.

ORTHODONTICS

Emphasis in this examination is on the design and function of orthodontic appliances, including materials and fabrication techniques, terminology and occlusion.

PARTIAL DENTURES

Subject matter includes the theory of survey and design; physical properties and correct handling of materials; fabrication procedures and techniques; and the design and use of restorations and appliances normally associated with the Partial Denture specialty.

PRACTICAL EXAM

The Practical examination is a hands-on exam that requires a candidate to demonstrate their competence over a range of procedures normally associated with their chosen specialty. The Practical exam consists of preliminary procedures that must be performed in the candidate's own laboratory prior to the examination date, plus specific steps which must be completed under the observation of the NBC Examiners at the exam site.

Materials and specific instructions for the examination will be mailed to candidates approximately four (4) weeks before the exam date. The candidate instruction booklet should be read by each candidate immediately upon receipt. All of the instructions should be followed carefully and completely.

The Practical examination candidate instruction booklet for each specialty is made up of four (4) parts:

1. A list of materials to bring to the exam site.
2. Instructions for pouring casts and other procedures which must be done in advance of the exam date.
3. A complete list of the procedures you will be asked to perform at the examination.
4. The standards that will be applied in evaluating the examination and the specific items that will be graded.

The NBC uses both the US Postal Service and parcel delivery services. This makes it imperative that all candidates maintain a correct, current street address and mailing address on file with the NBC Headquarters. If a candidate relocates and fails to notify the NBC on a timely basis, resulting delays and/or the cost of new exam materials will be the candidate's responsibility.

HOW TO TAKE A TEST

You have studied long, hard and conscientiously.

With your official admission card in hand, and your heart pounding, you have been admitted to the examination room.

You note that there are several hundred other applicants in the examination room waiting to take the same test.

They all appear to be equally well prepared.

You know that nothing but your best effort will suffice. The "moment of truth" is at hand: you now have to demonstrate objectively, in writing, your knowledge of content and your understanding of subject matter.

You are fighting the most important battle of your life—to pass and/or score high on an examination which will determine your career and provide the economic basis for your livelihood.

What extra, special things should you know and should you do in taking the examination?

I. YOU MUST PASS AN EXAMINATION

A. WHAT EVERY CANDIDATE SHOULD KNOW

Examination applicants often ask us for help in preparing for the written test. What can I study in advance? What kinds of questions will be asked? How will the test be given? How will the papers be graded?

B. HOW ARE EXAMS DEVELOPED?

Examinations are carefully written by trained technicians who are specialists in the field known as "psychological measurement," in consultation with recognized authorities in the field of work that the test will cover. These experts recommend the subject matter areas or skills to be tested; only those knowledges or skills important to your success on the job are included. The most reliable books and source materials available are used as references. Together, the experts and technicians judge the difficulty level of the questions.

Test technicians know how to phrase questions so that the problem is clearly stated. Their ethics do not permit "trick" or "catch" questions. Questions may have been tried out on sample groups, or subjected to statistical analysis, to determine their usefulness.

Written tests are often used in combination with performance tests, ratings of training and experience, and oral interviews. All of these measures combine to form the best-known means of finding the right person for the right job.

II. HOW TO PASS THE WRITTEN TEST

A. BASIC STEPS

1) Study the announcement

How, then, can you know what subjects to study? Our best answer is: "Learn as much as possible about the class of positions for which you've applied." The exam will test the knowledge, skills and abilities needed to do the work.

Your most valuable source of information about the position you want is the official exam announcement. This announcement lists the training and experience qualifications. Check these standards and apply only if you come reasonably close to meeting them. Many jurisdictions preview the written test in the exam announcement by including a section called "Knowledge and Abilities Required," "Scope of the Examination," or some similar heading. Here you will find out specifically what fields will be tested.

2) Choose appropriate study materials

If the position for which you are applying is technical or advanced, you will read more advanced, specialized material. If you are already familiar with the basic principles of your field, elementary textbooks would waste your time. Concentrate on advanced textbooks and technical periodicals. Think through the concepts and review difficult problems in your field.

These are all general sources. You can get more ideas on your own initiative, following these leads. For example, training manuals and publications of the government agency which employs workers in your field can be useful, particularly for technical and professional positions. A letter or visit to the government department involved may result in more specific study suggestions, and certainly will provide you with a more definite idea of the exact nature of the position you are seeking.

3) Study this book!

III. KINDS OF TESTS

Tests are used for purposes other than measuring knowledge and ability to perform specified duties. For some positions, it is equally important to test ability to make adjustments to new situations or to profit from training. In others, basic mental abilities not dependent on information are essential. Questions which test these things may not appear as pertinent to the duties of the position as those which test for knowledge and information. Yet they are often highly important parts of a fair examination. For very general questions, it is almost impossible to help you direct your study efforts. What we can do is to point out some of the more common of these general abilities needed in public service positions and describe some typical questions.

1) General information

Broad, general information has been found useful for predicting job success in some kinds of work. This is tested in a variety of ways, from vocabulary lists to questions about current events. Basic background in some field of work, such as sociology or economics, may be sampled in a group of questions. Often these are principles which have become familiar to most persons through exposure rather than through formal training. It is difficult to advise you how to study for these questions; being alert to the world around you is our best suggestion.

2) Verbal ability

An example of an ability needed in many positions is verbal or language ability. Verbal ability is, in brief, the ability to use and understand words. Vocabulary and grammar tests are typical measures of this ability. Reading comprehension or paragraph interpretation questions are common in many kinds of civil service tests. You are given a paragraph of written material and asked to find its central meaning.

IV. KINDS OF QUESTIONS

1. Multiple-choice Questions

Most popular of the short-answer questions is the "multiple choice" or "best answer" question. It can be used, for example, to test for factual knowledge, ability to solve problems or judgment in meeting situations found at work.

A multiple-choice question is normally one of three types:

- It can begin with an incomplete statement followed by several possible endings. You are to find the one ending which *best* completes the statement, although some of the others may not be entirely wrong.
- It can also be a complete statement in the form of a question which is answered by choosing one of the statements listed.
- It can be in the form of a problem – again you select the best answer.

Here is an example of a multiple-choice question with a discussion which should give you some clues as to the method for choosing the right answer:

When an employee has a complaint about his assignment, the action which will *best* help him overcome his difficulty is to

A. discuss his difficulty with his coworkers
B. take the problem to the head of the organization
C. take the problem to the person who gave him the assignment
D. say nothing to anyone about his complaint

In answering this question, you should study each of the choices to find which is best. Consider choice "A" – Certainly an employee may discuss his complaint with fellow employees, but no change or improvement can result, and the complaint remains unresolved. Choice "B" is a poor choice since the head of the organization probably does not know what assignment you have been given, and taking your problem to him is known as "going over the head" of the supervisor. The supervisor, or person who made the assignment, is the person who can clarify it or correct any injustice. Choice "C" is, therefore, correct. To say nothing, as in choice "D," is unwise. Supervisors have and interest in knowing the problems employees are facing, and the employee is seeking a solution to his problem.

2. True/False

3. Matching Questions

Matching an answer from a column of choices within another column.

V. RECORDING YOUR ANSWERS

Computer terminals are used more and more today for many different kinds of exams.

For an examination with very few applicants, you may be told to record your answers in the test booklet itself. Separate answer sheets are much more common. If this separate answer sheet is to be scored by machine – and this is often the case – it is highly important that you mark your answers correctly in order to get credit.

VI. BEFORE THE TEST

YOUR PHYSICAL CONDITION IS IMPORTANT

If you are not well, you can't do your best work on tests. If you are half asleep, you can't do your best either. Here are some tips:

1) Get about the same amount of sleep you usually get. Don't stay up all night before the test, either partying or worrying—DON'T DO IT!
2) If you wear glasses, be sure to wear them when you go to take the test. This goes for hearing aids, too.
3) If you have any physical problems that may keep you from doing your best, be sure to tell the person giving the test. If you are sick or in poor health, you relay cannot do your best on any test. You can always come back and take the test some other time.

Common sense will help you find procedures to follow to get ready for an examination. Too many of us, however, overlook these sensible measures. Indeed, nervousness and fatigue have been found to be the most serious reasons why applicants fail to do their best on civil service tests. Here is a list of reminders:

- Begin your preparation early – Don't wait until the last minute to go scurrying around for books and materials or to find out what the position is all about.
- Prepare continuously – An hour a night for a week is better than an all-night cram session. This has been definitely established. What is more, a night a week for a month will return better dividends than crowding your study into a shorter period of time.
- Locate the place of the exam – You have been sent a notice telling you when and where to report for the examination. If the location is in a different town or otherwise unfamiliar to you, it would be well to inquire the best route and learn something about the building.
- Relax the night before the test – Allow your mind to rest. Do not study at all that night. Plan some mild recreation or diversion; then go to bed early and get a good night's sleep.
- Get up early enough to make a leisurely trip to the place for the test – This way unforeseen events, traffic snarls, unfamiliar buildings, etc. will not upset you.

- Dress comfortably – A written test is not a fashion show. You will be known by number and not by name, so wear something comfortable.
- Leave excess paraphernalia at home – Shopping bags and odd bundles will get in your way. You need bring only the items mentioned in the official notice you received; usually everything you need is provided. Do not bring reference books to the exam. They will only confuse those last minutes and be taken away from you when in the test room.
- Arrive somewhat ahead of time – If because of transportation schedules you must get there very early, bring a newspaper or magazine to take your mind off yourself while waiting.
- Locate the examination room – When you have found the proper room, you will be directed to the seat or part of the room where you will sit. Sometimes you are given a sheet of instructions to read while you are waiting. Do not fill out any forms until you are told to do so; just read them and be prepared.
- Relax and prepare to listen to the instructions
- If you have any physical problem that may keep you from doing your best, be sure to tell the test administrator. If you are sick or in poor health, you really cannot do your best on the exam. You can come back and take the test some other time.

VII. AT THE TEST

The day of the test is here and you have the test booklet in your hand. The temptation to get going is very strong. Caution! There is more to success than knowing the right answers. You must know how to identify your papers and understand variations in the type of short-answer question used in this particular examination. Follow these suggestions for maximum results from your efforts:

1) Cooperate with the monitor

The test administrator has a duty to create a situation in which you can be as much at ease as possible. He will give instructions, tell you when to begin, check to see that you are marking your answer sheet correctly, and so on. He is not there to guard you, although he will see that your competitors do not take unfair advantage. He wants to help you do your best.

2) Listen to all instructions

Don't jump the gun! Wait until you understand all directions. In most civil service tests you get more time than you need to answer the questions. So don't be in a hurry. Read each word of instructions until you clearly understand the meaning. Study the examples, listen to all announcements and follow directions. Ask questions if you do not understand what to do.

3) Identify your papers

Civil service exams are usually identified by number only. You will be assigned a number; you must not put your name on your test papers. Be sure to copy your number correctly. Since more than one exam may be given, copy your exact examination title.

4) Plan your time

Unless you are told that a test is a "speed" or "rate of work" test, speed itself is usually not important. Time enough to answer all the questions will be provided, but this does not mean that you have all day. An overall time limit has been set. Divide the total time (in minutes) by the number of questions to determine the approximate time you have for each question.

5) Do not linger over difficult questions

If you come across a difficult question, mark it with a paper clip (useful to have along) and come back to it when you have been through the booklet. One caution if you do this – be sure to skip a number on your answer sheet as well. Check often to be sure that you have not lost your place and that you are marking in the row numbered the same as the question you are answering.

6) Read the questions

Be sure you know what the question asks! Many capable people are unsuccessful because they failed to *read* the questions correctly.

7) Answer all questions

Unless you have been instructed that a penalty will be deducted for incorrect answers, it is better to guess than to omit a question.

8) Speed tests

It is often better NOT to guess on speed tests. It has been found that on timed tests people are tempted to spend the last few seconds before time is called in marking answers at random – without even reading them – in the hope of picking up a few extra points. To discourage this practice, the instructions may warn you that your score will be "corrected" for guessing. That is, a penalty will be applied. The incorrect answers will be deducted from the correct ones, or some other penalty formula will be used.

9) Review your answers

If you finish before time is called, go back to the questions you guessed or omitted to give them further thought. Review other answers if you have time.

10) Return your test materials

If you are ready to leave before others have finished or time is called, take ALL your materials to the monitor and leave quietly. Never take any test material with you. The monitor can discover whose papers are not complete, and taking a test booklet may be grounds for disqualification.

VIII. EXAMINATION TECHNIQUES

1) Read the general instructions carefully. These are usually printed on the first page of the exam booklet. As a rule, these instructions refer to the timing of the examination; the fact that you should not start work until the signal and must stop work at a signal, etc. If there are any *special* instructions, such as a choice of questions to be answered, make sure that you note this instruction carefully.

2) When you are ready to start work on the examination, that is as soon as the signal has been given, read the instructions to each question booklet, underline any key words or phrases, such as *least*, *best*, *outline*, *describe*

and the like. In this way you will tend to answer as requested rather than discover on reviewing your paper that you *listed without describing*, that you selected the *worst* choice rather than the *best* choice, etc.

3) If the examination is of the objective or multiple-choice type – that is, each question will also give a series of possible answers: A, B, C or D, and you are called upon to select the best answer and write the letter next to that answer on your answer paper – it is advisable to start answering each question in turn. There may be anywhere from 50 to 100 such questions in the three or four hours allotted and you can see how much time would be taken if you read through all the questions before beginning to answer any. Furthermore, if you come across a question or group of questions which you know would be difficult to answer, it would undoubtedly affect your handling of all the other questions.

4) If the examination is of the essay type and contains but a few questions, it is a moot point as to whether you should read all the questions before starting to answer any one. Of course, if you are given a choice – say five out of seven and the like – then it is essential to read all the questions so you can eliminate the two that are most difficult. If, however, you are asked to answer all the questions, there may be danger in trying to answer the easiest one first because you may find that you will spend too much time on it. The best technique is to answer the first question, then proceed to the second, etc.

5) Time your answers. Before the exam begins, write down the time it started, then add the time allowed for the examination and write down the time it must be completed, then divide the time available somewhat as follows:
   - If 3-1/2 hours are allowed, that would be 210 minutes. If you have 80 objective-type questions, that would be an average of 2-1/2 minutes per question. Allow yourself no more than 2 minutes per question, or a total of 160 minutes, which will permit about 50 minutes to review.
   - If for the time allotment of 210 minutes there are 7 essay questions to answer, that would average about 30 minutes a question. Give yourself only 25 minutes per question so that you have about 35 minutes to review.

6) The most important instruction is to *read each question* and make sure you know what is wanted. The second most important instruction is to *time yourself properly* so that you answer every question. The third most important instruction is to *answer every question.* Guess if you have to but include something for each question. Remember that you will receive no credit for a blank and will probably receive some credit if you write something in answer to an essay question. If you guess a letter – say "B" for a multiple-choice question – you may have guessed right. If you leave a blank as an answer to a multiple-choice question, the examiners may respect your feelings but it will not add a point to your score. Some exams may penalize you for wrong answers, so in such cases *only*, you may not want to guess unless you have some basis for your answer.

7) Suggestions
   a. Objective-type questions
      1. Examine the question booklet for proper sequence of pages and questions
      2. Read all instructions carefully
      3. Skip any question which seems too difficult; return to it after all other questions have been answered
      4. Apportion your time properly; do not spend too much time on any single question or group of questions
      5. Note and underline key words – *all, most, fewest, least, best, worst, same, opposite,* etc.
      6. Pay particular attention to negatives
      7. Note unusual option, e.g., unduly long, short, complex, different or similar in content to the body of the question
      8. Observe the use of "hedging" words – *probably, may, most likely,* etc.
      9. Make sure that your answer is put next to the same number as the question
      10. Do not second-guess unless you have good reason to believe the second answer is definitely more correct
      11. Cross out original answer if you decide another answer is more accurate; do not erase until you are ready to hand your paper in
      12. Answer all questions; guess unless instructed otherwise
      13. Leave time for review

   b. Essay questions
      1. Read each question carefully
      2. Determine exactly what is wanted. Underline key words or phrases.
      3. Decide on outline or paragraph answer
      4. Include many different points and elements unless asked to develop any one or two points or elements
      5. Show impartiality by giving pros and cons unless directed to select one side only
      6. Make and write down any assumptions you find necessary to answer the questions
      7. Watch your English, grammar, punctuation and choice of words
      8. Time your answers; don't crowd material

8) Answering the essay question

Most essay questions can be answered by framing the specific response around several key words or ideas. Here are a few such key words or ideas:

M's: manpower, materials, methods, money, management

P's: purpose, program, policy, plan, procedure, practice, problems, pitfalls, personnel, public relations

a. Six basic steps in handling problems:
   1. Preliminary plan and background development
   2. Collect information, data and facts
   3. Analyze and interpret information, data and facts
   4. Analyze and develop solutions as well as make recommendations

5. Prepare report and sell recommendations
6. Install recommendations and follow up effectiveness

b. Pitfalls to avoid

1. *Taking things for granted* – A statement of the situation does not necessarily imply that each of the elements is necessarily true; for example, a complaint may be invalid and biased so that all that can be taken for granted is that a complaint has been registered
2. *Considering only one side of a situation* – Wherever possible, indicate several alternatives and then point out the reasons you selected the best one
3. *Failing to indicate follow up* – Whenever your answer indicates action on your part, make certain that you will take proper follow-up action to see how successful your recommendations, procedures or actions turn out to be
4. *Taking too long in answering any single question* – Remember to time your answers properly

EXAMINATION SECTION

EXAMINATION SECTION
TEST 1

DIRECTIONS: Each question or incomplete statement is followed by several suggested answers or completions. Select the one the BEST answers the question or completes the statement. *PRINT THE LETTER OF THE CORRECT ANSWER IN THE SPACE AT THE RIGHT.*

1. Of the following, the most appropriate use for impression wax is 1.____

   A. making custom trays for wash injections
   B. making dies for temporary crowns
   C. preliminary impressions of edentulous ridges for complete dentures
   D. making direct wax pattern inlays

2. In the ideal centric occlusion, the ______ teeth occlude. 2.____

   A. posterior
   B. anterior
   C. canine
   D. incisor

3. The principal advantage associated with the construction of two-piece impression trays over stock or one-piece custom trays is their 3.____

   A. greater dimensional stability
   B. shorter time requirements
   C. ability to be disassembled and reassembled
   D. lack of bulk

4. A technician is arranging 33-degree anatomic maxillary posterior teeth. Typically, each of the following teeth will contact the occlusal plane at some point, EXCEPT the 4.____

   A. first premolar
   B. second premolar
   C. first molar
   D. second molar

5. During mastication, the ______ keeps food on occlusal surfaces. 5.____

   A. orbicularis oris
   B. orbicularis oculi
   C. zygomaticus minor
   D. depressor anguli oris

6. A technician is carving the gingival margin around the anterior teeth of a trial maxillary denture. The technician should use a carver or #7 spatula, held at an angle of approximately ______ degrees. 6.____

   A. 30
   B. 45
   C. 60
   D. 90

7. Before flasking a denture with artificial stone, the interior of the flask is best lubricated with 7.____

   A. silicone lubricant
   B. mineral oil
   C. tinfoil substitute
   D. powdered talc

8. Which of the roots in on the maxillary first molar is longest? 8.____

   A. Mesiofacial
   B. Distal
   C. Lingual
   D. Facial

9. The last step in deflasking is usually to 9.____

   A. remove stone from the distobuccal corners
   B. tap away the stone enclosing the cast
   C. remove the denture base from the cast
   D. remove the sectioned lingual or palatal area

10. Which of the following is NOT a purpose of a baseplate? 10.____

   A. Carrying occlusal rims
   B. Checking the accuracy of previous records
   C. Holding the teeth for the try-in stage
   D. Establishing the occlusal plane

11. Often, the ______ cusp of the maxillary third molar is missing. 11.____

   A. distolingual
   B. distofacial
   C. mesiolingual
   D. mesiofacial

12. The most significant advantage offered by resin denture teeth is that they 12.____

   A. are chip-resistant
   B. can bond to most heat-cured denture base resins
   C. have great wear resistance
   D. can be re-polished

13. Of the following muscles, the movement of the temporomandibular joint is most directly affected by the 13.____

   A. masseter
   B. trapezius
   C. lateral pterygoid
   D. medial pterygoid

14. Which of the following is NOT a typical characteristic in a tapering maxillary arch? 14.____

   A. Incisal tips of the canines are slightly below the incisal edges of the lateral incisors.
   B. Lateral incisors are slightly above the occlusal plane.

C. Central incisors are farther forward of the canines than in other types of arches.
D. Central incisors are rotated inward at the distal aspect.

15. A patient has dental decay that has progressed into the tooth, exposing the dentin. Which is likely to happen as a result of this irritation? 15.____

A. The dentinal tubules will become sealed off.
B. The pulp will die as it is contacted by air.
C. Ameloblasts will attempt to cover the exposure with enamel.
D. Secondary dentin will form in an attempt to repair the tissue.

16. In a typical arrangement of Pilkington-Turner 30-degree posterior teeth, the 16.____

A. buccal cusps of the first and second premolars touch the occlusal plane
B. long axes of the premolars should be tilted slightly from vertical (in the buccal view)
C. lingual cusps of the first and second premolars touch the occlusal plane
D. long axes of the molars should be at right angles to the occlusal plane (in the buccal view)

17. The ______ muscle has two origins on the zygomatic arch. 17.____

A. sternocleidomastoid
B. masseter
C. lateral pterygoid
D. temporal

18. A technician is deflasking a denture. After the wax trial base and baseplate have been discarded, and no teeth are determined to have been dislodged, the next step is usually to. 18.____

A. flush each half-flask with boiling detergent water
B. scrub each half-flask with a brush and detergent
C. remove larger bits of remaining stone with a scalpel
D. paint tinfoil substitute on the exposed stone surfaces

19. Agar hydrocolloid impression materials 19.____

A. have high tear strength in narrow spaces
B. are hydrophobic
C. can be poured after several hours if kept in water
D. are compatible with a moist field

20. Usually, ______ g of dental stone is adequate for most impressions. 20.____

A. 50
B. 100
C. 200
D. 350

21. All other factors aside, the quickest and easiest method of making a usable baseplate is to 21.____

A. vacuum mold a sheet of thermoplastic resin to the cast
B. hand-adapt a rolled resin sheet

C. sprinkle on polymer and add monomer
D. confine resin in a stone index for curing

22. Heat-cured acrylic resin is packed into the denture flask to form the denture base during the ______ stage of polymerization. 22.____

A. ropy
B. sandy
C. stringy
D. dough

23. Rebasing a denture is most often due to dissatisfaction with the ______ of the denture. 23.____

I. color
II. teeth
III. porosity
IV. fit

A. I only
B. I or III
C. I, III or IV
D. II, III or IV

24. A technician has received a transfer fork that registers the occlusal relationships of a patient's teeth. The technician coats the indentations with a thin layer of zinc oxide/ eugenol impression paste, for the purpose of 24.____

A. making the wax less porous
B. fastening the transfer fork to the articulator
C. preventing the wax from distorting
D. keeping the cast from sticking to the wax during articulation

25. Which of the following is NOT an advantage associated with the use of metal denture bases? 25.____

A. Ease in relining
B. No warpage
C. Less tissue change under the base
D. Increased accuracy

KEY (CORRECT ANSWERS)

1. C
2. A
3. D
4. D
5. B
6. C
7. A
8. C
9. B
10. D
11. A
12. B
13. C
14. A
15. D
16. C
17. B
18. A
19. D
20. C
21. A
22. D
23. B
24. C
25. A

TEST 2

DIRECTIONS: Each question or incomplete statement is followed by several suggested answers or completions. Select the one the BEST answers the question or completes the statement. *PRINT THE LETTER OF THE CORRECT ANSWER IN THE SPACE AT THE RIGHT.*

1. A heat-processed denture is NOT ______ than a chemically cured denture. 1.____

   A. harder
   B. less dimensionally accurate
   C. more porous
   D. stronger

2. Which of the following impression materials is transformed from a liquid to a gel when set? 2.____

   A. Zinc oxide/eugenol
   B. Polysulfide
   C. Condensation silicone
   D. Alginate

3. A technician is constructing a baseplate out of autopolymerizing resin. He has used soft-curing resin to block out several undercuts. Occasionally, this soft-curing resin can flow out of the undercuts instead of remaining in place. The technician can prevent this problem by 3.____

   A. warming the cast in hot water, or with a chip blower
   B. using hard-curing resin
   C. chilling the cast slightly
   D. using baseplate wax

4. In recent years, many technicians have switched from reversible hydrocolloid impression material to newer elastomeric impression materials. Which of the following is NOT a reason for this? 4.____

   A. Elastomers are more accurate
   B. Impressions don't have to be poured immediately
   C. Surfactants are usually not required
   D. Elastomers don't require as much equipment

5. When arranging the maxillary anterior teeth, the cervical third of the canines should be tilted 5.____

   A. mesially
   B. lingually
   C. distally
   D. buccally

6. Which of the following premolars is commonly bifurcated? 6.____

   A. Maxillary first
   B. Maxillary second

C. Mandibular first
D. Mandibular second

7. Boxing final impressions before pouring 7.____
   I. controls the form and thickness of the base of the cast
   II. facilitates the placement of remounting plates
   III. preserves the extension and thickness of borders
   IV. conserves dental stone

   A. I and III
   B. I, II and III
   C. II only
   D. I, II, III and IV

8. When packing a denture, resin flash should be trimmed with a 8.____

   A. sharp scalpel
   B. dull spatula
   C. carbide bur
   D. PKT #2 tool

9. The suprahyoid muscles include each of the following, EXCEPT the 9.____

   A. stylohyoid
   B. thyrohyoid
   C. digastric
   D. geniohyoid

10. When repairing a plastic anterior denture tooth, which of the following is done FIRST? 10.____

   A. Grinding the labial gingival margin
   B. With a bur, placing shallow indentations in the denture-tooth ridge lap
   C. Pouring a plaster index on the labial surface of the tooth to be replaced
   D. Securing a replacement tooth in the base with sticky wax

11. In making a custom tray from chemical-cured resin, some technicians place three or four 2-mm holes in the anterior and posterior ridge regions of the wax spacer before adapting the tray material over it. Ultimately, this technique results in 11.____

   A. the stabilization of wax rims during a try-in
   B. insulating the patient from the heat of the exothermic reaction
   C. blocking out tissue undercuts before the final construction
   D. the prevention of large areas of tissue being compressed during the taking of an impression

12. The tint for a denture base's basic pink color is distributed in bottles labeled 12.____

   A. A
   B. B
   C. E
   D. H

13. Which of the following is NOT a guideline to be followed in constructing metal occlusals for denture teeth? 13.____

    A. When flasking the occlusals and teeth, the buccal surfaces should be depressed slightly toward the cervical aspect.
    B. Before forming the castings, maxillary and mandibular teeth should be reduced to provide about 4 mm of interocclusal space.
    C. Castings should be about 2 mm thick.
    D. Incisal shade resin should be sifted into the mold last when occlusals and resin teeth are cured in the flask.

14. Which of the following nerves innervates the lingual gingiva of the maxillary central incisor? 14.____

    A. Nasopalatine
    B. Posterior superior alveolar
    C. Inferior alveolar
    D. Trigeminal

15. A technician is articulating a 33-degree anatomic mandibular second premolar. In centric occlusion, the tip of the buccal cusp will typically contact the 15.____

    A. buccal groove of the maxillary first molar
    B. distal slope of the lingual cusp of the maxillary first premolar
    C. mesial marginal ridge of the maxillary second premolar
    D. the mesiobuccal slope of the maxillary second premolar

16. The main disadvantage associated with the use of thermoplastic shellac baseplate materials for making impression trays is their 16.____

    A. intense exothermic reaction
    B. dimensional instability
    C. difficulty in trimming
    D. complexity

17. Which of the following is NOT an advantage associated with heat-cured compression-molded resin baseplates? 17.____

    A. Bases can become part of the denture themselves
    B. Excellent preservation of master casts
    C. Minimal finishing and polishing requirements
    D. Thickness can be controlled during wax-up

18. Which of the following is associated with a Class III occlusion? 18.____

    A. Prognathic lower jaw
    B. Retrognathic lower jaw
    C. Enlarged lower jaw
    D. Lateral mandibular glide

19. Finished complete dentures should have a palate thickness of about ______ . 19.____

    A. 1
    B. 2

C. 3
D. 4

20. Cracks in dental enamel are called 20.____

A. spindles
B. imbrications
C. lamellae
D. villi

21. When finishing and polishing a denture, the first area to receive attention is usually the 21.____

A. outer border
B. gingival margins
C. palate or lingual border
D. incisal or occlusal surfaces

22. In the ideal protrusive movement, the ______ teeth touch. 22.____

A. canine and posterior
B. anterior
C. canine
D. anterior and posterior

23. Each of the following is a typical procedure involved in the waxing of a trial maxillary denture, EXCEPT 23.____

A. forming a slight bulge over the maxillary premolars, from the canine eminence to the molar process
B. developing a slight root prominence over the maxillary central incisors
C. developing a gingival bulge that is approximately 5 to 6 mm wide over the second molar
D. carving a slight fossa between the root of the central incisor and the canine eminence

24. The superior aspect of the external auditory meatus, often used as a reference point in dental work, is known as the 24.____

A. porion
B. nasion
C. A-point
D. B-point

25. A technician plans to make a denture base out of fluid resin. The most important adjustment to make in this procedure is to 25.____

A. add more water to the flasking material
B. leave at least a 0.5 mm diastema between each canine and first premolar
C. increase the interocclusal distance about 0.5 mm in the incisal guide-pin area of the articulator
D. apply a coat of separating fluid to the incisal or occlusal surfaces of the teeth

KEY (CORRECT ANSWERS)

1. C
2. D
3. A
4. C
5. D
6. A
7. D
8. B
9. B
10. D
11. D
12. D
13. A
14. A
15. C
16. B
17. B
18. A
19. B
20. C
21. A
22. B
23. A
24. A
25. C

TEST 3

DIRECTIONS: Each question or incomplete statement is followed by several suggested answers or completions. Select the one the BEST answers the question or completes the statement. *PRINT THE LETTER OF THE CORRECT ANSWER IN THE SPACE AT THE RIGHT.*

1. On the facial surface of the anterior teeth, the greatest convexity will be found at the 1.____

   A. junction of the middle and incisal thirds
   B. incisal third
   C. middle third
   D. cervical third

2. A technician is trimming a diagnostic cast. The simplest and most effective way to align the back cuts of the maxillary and mandibular portions of the cast is to 2.____

   A. articulate the casts with pins and then trim them simultaneously
   B. articulate the casts with a wax bite and then trim them simultaneously
   C. trim the longer cast first and then articulate the casts with a wax bite
   D. trim the shorter cast first and then articulate the casts with a wax bite

3. Characteristics typical of a Class II, division II occlusion include 3.____
   I. mesioclusion
   II. crowded maxillary incisors
   III. a deep overbite
   IV. an abnormal overjet

   A. I and II
   B. II and III
   C. I, II and IV
   D. I, II, III and IV

4. Which of the following is NOT a significant problem associated with the flask method of rebasing a denture? 4.____

   A. Air inclusions in the flasking material producing nodules on the rebased denture
   B. Risk of dislodging a tooth from the flasking material when packing
   C. Breaking the cast while separating the denture
   D. Occlusal errors

5. Before making a wax baseplate, it is advisable to apply a separating layer of _______ on the cast surfaces. 5.____

   A. powdered talc
   B. Super-Sep fluid
   C. mineral oil
   D. slurry water

6. In centric occlusion, the lingual cusps of the maxillary molars strike their antagonists 6.____

   A. facial to the facial cusps of the mandibular teeth
   B. lingual to the lingual cusps of the mandibular teeth

C. on the facial portion of the facial cusps
D. on the central portion of the mandibular occlusal surface

7. A technician is boxing an impression with wax. The height of the wax should generally be adjusted so that it extends approximately ______ mm above the highest point on the impression. 7.____

A. 4
B. 7
C. 13
D. 22

8. The first step in removing a denture from a cast is to 8.____

A. direct a blast of air between the denture and the cast base
B. divide the cast base into several sections
C. make a saw cut opposite the central incisors
D. thin the cast base as much as possible with a cast trimmer

9. Which of the following is a term that denotes the dislocation of the temporomandibular joint? 9.____

A. Prognathicism
B. Malocclusion
C. Glide
D. Subluxation

10. What is the term for the area where the head of the mandible lies? 10.____

A. Glenoid fossa
B. Emenentia
C. External auditory meatus
D. Articular eminence

11. Metal occlusal surfaces for denture teeth may be indicated when 11.____
I. their use is needed to reinforce and strengthen the denture
II. constructing a denture that will be opposed by a reconstructed dentition with gold occlusal surfaces
III. constructing a denture with a functionally generated path concept in which considerable modification of the teeth is necessary
IV. special wax carving techniques are completed on a fully adjustable articulator

A. I and II
B. I and III
C. II, III and IV
D. I, II, III and IV

12. A technician discovers a lack of space for setting the mandibular first premolar in a complete denture. Each of the following is a possible solution, EXCEPT 12.____

A. leaving a 1 mm space between the mandibular canine and the first premolar
B. grinding the lower premolar carefully on mesial and distal surfaces

C. leaving out the lower central or lateral incisor
D. leaving out the mandibular second premolar

13. The most commonly used impression tray materials are 13.____

A. special autopolymerizing acrylic resins
B. thermoplastic resin sheets
C. hard thermoplastic waxes
D. thermoplastic shellac baseplate materials

14. A technician wants to add a plastic palate form to a trial denture before flasking. With a fissure bur, the existing palate should be cut at a distance of about ______ from the denture teeth. 14.____

A. 3 to 4
B. 5 to 6
C. 7 to 8
D. 9 to 10

15. Which of the following arteries supplies the muscles of mastication? 15.____

A. pterygoid plexus
B. superficial temporal
C. mental
D. maxillary

16. In the ______ arch configuration, the long axes of the anterior teeth generally deviate most noticeably from the sagittal plane, or midline. 16.____

A. Square
B. Square-tapering
C. Tapering
D. Ovoid

17. Gold alloys of Type(s) ______ are sufficiently rigid for use as cast metal denture bases. 17.____

A. I only
B. I and II
C. III and IV
D. V only

18. ______ exists where the premolars occlude during a lateral mandibular glide. 18.____

A. Group function
B. The balancing side
C. The working side
D. Posterior coupling

19. If a technician makes a denture base out of poured fluid resin, the denture will be flasked in 19.____

A. dental plaster
B. dental stone

C. silicone
D. hydrocolloid

20. Occlusal trauma is characterized by 20.____

A. healing occurring with the inflammation
B. thinning of principal fibers due to tension
C. reparation after the inflammation is removed
D. bone resorption from obstruction of blood flow to principal fibers

21. A technician is constructing a baseplate out of autopolymerizing resin using the sprinkle-on method. When relief is applied to the cast, 21.____

A. soft-curing resin should be used to block out only the severest undercuts
B. baseplate wax should be used to block out only the severest undercuts
C. soft-curing resin should be used to block out all the undercuts
D. baseplate wax should be used to block out all the undercuts

22. After deflasking, a technician is painting tinfoil substitute over the cast and stone. The technician should be careful to avoid applying tinfoil substitute to the 22.____

A. ridgelaps of resin teeth
B. distolingual area
C. interproximal areas
D. peripheral roll

23. Which of the following gypsum products requires the highest water-to-powder ratio? 23.____

A. High strength dental stone
B. High strength/high expansion dental stone
C. Dental stone
D. Model plaster

24. In centric occlusion, the mesiobuccal inclined plane of the mandibular second molar contacts the 24.____

A. central fossa of the maxillary second molar
B. marginal ridge of the mesiolingual cusp of the maxillary first molar
C. mesiobuccal cusp of the maxillary second molar
D. marginal ridge of the distobuccal cusp of the maxillary first molar

25. Most dentists agree that for most patients, the average period of satisfactory service for a denture is about ______ years. 25.____

A. 2
B. 5
C. 7
D. 10

KEY (CORRECT ANSWERS)

1. D
2. C
3. B
4. C
5. A

6. D
7. C
8. D
9. D
10. A

11. D
12. D
13. A
14. B
15. D

16. C
17. C
18. A
19. D
20. D

21. B
22. A
23. D
24. D
25. C

TEST 4

DIRECTION: Each question or incomplete statement is followed by several suggested answers or completions. Select the one the BEST answers the question or completes the statement. *PRINT THE LETTER OF THE CORRECT ANSWER IN THE SPACE AT THE RIGHT.*

1. A technician is using the double-pour method to make a working cast. Most often, this means that the anatomic portion 1.____

   A. and the art portion will be poured in stone, each separately
   B. and the art portion will be poured in plaster, each separately
   C. plaster; the base in dental stone
   D. dental stone; the base in plaster

2. Which of the following is MOST likely to have a transverse ridge? 2.____

   A. Maxillary first premolar
   B. Mandibular first premolar
   C. Maxillary second premolar
   D. Mandibular second premolar

3. Boxing with wax is usually most appropriate for impressions that are made from 3.____

   A. silicone
   B. alginate
   C. zinc oxide/eugenol impression paste
   D. rubber

4. A technician is placing the maxillary anterior teeth of a denture. Which of the following is typically FALSE? 4.____

   A. The central incisor is inclined slightly from the vertical.
   B. The incisal edge of the lateral incisor touches the occlusal plane.
   C. The canine is set at a right angle to the occlusal plane.
   D. The incisal edge of the central incisor touches the occlusal plane

5. Typically, ______ dental modeling compound softens at a higher temperature than other colors. 5.____

   A. white
   B. red
   C. green
   D. black

6. Flat tooth forms for a denture, such as Rational 0-degree posterior teeth, are appropriate for 6.____

   I. flat or heavily resorbed ridges
   II. crossbites
   III. patients with uncoordinated jaw movements
   IV. severe overbites

A. I and II
B. II and IV
C. I, II and III
D. I, II, III and IV

7. The mandible may be retruded or depressed by the ______ muscle. 7.____

A. thyrohyoid
B. masseter
C. medial pterygoid
D. digastric

8. A technician is rebasing a denture. If the teeth are porcelain, they will be removed by 8.____

A. heating them with a hot spatula
B. chilling with a cold spatula
C. grinding them down to near the margin
D. grinding them down to the retaining holes

9. A technician is mounting a mandibular cast on an articulator. The FIRST step in this process is usually to 9.____

A. fit the occlusal registration to the maxillary cast
B. invert the articulator with the maxillary cast in place
C. remove the maxillary cast from the articulator
D. set the incisal guide pin to the appropriate height

10. A technician is constructing a baseplate out of autopolymerizing resin using the sprinkle-on method. It is essential that the technician 10.____

A. adapt the resin by hand after it has been applied
B. have polymer and monomer ready in premeasured amounts
C. cure the baseplate in a pressure pot
D. perform the construction in a hood or well-ventilated area

11. Which of the following primary teeth has a lingual ridge on its lingual surface? 11.____

A. Mandibular central
B. Maxillary central
C. Mandibular canine
D. Maxillary canine

12. The most distinct feature of the maxillary first deciduous molar is its 12.____

A. mesial profile
B. transverse ridge
C. occlusion
D. buccal cervical ridge

13. Baseplate wax should NOT be used to block out undercuts in the construction of ______ baseplates. 13.____

A. vacuum-molded resin
B. sprinkle-on resin

C. hand-adapted resin
D. thermoplastic shellac

14. The starting point or "anchor" in the placement of mandibular posterior teeth is typically the 14.____

A. first premolar
B. second premolar
C. first molar
D. third molar

15. The soft palate is pulled into contact with the posterior pharyngeal wall by the _______ muscle. 15.____

A. uvula
B. styloglossus
C. levator veli palatini
D. procerus

16. Porcelain prosthetic teeth have retentive recesses known as _______ in the ridge laps that can retain the teeth in the denture base. 16.____

A. diastemas
B. pinholes
C. diatorics
D. obstinators

17. When waxing a mandibular trial denture, wax should be flowed onto the lingual surface and the gingival margins carved to produce a gingival marginal angle of about _______ below the horizontal. 17.____

A. 20
B. 35
C. 45
D. 60

18. A technician wants to make an acrylic resin soft and pliable. The technician should 18.____

A. use less monomer in the mix
B. use less powder in the mix
C. add benzoyl peroxide
D. add aromatic esters

19. Viewed from above, the narrowest part of the maxillary arch of a denture would typically be in the area of the 19.____

A. canines
B. first premolars
C. second premolars
D. first molar

20. What is the term used to denote carving of the denture base to simulate the contours of the natural tissues that are to be replaced by the denture? 20.____

A. Garnishment
B. Mimicry
C. Anatomizing
D. Festooning

21. ______ impression materials produce alcohol during setting and are subject to distortion as the alcohol evaporates. 21.____

A. Reversible hydrocolloid
B. Addition silicone
C. Zinc oxide/eugenol
D. Condensation silicone

22. A technician has remounted a denture on an articulator for adjustments. Which of the following is NOT a guideline to be followed in making these adjustments? 22.____

A. When adjusting the working position, adjust the buccal cusps of the upper teeth and the lingual cusps of the mandibular teeth to eliminate defective contacts.
B. In the working position, adjust maxillary buccal cusps and lingual cusps of mandibular teeth.
C. In the centric relation, grind the cusp tips rather than the fossae.
D. If possible, grind the inclines of the maxillary lingual cusps on the balancing side rather than the buccal cusps of mandibular dentures.

23. Another term for a Class II occlusion is 23.____

A. mesioclusion
B. distoclusion
C. neutroclusion
D. lateral excursion

24. The floor of the mouth is formed by the ______ muscle. 24.____

A. omohyoid
B. gastric
C. mylohyoid
D. stylohyoid

25. Cast metal denture bases should be each of the following, EXCEPT 25.____

A. dense
B. accurate enough to seat on the master cast without rocking
C. as thick as possible for maximum rigidity
D. of a biologically compatible alloy

KEY (CORRECT ANSWERS)

1. D
2. B
3. C
4. B
5. D
6. C
7. D
8. A
9. D
10. D
11. D
12. D
13. A
14. C
15. C
16. C
17. A
18. D
19. B
20. D
21. D
22. C
23. B
24. C
25. C

EXAMINATION SECTION
TEST 1

DIRECTIONS: Each question or incomplete statement is followed by several suggested answers or completions. Select the one the BEST answers the question or completes the statement. *PRINT THE LETTER OF THE CORRECT ANSWER IN THE SPACE AT THE RIGHT.*

1. The manipulation of each of the following dental materials is likely to generate particulate matter, EXCEPT 1.____

   A. amalgam
   B. alginate
   C. porcelain
   D. gypsum

2. Which of the following types of ceramics participates actively in osseointegration? 2.____

   A. Calcium phosphate
   B. Titanium
   C. Aluminum oxide
   D. Vanadium

3. Metabolic disturbances affect enamel deposition so that incremental growth lines, known as ______, analogous to tree rings, generally can be seen in sections of undecalcified enamel. 3.____

   A. strata corneum
   B. strata intermedium
   C. lines of Retzius
   D. rests of Malassez

4. Medicare is a health care program designed for ______ patients. 4.____

   A. institutionalized
   B. senior or elderly
   C. homeless
   D. unemployed

5. Certification for dental technicians 5.____

   A. has been in effect since the early 20th century
   B. is voluntary
   C. requires only a written examination
   D. is mandated by most statutes

6. Which portion of the gingiva attaches directly to the tooth? 6.____

   A. Sulcular epithelium
   B. Alveolar mucosa
   C. Tranvserse gingiva
   D. Articulated gingiva

7. Outgoing items from the dental laboratory should be stored in 7.___

    A. a mild bleach solution
    B. a complex phenol
    C. diluted mouthwash
    D. iodophor

8. Which of the following conditions would make it necessary for a curing light in the laboratory to be repaired? 8.___

    A. The light appears slightly blue
    B. The light appears slightly yellow
    C. The light cases a slower set of dark composite
    D. A 2-mm layer of composite material does not cure completely at the recommended exposure time

9. ______ wax is the wax used to form a base for pouring a gypsum model. 9.___

    A. Pattern
    B. Inlay
    C. Boxing
    D. Baseplate

10. A technician wants to decrease the working time of a gypsum cast, but doesn't want to alter its physical properties. The technician should 10.___

    A. increase the rate of spatulation
    B. increase the water temperature
    C. decrease the water-to-powder ratio
    D. decrease the water temperature

11. The first civilization to designate a doctor that specializes in treating teeth were the 11.___

    A. Sumerians
    B. Chinese
    C. Egyptians
    D. Romans

12. Which of the following, because it retards the rate at which resin sets, cannot be used under composite materials? 12.___

    A. Zinc polycarboxylate
    B. Copal varnish
    C. Zinc phosphate
    D. Primer

13. Surface disinfectants used for workbenches and receiving areas in a dental laboratory typically include 13.___

    I. glutaraldehydes
    II. chlorine compounds
    III. phenolic compounds
    IV. iodophors

    A. I and III
    B. II only
    C. II and III
    D. II, III and IV

14. Tooth number ______ is nonsuccedaneous. 14.____

A. 8
B. 12
C. 26
D. 30

15. In the ______ dentition, the ratio of root length to crown length is greatest. 15.____

A. mandibular
B. maxillary
C. permanent
D. primary

16. Which of the following would be used for a temporary direct restoration? 16.____

A. Zinc oxide/eugenol
B. Zinc phosphate
C. Zinc polycarboxylate
D. Glass ionomer

17. The infrahyoid muscles include each of the following, EXCEPT the 17.____

A. genihyoid
B. omohyoid
C. thyrohyoid
D. sternohyoid

18. A patient has just received a new denture. He should be told to keep the wet when they are removed, in order to avoid 18.____

A. discoloration
B. plasticizing
C. loss of thermal sensation
D. shrinkage

19. Solder is NOT typically used to 19.____

A. join a wire loop to a band in a space retainer
B. repair holes in crowns
C. join a bridge retainer to a pontic
D. add a contact to a crown

20. In a Class II, division II occlusion, the maxillary incisors are 20.____

A. impacted
B. protruded
C. edge to edge
D. retruded

21. The periodontal ligament is attached to the tooth by ______ fibers. 21.____

A. Sharpey's
B. sulcular
C. reticular
D. gingival

22. When impressions are not disinfected before they are poured, microorganisms can get into the gypsum and survive 22.____

A. for 3 to 6 hours
B. for 24 to 48 hours
C. for a week or more
D. indefinitely

23. Tooth number 9 has a greater height of contour on the facial and lingual in the ______ third portion of the tooth. 23.____

A. occlusal
B. incisal
C. middle
D. cervical

24. A technician reads an order for a restoration to be made to a tooth that is designated "9" on the work order. The code system being used is ______; the tooth designated is ______. 24.____

A. FDI; mandibular left canine
B. FDI; mandibular right central incisor
C. Universal; mandibular left second premolar
D. Universal; maxillary left central incisor

25. A scalpel is typically used in a dental laboratory to 25.____

I. remove excess stone below the gingival margin of a die
II. trim the palatal portion of a cast
III. remove a die from a full-arch working cast
IV. define the gingival margins on a cast or die

A. I and II
B. II, III and IV
C. IV only
D. I, II, III and IV

KEY (CORRECT ANSWERS)

1. A
2. A
3. C
4. B
5. B
6. A
7. C
8. D
9. C
10. B
11. C
12. B
13. C
14. D
15. D
16. A
17. A
18. D
19. B
20. D
21. A
22. C
23. D
24. D
25. C

TEST 2

DIRECTIONS: Each question or incomplete statement is followed by several suggested answers or completions. Select the one the BEST answers the question or completes the statement. *PRINT THE LETTER OF THE CORRECT ANSWER IN THE SPACE AT THE RIGHT.*

1. Which of the following metals is/are typically used to add strength to a high noble alloy? 1.____

   I. Silver
   II. Copper
   III. Nickel
   IV. Aluminum

   A. I or II
   B. I, II or III
   C. III or IV
   D. I, II, III or IV

2. Guidelines for polishing each case in a dental laboratory include 2.____

   I. using unit doses of pumice wet with disinfectant
   II. discarding the pumice slurry after each use
   III. wearing safety glasses and a mask, or a full-face shield
   IV. trimming appliances with a sterile acrylic bur

   A. I and III
   B. I, III and IV
   C. III only
   D. I, II, III and IV

3. The mesiofacial cusp of tooth number 3 falls between teeth numbers 30 and 31. This describes the occlusion known as Class 3.____

   A. I
   B. II, Division I
   C. II, Division II
   D. III

4. Material that does not flow well is described as having 4.____

   A. low cure
   B. low strain
   C. high adhesion
   D. high viscosity

5. Malpractice may be considered a tort because it 5.____

   A. causes harm to an individual
   B. is a breach of faithfulness to the professional's promises and obligations
   C. is a violation of a health care professional's code of ethics
   D. involves touching an individual with the intention to harm

6. Which of the following terms is used to describe the lymph nodes that drain the lower anterior teeth? 6.____

   A. Cervical
   B. Submandibular
   C. Facial
   D. Submental

7. Acrylic denture bases began to replace older Vulcanite bases in the 7.____

   A. 1890s
   B. 1910s
   C. 1940s
   D. 1970s

8. Which of the following is the smallest permanent tooth? 8.____

   A. Mandibular central incisor
   B. Maxillary central incisor
   C. Mandibular lateral incisor
   D. Maxillary lateral incisor

9. The periodontal ligament is composed of each of the following, EXCEPT 9.____

   A. collagen fibers
   B. nerve fibers
   C. odontoblasts
   D. blood vessels

10. Which of the following techniques is NOT recommended for disinfecting impressions? 10.____

   A. Immersing
   B. Dipping
   C. Spraying
   D. Sterilizing

11. The gingiva that occupies the space between teeth is described as 11.____

   A. papillary
   B. apical
   C. marginal
   D. free

12. A technician is preparing a wax pattern. To place melted wax near the occlusal fossa extending to the cusp tip, the technician should use a(n) 12.____

   A. wax bur
   B. PKT #1 instrument
   C. burnisher
   D. PKT #3 instrument

13. What is the tooth with the longest root in the dental arch? 13.____

   A. Mandibular canine
   B. Maxillary canine
   C. Mandibular central
   D. Maxillary central

14. The point at which dental wax softens is described as the 14.____

A. dimensional change
B. melting range
C. residual
D. flow

15. The nerve supply to the muscles of mastication is provided by cranial nerve 15.____

A. IV
B. VI
C. VIII
D. X

16. Which of the following dental tissues provides nutrients to odontoblasts, removes wastes, and acts as a sensor for the tooth? 16.____

A. Enamel
B. Pulp
C. Dentin
D. Gingiva

17. To qualify for certification, dental technicians must have either a dental technology degree or a minimum of ______ years of on-the-job training 17.____

A. 2 B. 3 C. 4 D. 5

18. The bonding agent used for endodontic posts in root canals should be 18.____

I. light-curing
II. self-curing
III. dual-curing
IV. applied thinly

A. I and IV
B. I and III
C. II, III and IV
D. I, II, III and IV

19. Bonded joints between teeth and materials are formed by ______ cements. 19.____

A. metal oxide
B. resin
C. polymer
D. zinc phosphate

20. A technician has mixed luting cement in the laboratory by hand. Which of the following is an advantage associated with hand-mixing? 20.____

A. Shades can be mixed if necessary
B. Less cleanup required
C. More consistent mixture
D. Convenience

21. In order to be certified, a dental laboratory must do each of the following, EXCEPT 21.____

A. employ certified dental technicians in supervisory positions
B. renew certification periodically after undergoing a review
C. document compliance with accepted health and safety standards
D. maintain high levels of training and practice in infection control

22. Gypsum models usually reach full strength about ______ hour(s) after they are poured. 22.____

A. 1
B. 12
C. 24
D. 48

23. A material that has become permanently deformed is said to have exceeded its 23.____

A. ultimate strength
B. hardness
C. tensile strength
D. resiliency

24. For what purpose are bioactive ceramic materials used to coat implant fixtures? 24.____

A. Increasing implant passivity
B. Maximizing abutment mobility
C. Forming strong bonds with bone
D. Plasticizing the acrylic

25. When making casts, advantages associated with the use of a solid working cast with individual dies of prepared teeth include 25.____

I. Overall pattern accuracy is maintained as the wax pattern is transferred from the dies to the solid cast.
II. The positional relationship between the prepared teeth is maintained.
III. The gingival contours of the wax pattern are readily accessible on the die.
IV. It is easier for the technician to develop occlusal and axial contours.

A. I and II
B. I, II and III
C. II and III
D. I, II and III

KEY (CORRECT ANSWERS)

1. A
2. D
3. D
4. D
5. A
6. D
7. C
8. A
9. C
10. D
11. A
12. B
13. B
14. B
15. B
16. B
17. D
18. C
19. C
20. A
21. B
22. C
23. A
24. C
25. C

TEST 3

DIRECTIONS: Each question or incomplete statement is followed by several suggested answers or completions. Select the one the BEST answers the question or completes the statement. *PRINT THE LETTER OF THE CORRECT ANSWER IN THE SPACE AT THE RIGHT.*

1. Which of the following gypsum products has the highest compressive strength? 1.____

   A. High strength dental stone
   B. High strength/high expansion dental stone
   C. Dental stone
   D. Model plaster

2. A dental technician is sending an impression back to a dental office. Before packing the impression, the technician should remember that 2.____

   A. polyether impressions should be immersed for at least 30 minutes in disinfectant before transport
   B. the impression should be dried thoroughly before transport
   C. alginate impressions require climate-controlled transport
   D. impressions should never be transported in a disinfectant solution

3. The curvature of the cervical line of a tooth is greatest on the ______ surface. 3.____

   A. distal
   B. mesial
   C. lingual
   D. facial

4. Before they are autoclaved, placement instruments should have all remnants of amalgam removed from them. The reason for this is because 4.____

   A. steam may cause the amalgam to fuse to the instrument
   B. the heat of autoclaving can melt silver and clog the drain
   C. steam may cause the amalgam to corrode
   D. the heat of autoclaving can release mercury vapor

5. In a class I occlusion, the mandibular lateral incisor 5.____

   A. opposes only the maxillary canine
   B. opposes the maxillary central and lateral incisors
   C. does not contact the opposing teeth
   D. opposes the maxillary lateral incisor and canine

6. Which of the following is a masticating muscle that does NOT have the primary action of elevating the mandible? 6.____

   A. Temporalis
   B. Masseter
   C. Medial pterygoid
   D. Lateral pterygoid

7. Which of the following cements undergoes an exothermic reaction during mixing? 7.___

   A. Calcium hydroxide
   B. Zinc phosphate
   C. Glass ionomer
   D. Resin

8. Under OSHA's Bloodborne Pathogens Standard, dental laboratory personnel must be offered 8.___

   A. a hepatitis B vaccine
   B. a smallpox vaccine
   C. hazardous chemicals training
   D. eyewash station training

9. The placement of a completed alginate impression on a flat surface, impression side down, may tend to flatten the impression. Which of the following is a reason for this? 9.___

   A. Water retention
   B. Compression
   C. Elasticity
   D. Void reduction

10. A technician reads an order for a restoration to be made to a tooth that is designated "48" on the work order. The code system being used is ______; the tooth designated is ______. 10.___

   A. FDI; maxillary left second molar
   B. FDI; mandibular right third molar
   C. Universal; maxilllary right second premolar
   D. Universal; mandibular left central incisor

11. Which of the following is NOT a layer of the enamel organ? 11.___

   A. Strata corneum
   B. Stratum intermedium
   C. Inner enamel epithelium
   D. Stellate reticulum

12. Which of the following is a term that means "a civil wrong or action that brings harm to an individual's person, property, or reputation"? 12.___

   A. Malpractice
   B. Breach
   C. Tort
   D. Malfeasance

13. What is the term for a cohesive layer on the dentin surface that consists of cut tooth debris and salivary contaminants? 13.___

   A. Strue
   B. Hybrid layer
   C. Smear layer
   D. Microleakage

14. Calcium hydroxide may need to be placed under ______ to protect the pulp from acid. 14.____

    I. glass ionomer
    II. resin
    III. zinc phosphate
    IV. zinc polycarboxylate

    A. I only
    B. I and III
    C. II, III and IV
    D. I, II, III and IV

15. In the international code, tooth 8-5 denotes the 15.____

    A. permanent mandibular left second molar
    B. permanent mandibular right second molar
    C. primary mandibular left second molar
    D. primary mandibular right second molar

16. Which of the following were declared illegal in the United States in 1939? 16.____

    A. Dental amalgams containing more than 50 percent mercury
    B. Mail-order dentures
    C. Dentists who practiced without a license
    D. Anesthetics containing ether

17. Each of the following are hypocalcified areas in enamel, EXCEPT 17.____

    A. lines of Retzius
    B. enamel rods
    C. tufts
    D. spindles

18. In the United States, the first material to be widely used for the purpose of filling tooth cavities was ______, which dates to the Civil War era. 18.____

    A. silver amalgam
    B. gold
    C. baked porcelain
    D. composite

19. Solder joints in crowns, bridges and veneers are typically smoothed with a 19.____

    A. fine rubber disc
    B. carboniferous disc
    C. silicon impregnated rubber tip
    D. tapered stone

20. The excess space available for the permanent canine and premolars is known as the ______ space. 20.____

    A. macrodontic
    B. leeway
    C. gratuitous
    D. primate

21. What is another term for the cementoenamel junction (CEJ)? 21.____

A. Gingival margin
B. Line of Retzius
C. Sulcus
D. Cervical line

22. Which of the following is LEAST typically an indirect restorative material? 22.____

A. Porcelain
B. Gold
C. Amalgam
D. Porcelain

23. Ceramic is used on metal structures for the purpose of 23.____

A. reducing tarnish
B. veneering
C. preventing corrosion
D. strengthening

24. The biggest problem facing the early pioneers in denture fabrication was 24.____

A. the lack of a durable and affordable denture base material
B. an overemphasis by practitioners on tooth extraction
C. the difficulty in making accurate dental impressions
D. infection control

25. A tapered brush is often used in a dental laboratory for each of the following, EXCEPT 25.____

A. dusting powdered wax on the occlusal surface of a pattern
B. applying dentin powder to the surface of a pontic
C. applying wax separating medium to a working cast
D. applying a hard wax layer over a soft wax layer

KEY (CORRECT ANSWERS)

1. D
2. B
3. A
4. B
5. C

6. A
7. A
8. B
9. C
10. A

11. A
12. C
13. B
14. A
15. A

16. C
17. A
18. D
19. D
20. D

21. B
22. D
23. A
24. D
25. D

TEST 4

DIRECTIONS: Each question or incomplete statement is followed by several suggested answers or completions. Select the one the BEST answers the question or completes the statement. *PRINT THE LETTER OF THE CORRECT ANSWER IN THE SPACE AT THE RIGHT.*

1. Some of the continuing education testing that may be used to satisfy renewal requirements for dental technicians is provided by the 1.____

   A. *Journal of Prosthodontics*
   B. *Journal of the American Dental Association*
   C. *Journal of Dental Education*
   D. *Journal of Dental Technology*

2. In order to be considered a "high noble" material, an alloy must contain ______ percent gold by weight. 2.____

   A. 20
   B. 40
   C. 60
   D. 80

3. The concept of informed consent upholds the ethical principle of ______ in health care decision-making. 3.____

   A. autonomy
   B. paternalism
   C. confidentiality
   D. documentation

4. The receiving area of a dental laboratory should be treated with surface disinfectant 4.____

   A. at the beginning and the end of every work day
   B. at the end of every work day
   C. every other day
   D. weekly

5. The reason newly-poured gypsum models contain excess water is because 5.____

   A. more water insures fewer voids
   B. thick gypsum mixes set too quickly
   C. more water is needed for mixing and pouring than for setting
   D. thinner mixes set more quickly

6. In terms of occlusion, an overbite would be classified as a(n) 6.____

   A. vertical overlap
   B. neutroclusion
   C. overjet
   D. mesioclusion

7. The main disadvantage associated with the early Vulcanite denture bases was that they 7.____

   A. had an unattractive dark red color
   B. often caused allergic reactions
   C. were too costly for most people
   D. relied on springs for retention

8. Because latex retards the set of ______ impression materials, technicians should be careful to use non-latex gloves when preparing them. 8.____

   A. gypsum
   B. silicone
   C. polysulfide
   D. hydrocolloid

9. Dental cements that bond before placement include 9.____
   I. polycarboxylate
   II. zinc oxide/eugenol
   III. composite resin
   IV. glass ionomer

   A. I only
   B. I and III
   C. III and IV
   D. II, III and IV

10. Which of the following is a procedure that will create a high-impact resin? 10.____

   A. Adding rubber to acrylic
   B. Removing free monomer
   C. Heat treating polymerized resin
   D. Adding plasticizers

11. What is the collective term for the areas of oral ectoderm that thicken and grow down into the mesoderm of the developing jaws? 11.____

   A. Enamel organs
   B. Mucosa
   C. Meatae
   D. Dental papillae

12. In the universal code, tooth "I" would be replaced by tooth number 12.____

   A. 4
   B. 9
   C. 12
   D. 15

13. The bonding of materials to dentin is best accomplished by 13.____

   A. eliminating the formation of a hybrid layer
   B. keeping the dentin moist after etching
   C. etching with 30% acid for 30 seconds
   D. keeping the dentin dry after etching

14. Which of the following could be described as a trail of cells left by the enamel organ as a guide for root development of the tooth? 14.____

   A. Hertwig's epithelial root sheath
   B. Rests of Malassez
   C. Lines of Retzius
   D. Ducts of Rivinus

15. Early fillings to restore decayed teeth date back to the _______, who pressed gold into teeth over 2000 years ago. 15.____

   A. Phoenicians
   B. Greeks
   C. Chinese
   D. Egyptians

16. How many pulp horns are on the roof of the pulp chamber in the primary mandibular first molar? 16.____

   A. 2
   B. 3
   C. 4
   D. 5

17. Which of the following teeth is wider on the lingual surface than the buccal? 17.____

   A. Maxillary first molar
   B. Mandibular first molar
   C. Maxillary central incisor
   D. Mandibular first premolar

18. An alginate impression should be removed from the mouth in one long, continuous pull, in order to prevent 18.____

   A. warp
   B. suction
   C. syneresis
   D. tearing

19. A carbide bur would be used for which of the following procedures? 19.____

   A. Removing utility wax from the area surrounding a dowel pin
   B. Separating a die from a solid cast
   C. Trimming sectioned dies with a tapered root form
   D. Removing excess stone from below the gingival margin of a cast

20. Which of the following is NOT a bone of the zygomatic process? 20.____

   A. Maxillary
   B. Zygoma
   C. Temporal
   D. Parietal

21. Solid materials that flow under mechanical forces are described as 21.____

A. starchy
B. thixotropic
C. colloidal
D. viscous

22. Which of the following is a jacket crown material with high aesthetic appeal, but is also susceptible to fracture? 22.____

A. Composite resin
B. Cast ceramic
C. Gold alloy (noble)
D. Porcelain

23. The certifying organization for U. S. prosthodontists is the 23.____

A. American Board of Prosthodontics
B. American Dental Association
C. Academy of American Prosthodontics
D. National Association of Dental Laboratories

24. Which of the anterior teeth is MOST likely to have a lingual ridge? 24.____

A. Mandibular canine
B. Mandibular central
C. Maxillary central
D. Maxillary canine

25. The apex of a properly made Gothic arch tracing indicates 25.____

A. condylar path inclination
B. protrusive occlusion
C. overjet
D. centric occlusion

KEY (CORRECT ANSWERS)

1. B
2. D
3. B
4. D
5. B

6. C
7. B
8. A
9. B
10. B

11. A
12. C
13. C
14. B
15. D

16. B
17. B
18. A
19. A
20. D

21. C
22. B
23. B
24. A
25. D

ANATOMIC SCIENCES
EXAMINATION SECTION
TEST 1

DIRECTIONS: Each question or incomplete statement is followed by several suggested answers or completions. Select the one that BEST answers the question or completes the statement. *PRINT THE LETTER OF THE CORRECT ANSWER IN THE SPACE AT THE RIGHT.*

1. The two muscles which use the pterygomandibular raphe for part of their attachment receive their innervation from the 1.____

   A. vagus nerve
   B. facial nerve
   C. mandibular nerve
   D. facial and vagus nerves
   E. mandibular and vagus nerves

2. Preganglionic nerve cell bodies for fibers which go to the otic ganglion are located in the 2.____

   A. inferior salivatory nucleus
   B. superior salivatory nucleus
   C. dorsal motor nucleus of vagus nerve
   D. accessory nucleus of oculomotor nerve
   E. mesencephalic nucleus of trigeminal nerve

3. The lingula of the mandible serves as an attachment for the 3.____

   A. temporalis muscle
   B. stylomandibular ligament
   C. sphenomandibular ligament
   D. temporomandibular ligament
   E. tendon of the digastric muscle

4. The dental pulp may react to peripheral stimulation by 4.____
   I. inflammation
   II. dentin deposition
   III. growth of pain endings
   IV. elastic fiber production
   V. odontoblastic proliferation

   The CORRECT combination is:

   A. I or II
   B. I or III
   C. II, III, or V
   D. III or IV
   E. IV or V

5. Which of the following does cementum repair in an adult tooth? 5.____
   I. Resorbed bone
   II. Resorbed dentin
   III. Resorbed enamel
   IV. Resorbed cementum

   The CORRECT answer is:

   A. I, II
   B. I, III
   C. II, III
   D. II, IV
   E. III, IV

6. The pterygoid plexus is *usually* formed by veins which are tributaries of the 6.___

   A. facial vein
   B. angular vein
   C. maxillary vein
   D. retromandibular vein
   E. jugular vein

7. The chorda tympani carries preganglionic parasympathetic fibers from the facial nerve to the 7.___

   A. pterygopalatine ganglion
   B. otic ganglion
   C. inferior alveolar nerve
   D. submandibular ganglion
   E. optic nerve

8. Cementum differs from dentin in that cementum 8.___

   A. contains more inorganic material than dentin
   B. may contain cells, whereas dentin contains cells as well as cell processes
   C. contains some elastic fibers, whereas dentin contains only collagenous fibers
   D. is produced by cells of the periodontal ligament, but dentin is produced by pulp cells
   E. there is no difference

9. The insertion of the lateral pterygoid muscle is into the 9.___

   A. articular disk of the temporomandibular joint and mandibular neck
   B. medial surface of the mandibular angle
   C. coronoid process of the mandible
   D. pterygomandibular raphe
   E. none of the above

10. Which of the following is *never* found at the outer surface of the enamel? 10.___

   A. Perikymata
   B. Enamel tufts
   C. Enamel matrix
   D. Enamel lamella
   E. All of the above

11. A muscle that acts to protrude the mandible is the 11.___

   A. masseter
   B. mylohyoid
   C. digastric
   D. temporalis
   E. lateral pterygoid

12. A calcified body located in the periodontal ligament is called 12.___

   A. denticle
   B. cementicle
   C. isle of Langerhans
   D. deciduous root fragment
   E. epithelial rest of Malassez

13. Incremental lines of Retzius appear 13.____

A. in dentin and follow the appositional pattern
B. in enamel and follow the appositional pattern
C. as lines in the dentin running at right angles to the dentino-enamel junction
D. between bundle bone and lamellated bone of the alveolus
E. only on x-rays

14. The embryonic vestibular lamina gives rise to the 14.____

A. space between the alveolar portion of the jaws, and the lips and cheeks
B. deciduous teeth
C. outer dental epithelium
D. buccopharyngeal membrane
E. premaxilla

15. The tendon of the tensor veli palatini muscle curves around the 15.____

A. angular spine
B. styloid process
C. pterygoid hamulus
D. lateral pterygoid plate
E. neck of the condyle of the mandible

16. Which of the following cranial nerves contain a complete combination of autonomic efferent, somatic efferent and special taste afferent fibers? 16.____

I. Vagus
II. Facial
III. Trigeminal
IV. Oculomotor
V. Vestibulocochlear

The CORRECT answer is:

A. I, II
B. I, III
C. I, IV
D. II, III
E. II, V

17. Hypomineralized structures which extend from the dentino-enamel junction to the surface of the enamel are called 17.____

A. enamel rods
B. enamel lamellae
C. enamel spindles
D. Hunter-Schreger bands
E. incremental lines of Retzius

18. Infection spreading via lymphatics from the lower lip would FIRST enter the bloodstream at the 18.____

A. brachiocephalic vein
B. inferior labial vein
C. inferior labial artery
D. pterygoid venous plexus
E. none of the above

19. The palatine tonsil lies between arches formed by the 19.____

A. levator veli palatini and tensor veli palatini muscles
B. palatoglossus and palatopharyngeus muscles
C. levator veli palatini and salpingopharyngeus muscles
D. salpingopharyngeus and palatopharyngeus muscles
E. none of the above

20. Bone of the lingual alveolar process of the maxillary incisor consists of 20.____

A. an intervening layer of supporting spongiosa
B. an inner cribriform plate
C. an outer cortical plate
D. all of the above
E. none of the above

21. Which of the following arteries does NOT accompany the corresponding nerve throughout its course? 21.____

A. Lingual
B. Infraorbital
C. Inferior alveolar
D. Posterior superior alveolar
E. All of the above

22. As seen in a buccolingual section through a tooth and its related gingiva, the separation between free gingiva and attached gingiva extends between the 22.____

A. alveolar crest and the free gingival groove
B. bottom of the gingival sulcus and the free gingival groove
C. apical margin of the epithelial attachment and the alveolar crest
D. apical margin of the epithelial attachment and the free gingival groove
E. alveolar crest and the free gingival groove

23. The remnants of the epithelial sheath of Hertwig are called the epithelial rests of Malassez. The fate of these is that they 23.____

I. may undergo calcification
II. may form into cementicles
III. become fibrous
IV. always disappear

The CORRECT answer is:

A. I, II, III
B. I, II
C. II, III
D. II, III, IV
E. III, IV

24. During the functional life of a tooth, certain changes occur, which include: 24.____

I. Enamel permeability decreases and length of anatomic root increases
II. Pulp stones are acquired and height of alveolar bone increases
III. Pulp cellularity decreases and amount of sclerotic dentin increases
IV. Interglobular dentin increases and perikymata decreases

The CORRECT answer is:

A. I, II
B. I, III
C. I, IV
D. II, III
E. II, IV

25. To expose the submandibular duct by an intraoral approach, one must cut through 25.____

A. mucous membrane
B. mylohyoid muscle
C. buccinator muscle
D. geniohyoid muscle
E. all of the above

KEY (CORRECT ANSWERS)

1. D
2. A
3. C
4. A
5. D
6. C
7. D
8. D
9. A
10. B
11. E
12. B
13. B
14. A
15. C
16. A
17. B
18. A
19. B
20. D
21. A
22. B
23. B
24. B
25. A

TEST 2

DIRECTIONS: Each question or incomplete statement is followed by several suggested answers or completions. Select the one that BEST answers the question or completes the statement. *PRINT THE LETTER OF THE CORRECT ANSWER IN THE SPACE AT THE RIGHT.*

1. Which of the following items are components of the tooth germ?
   I. Meckel's cartilage
   II. Enamel organ
   III. Successional lamina
   IV. Dental papilla
   V. Vestibular lamina
   VI. Dental sac
   VII. Rathke's pouch
   The CORRECT answer is:

   A. I, III, V, VII
   B. II, IV, VI
   C. II, IV, VI, VII
   D. IV, V, VI, VII
   E. IV, VI

2. In the development of the face, what brings about a separation between lips and cheeks, externally, and the jaw structures, internally?

   A. Lamina dura
   B. Dental lamina
   C. Lamina propria
   D. Vestibular lamina
   E. None of the above

3. The superior portion of the genioglossal muscle joins

   A. mandible to styloid process of the skull
   B. mandible to tongue
   C. mandible to hyoid
   D. hyoid to tongue
   E. tongue to hyoid

4. The submental lymph nodes receive lymphatic vessels from all of the following EXCEPT the

   A. mandibular molars
   B. tip of the tongue
   C. middle of the lower lip
   D. mandibular lateral incisors
   E. mandibular central incisors

5. The gingival area where non-keratinized epithelium is MOST frequently seen and which, therefore, may be considered most vulnerable to inflammation is the

   A. sulcular surface of the free gingiva
   B. attached gingiva
   C. palatal gingiva
   D. all of the above
   E. none of the above

6. Which feature of cellular cementum BEST differentiates it from acellular cementum? 6.____

   A. Lacunae
   B. Embedded Sharpey's fibers
   C. An incremental growth pattern
   D. Separate and distinct functions
   E. None of the above

7. Compact bone as found in the cribriform plate (lamina dura) of the wall of the alveolar socket is characterized by 7.____

   A. containing a collagenous fiber background, and by resisting resorption when placed under pressure as in orthodontic movement of teeth
   B. forming the crest of the alveolar socket at which place transseptal fibers of the periodontal ligament are attached
   C. containing Sharpey's fibers which are extensions of the reticular fibers of the periodontal ligament
   D. being perforated by vascular canals and by possessing numerous lamellae
   E. none of the above

8. Which muscle of the soft palate is NOT supplied by the pharyngeal plexus? 8.____

   A. Palatoglossus
   B. Palatopharyngeus
   C. Musculus uvulae
   D. Tensor veli palatini
   E. Levator veli palatini

9. All of the following structures may be found in oral mucous membrane EXCEPT the 9.____

   A. basal lamina
   B. lamina propria
   C. muscularis mucosae
   D. keratohyaline granules
   E. stratified squamous epithelium

10. Which of the following bony changes dominate during tooth eruption? 10.____

   A. Apposition on the surface of the alveolar crest and apposition on the socket fundus
   B. Apposition on the surface of the alveolar crest and resorption on the socket fundus
   C. Resorption on the surface of the alveolar crest and apposition on the socket fundus
   D. Resorption on the surface of the alveolar crest and resorption on the socket fundus
   E. None of the above

11. Apical abscesses on certain teeth have a marked tendency to produce cervical spread of infection which occurs most rapidly in abscesses of 11.____

   A. maxillary incisors
   B. mandibular canines
   C. maxillary premolars
   D. mandibular second and third molars
   E. none of the above

12. At the time enamel matrix is first formed in a given tooth,

    A. no predentin has yet been formed
    B. the nuclei of the ameloblasts move to the nonsecreting end of the cell
    C. the root of the tooth is largely covered with acellular cementum
    D. the cells of the stellate reticulum near the cervical portion of the tooth have lost their nuclei
    E. none of the above

13. The mandibular foramen is located

    A. nearest the premolars
    B. nearest the incisors
    C. medial to the lingual borders of the molars
    D. below the occlusal plane of the mandibular molars and posterior to them
    E. above the occlusal plane of the mandibular molars and posterior to them

14. Development of the body of the mandible involves

    A. Reichert's cartilage
    B. a complete cartilage model
    C. intramembranous bone development
    D. all of the above
    E. none of the above

15. When a tooth first erupts into the oral cavity, the attached epithelial cuff is composed of epithelium derived from

    A. oral mucosa
    B. reduced dental epithelium
    C. epithelial rests of Malassez
    D. Hertwig's epithelial root sheath
    E. increased dental epithelium

16. Which of the following statements about the mandible is(are) CORRECT?
    I. The mandible is the largest bone in the face.
    II. It is the only freely movable bone in the face.
    III. The right and left mandibles are joined at the chin by an invisible suture.
    IV. The right and left mandibles appear to be one bone and are referred to as one bone.
    V. The mandible consists of a body and two vertical extensions of the body, rami-one ramus on each side.

    The CORRECT answer is:

    A. I *only*
    B. I, II
    C. I, II, III
    D. I, II, III, IV
    E. I, II, III, IV, V

17. Which of the following statements about the temporomandibular joint is(are) CORRECT? 17.____

    I. The temporomandibular joint derives its name from the two bones involved in the joint.
    II. The temporomandibular joint makes possible the movements of the mandible.
    III. All movements of the mandible and the function of the teeth are closely associated with the temporomandibular joint.
    IV. The structures which form the joint include four ligaments.
    V. The temporomandibular joint varies widely from person to person

    The CORRECT answer is:

    A. I *only*
    B. I, II
    C. I, II, III
    D. I, II, III, IV
    E. I, II, III, IV, V

18. Which of the following CORRECTLY describes the structure of the major salivary glands? 18.____

    A. Simple tubular gland
    B. Compound acinar gland
    C. Simple tubuloalveolar gland
    D. Compound tubuloalveolar gland
    E. Simple acinar gland

19. In the mandibular block anesthesia, which of the following muscles is penetrated if the tip of the needle is resting well below the mandibular foramen? 19.____

    A. Temporal
    B. Masseter
    C. Medial pterygoid
    D. Lateral pterygoid
    E. Sternocleidomastoid

20. The arterial supply of the submandibular gland is from which branch of the external carotid artery? 20.____

    A. Ascending pharyngeal
    B. Superior thyroid
    C. Maxillary
    D. Facial
    E. Descending pharyngeal

21. The enamel has no possibility of self-repair because 21.____

    A. it has only a small percent of organic content
    B. its formative cells are lost once it is completely formed
    C. it is essentially a keratin tissue and has no blood vessels
    D. it has no direct connection with the active cells of the dental pulp
    E. it has a large percent of organic content

22. The periodontal ligament consists of groups of collagenous fiber bundles. The group of fibers which gives the GREATEST support against masticatory forces is the 22.____

    A. apical
    B. oblique
    C. horizontal
    D. alveolar crest
    E. interradicular

23. The superior orbital fissure is located between the

    A. greater and lesser wings of the sphenoid
    B. greater wing of the sphenoid and the maxilla
    C. lesser wing of the sphenoid and the palatine bone
    D. greater wing of the sphenoid and the pterygoid process of the sphenoid
    E. pterygoid process of the sphenoid and the maxilla

24. Gingival massage through toothbrushing increases the circulation of blood in vessels of the

    A. epithelial covering of the gingiva
    B. basal layer of the epithelium
    C. lamina propria
    D. dental pulp
    E. none of the above

25. The expected effect on the periodontal ligament following the loss of tooth function would be

    A. a slight edema
    B. formation of numerous cementicles
    C. an increase in thickness and fiber density
    D. a reduction in width and loss of regular arrangement of principal fibers
    E. a large edema

KEY (CORRECT ANSWERS)

1. B
2. D
3. B
4. A
5. A
6. A
7. D
8. D
9. C
10. A
11. D
12. B
13. E
14. C
15. B
16. E
17. E
18. D
19. C
20. D
21. B
22. B
23. D
24. C
25. D

ANATOMIC SCIENCES
EXAMINATION SECTION
TEST 1

DIRECTIONS: Each question or incomplete statement is followed by several suggested answers or completions. Select the one that BEST answers the question or completes the statement. *PRINT THE LETTER OF THE CORRECT ANSWER IN THE SPACE AT THE RIGHT.*

1. The sublingual gland is located 1.____

   A. in the oral vestibule
   B. deep to the genioglossal muscle
   C. inferior to the mylohyoiti muscle
   D. superior to the mylohyoid muscle
   E. next to the inferior meatus

2. The mucosa of the floor of the mouth is characterized by 2.____

   A. being non-keratinized, and by having no glands in the lamina propria
   B. having a thin elastic layer, and by having a stratified cuboidal epithelium
   C. being covered with a thin epithelial layer, and by possessing some serous salivary glands
   D. containing some lymph nodes in its lamina propria, and by being loose in texture
   E. being keratinized, and by having glands in the lamina propria

3. In considering the process of eruption, the prefunctional eruptive stage of a tooth begins when the 3.____

   A. bud stage begins
   B. cap stage begins
   C. bell stage begins
   D. dental lamina begins forming
   E. none of the above

4. The free gingival groove divides the 4.____

   A. free gingiva and the alveolar mucosa
   B. free gingiva and the attached gingiva
   C. attached gingiva and the alveolar mucosa
   D. interdental papillae and the marginal gingiva
   E. free gingiva and the marginal mucosa

5. The posterior border of the buccinator muscle fibers terminates, or is attached to, the 5.____

   A. stylohyoid ligament
   B. pterygomandibular raphel
   C. stylomandibular ligament
   D. sphenomandibular ligament
   E. none of the above

6. A calcified body located in the periodontal ligament is called a(n) 6.____

   A. denticle
   B. cementicle
   C. islet of Langerhans
   D. deciduous root fragment
   E. epithelial rest of Malassez

7. Pain originates in the pulp due to

   A. free nerve endings primarily located in the center of the pulp
   B. free nerve endings about the odontoblastic cells
   C. free nerve endings in the cell-rich layer of the pulp
   D. myelinated nerve fibers in the adjacent part of the dentin
   E. free nerve endings in the adjacent part of the dentin

8. The gingiva offers protection against bacterial invasion, the most important factor in this protection being that the

   A. lymph supply is good
   B. surface epithelium is highly impervious
   C. crest of the alveolar bone is highly impervious
   D. lamina propria contains heavy collagenous fibers
   E. lamina propria contains light collagenous fibers

9. Meckel's cartilage of the first branchial arch is characterized by

   A. forming from mesenchyme; chondrocytes in this cartilage elaborate inorganic salts which cause the cartilage to become calcified, after which the cartilage resorbs
   B. serving as a model for the future mandible; in midline, bilateral cartilages fuse to yield symphysis which forms by endochondral bone formation
   C. giving rise to hyaline cartilage which covers the articular surface of the condyle; eventually, this cartilage covering is replaced by a thin layer of compact bone
   D. being a model for the mandible but not participating in the formation of any part of the mandible; cartilage does, however, give rise to the malleus
   E. none of the above

10. Compared with intertubular dentin, peritubular dentin is characterized by having

    A. more inorganic salt content and a finer collagenous matrix
    B. less inorganic salt content and a heavier collagenous matrix
    C. more fluid content and a different refractive index
    D. fewer fibers and by being more stainable
    E. none of the above

11. Retraction of the mandible is achieved by the

    A. medial and lateral pterygoid muscles
    B. lateral pterygoid, geniohyoid, and digastric muscles
    C. lateral pterygoid and deep portion of masseter muscles
    D. posterior fibers of temporalis, geniohyoid, and digastric muscles
    E. none of the above

12. If there is a granular layer in the epithelium of oral mucosa, the granules are *primarily*

    A. vermilion granules which aid in imparting red color to mucosa
    B. keratohyalin granules which play a role in keratinization of mucosa
    C. melanin granules which, when sufficiently abundant, impart dark pigment to mucosa
    D. all of the above
    E. none of the above

13. Which of the following does NOT apply to the temporomandibular joint? 13.____

A. The retrodiscal pad is highly vascular.
B. A synovial fluid is found in the articular spaces.
C. Large numbers of collagenous fibers are found in the articular disk.
D. Compact bone in the articular fossa is especially thick and resistant to trauma.
E. The fibrous coverings of the articular surfaces are devoid of blood vessels.

14. The nerve supply to the muscles of mastication indicates that these muscles are derived from the 14.____

A. first branchial arch
B. second branchial arch
C. third branchial arch
D. fourth branchial arch
E. all of the above

15. Comparison among tonsils of humans shows that 15.____

A. the lingual tonsil is located posterior to the V-shaped row of the vallate papillae; mucosa of this area of the tongue is innervated by the glossopharyngeal nerve
B. the pharyngeal tonsil is covered on its free surface by respiratory and stratified squamous epithelia; this tonsil possesses crypts that are the deepest of all tonsil masses
C. the palatine tonsil is covered on its free surface by stratified squamous epithelium which is keratinized; nodules in this tonsil lack germinal centers
D. all masses of tonsillar tissue are subepithelial in location and all tonsil masses have crypts into which lymphocytes migrate to become salivary corpuscles
E. none of the above

16. The mental foramen is normally located below the apices of the mandibular 16.____

A. first and second molars
B. canine and first premolar
C. first and second premolars
D. second premolar and first molar
E. none of the above

17. Lymph vessels from the posterior portion of the nasal cavity end in the 17.____

A. submental nodes
B. submandibular nodes
C. superficial cervical nodes
D. deep cervical nodes and retropharyngeal nodes
E. none of the above

18. The rests of Malassez in the periodontal ligament derive from 18.____

A. dental pulp
B. lamina propria
C. vestibular lamina
D. odontogenic epithelium
E. none of the above

19. Dentin is a type of connective tissue 19.

A. with the same structural features as bone
B. best considered as dead tissue rather than living tissue
C. which is softer than enamel but harder than bone
D. which, except for location, is identical with cementum
E. which contains numerous, easily demonstrated nerve endings making it very sensitive

20. The portion of the medial wall of the infratemporal fossa is formed by the 20.

A. temporal surface of the frontal bone
B. lateral pterygoid plate of the sphenoid bone
C. zygomatic arch and ascending ramus of the mandible
D. infratemporal crest of the greater wing of the sphenoid
E. posterior surface of the zygomatic process of the maxillary bone

21. In the human embryo, the upper lip is formed by fusion of the 21.

A. median nasal process with maxillary processes
B. median nasal process with the second branchial arch
C. premaxilla with maxillary processes
D. first branchial arch with the second branchial arch
E. median nasal process with lateral nasal processes

22. The body of the mandible is formed by 22.

A. replacement of a cartilage model by bone
B. intramembranous ossification similar to that of the bones of the cranial vault
C. ordinary endochondral ossification similar to that of most long bones
D. conversion of cartilage directly into bone
E. none of the above

23. The eventual products of the dental papilla are 23.

A. pulp only
B. pulp and dentin only
C. pulp, dentin and cementum only
D. pulp, dentin, cementum, and the periodontal ligament
E. all of the above

24. Alveolar bone proper of the socket of a tooth is characterized by 24

A. consisting of compact bone, by showing dark on a radiograph, and by containing Sharpey's fibers
B. resorbing when subjected to pressure, by containing numerous openings through which vessels pass, and by often being called the cribriform plate
C. containing haversian systems, by having collagen fibers in its matrix, and by being about 96 percent inorganic salts
D. serving to attach free gingival periodontal ligament fibers, and by being a part of the total tooth attachment apparatus
E. all of the above

25. The gingival sulcus is bounded by the 25.____

A. tooth surface and epithelial covering of attached gingiva
B. tooth surface and epithelial covering of free gingiva
C. epithelial covering of free and attached gingiva
D. free gingival groove and mucogingival junction
E. none of the above

KEY (CORRECT ANSWERS)

1. D
2. A
3. E
4. B
5. B
6. B
7. B
8. B
9. D
10. A
11. D
12. B
13. D
14. A
15. A
16. C
17. D
18. D
19. C
20. B
21. A
22. B
23. B
24. B
25. B

TEST 2

DIRECTIONS: Each question or incomplete statement is followed by several suggested answers or completions. Select the one that BEST answers the question or completes the statement. *PRINT THE LETTER OF THE CORRECT ANSWER IN THE SPACE AT THE RIGHT.*

1. The PRINCIPAL fibers of the periodontal ligament, which resist apically-directed pressures on the tooth, extend from the cementum to the bone 1.

   A. apically
   B. occlusally
   C. horizontally
   D. all of the above
   E. only A and B above

2. The space between the jaws into which the teeth erupt is generally considered to be provided by growth at the 2.

   A. alveolar processes
   B. mandibular condyles
   C. sphenomaxillary, frontomaxillary, and zygomaticomaxillary sutures
   D. intermaxillary suture and mental symphysis
   E. none of the above

3. The temporalis muscle originates along the sides of the skull and passes 3

   A. *medial* to the zygomatic arch and inserts into the coronoid process of the mandible
   B. *lateral* to the zygomatic arch and inserts into the coronoid process of the mandible
   C. *medial* to the zygomatic arch and inserts into the medial side of the angle of the ramus
   D. *lateral* to the zygomatic arch and inserts into the medial side of the angle of the ramus
   E. none of the above

4. What does the glossopharyngeal nerve supply? 4

   I. Motor innervation to the tongue
   II. Taste sensation to the posterior third of the tongue
   III. Sensory innervation to the anterior two-thirds of the tongue
   IV. Motor innervation to the constrictors of the pharynx and the stylopharyngeus muscle

   The CORRECT answer is:

   A. I, II
   B. I, III
   C. I, IV
   D. II, IV
   E. III, IV

5. Infections of dental origin may reach the thorax by traversing a fascial space between the 5.

   A. prevertebral and parotid fascia
   B. pterygoid and pretracheal fascia
   C. superficial cervical and buccopharyngeal fascia
   D. carotid and masseteric fascia
   E. buccopharyngeal and prevertebral fascia

6. The mandibular fossa is divided into two parts by the 6.____

A. glenoid fissure
B. articular tubercle
C. petrotympanic fissure
D. zygomaticomaxillary suture
E. none of the above

7. Two muscles which attach to the pterygomandibular raphe are the 7.____

A. buccinator and the stylopharyngeus
B. buccinator and the superior pharyngeal constrictor
C. tensor veli palatini and the glossopalatinus
D. levator veli palatini and the palatopharyngeus
E. superior pharyngeal constrictor and the palatoglossus

8. Which of the following statements MOST accurately describes the mineralization process of enamel matrix? 8.____

A. Complete mineralization occurs in one phase concurrent with matrix formation.
B. Complete mineralization occurs in one phase which begins after the entire enamel matrix is fully formed. It progresses from the crown surface toward the dentinoenamel junction.
C. Mineralization occurs in two phases: first, an initial 25-30 percent calcification occurs concurrent with matrix formation; second, mineralization is completed by a wave of calcification which begins at the dentinoenamel junction and progresses toward the coronal surface
D. Mineralization occurs in two phases: first, an initial 80 percent calcification begins after the formation of matrix has ended; second, mineralization is completed long after the first phase and progresses from the surface of the crown toward the dentinoenamel junction.
E. None of the above

9. The sphenomandibular ligament is attached to the 9.____

A. lesser wing of the sphenoid bone and the neck of the mandible
B. spine of the sphenoid bone and the lingula of the mandible
C. spine of the sphenoid bone and the angle of the mandible
D. none of the above
E. all of the above

10. A needle for a mandibular injection passes posterior at the level of the mandibular foramen and enters the substance of the parotid.
Which of the following structures might it strike in the gland? 10.____

A. Lingual nerve
B. Mylohyoid nerve
C. External carotid artery
D. Internal carotid artery
E. None of the above

11. Immediately before the crown tip emerges clinically into the oral cavity, the status of the erupting tooth shows that the 11.____

A. coronal two-thirds of the root has been established; in the apical area of the root, the coronal end of Hertwig's sheath is yielding cell rests of Malassez
B. gingival lamina propria occlusal to the crown tip presents ingrowth of vascular capillaries; these capillaries are needed to provide nutrients to ameloblasts which are laying down the enamel matrix

C. alveolar crest fibers are present, but they are in a relaxed condition; such relaxation is needed in order to allow the erupting tooth to have cementum laid down in the cervical root area
D. bone in the fundus of the socket is being laid down under the influence of the hammock ligament; this bone consists of trabeculae whose long axes parallel the long axis of the forming tooth
E. none of the above

12. Salivary glands receive inputs
    I. by way of general visceral efferent nerve cells of the salivatory nuclei
    II. by way of spinal cord general visceral efferent nerve cells
    III. from preganglionic cells located in the midbrain
    IV. from the vagus nerve

    The CORRECT answer is:

    A. I *only*
    B. I, II
    C. I, II, IV
    D. III *only*
    E. III, IV

13. The oral mucous membrane of the hard palate differs from that of the cheek in that the former
    I. is covered with keratinized, stratified squamous epithelium
    II. is redder
    III. has well-marked epithelial ridges
    IV. has long papillae indenting the epithelium
    V. contains no glands

    The CORRECT answer is:

    A. I *only*
    B. I, II
    C. I, III
    D. I, III, IV
    E. I, III, IV, V

14. In tooth development, the morphology of the dentinoenamel junction is determined at the

    A. bud stage
    B. cap stage
    C. bell stage
    D. maturation stage
    E. dental lamina stage

15. The submandibular duct opens close to the

    A. mandibular second molar
    B. root of the tongue
    C. base of the tonsil
    D. maxillary second molar
    E. side of the frenulum of the tongue

16. Pulp capping is *likely* to be MORE successful in young teeth because
    I. the apical foramen is large, and the pulp contains relatively more cells
    II. there are less fibrous elements, and the vascularity is better
    III. the nerve supply is greater, and the odontoblastic cells are more columnar
    IV. there are more odontoblastic cells, and there is more tissue fluid

    The CORRECT answer is:

    A. I, II, III
    B. I, II, IV
    C. I, III, IV
    D. II, III, IV
    E. All of the above

17. Cells of the periodontal ligament associated with the formation of mineralized tissue include 17.____

I. fibroblasts
II. osteoblasts
III. cementoblasts
IV. chondroblasts

The CORRECT answer is:

A. I, II
B. I, III
C. I, IV
D. II, III
E. II, IV

18. If the chorda tympani is severed, there is 18.____

A. loss of taste in anterior two-thirds of tongue
B. loss of touch sense and taste from anterior two-thirds of tongue
C. paralysis of muscles of expression on same side
D. paralysis of muscles of expression on contralateral side
E. loss of taste in the posterior one-third of tongue

19. Glands of the oral cavity all have major basic components. 19.____
One component that is NOT a constant feature of all such glands is the

A. stroma
B. capsule
C. vascular element
D. parenchymal cells
E. none of the above

20. In placing a film for a periapical view of the mandibular molars, relaxation of which of the following muscles would aid most? 20.____

A. Mylohyoid
B. Geniohyoid
C. Buccinator
D. Palatoglossus
E. Submandibular

21. The cross striations characteristic of enamel rods represent 21.____

A. Hunter-Schreger bands
B. the junctional complex of ameloblasts
C. the area where enamel rods branch
D. incremental growth pattern
E. none of the above

22. During active tooth eruption, bone formation is often seen at the base of the socket. This newly formed bone is usually in the form of 22.____

A. vertical plates
B. compact bone
C. random trabeculae
D. horizontal plates
E. a honeycomb-like structure

23. Lymphatic vessels from the teeth of the maxilla drain *directly* into which of the following nodes? 23.

A. Buccal
B. Submental
C. Infraorbital
D. Submandibular
E. All of the above

24. Cementocytes morphologically resemble 24.

A. odontoblasts
B. fibroblasts
C. ameloblasts
D. osteocytes
E. none of the above

25. The space in the posterior part of the upper vestibule of the oral cavity will be reduced by which bony structure when the mouth is opened? 25.

A. Styloid process
B. Coronoid process
C. Condylar process
D. Maxillary tuberosity
E. None of the above

KEY (CORRECT ANSWERS)

1. B
2. B
3. A
4. D
5. E
6. C
7. B
8. C
9. B
10. C
11. A
12. B
13. D
14. C
15. A
16. B
17. D
18. A
19. B
20. A
21. D
22. D
23. D
24. D
25. B

DENTAL SCIENCE

EXAMINATION SECTION

TEST 1

DIRECTIONS: Each question or incomplete statement is followed by several suggested answers or completions. Select the one that BEST answers the question or completes the statement. *PRINT THE LETTER OF THE CORRECT ANSWER IN THE SPACE AT THE RIGHT.*

1. The setting of zinc oxide-eugenol impression pastes can be accelerated by the addition of a small amount of 1.____
   A. water B. glycerin
   C. plaster of paris D. petrolatum

2. As the gold content of a dental solder decreases, the 2.____
   A. hardness decreases B. ductility increases
   C. corrosion resistance decreases D. ultimate tensile strength decreases

3. When a liquid wets a solid completely, the contact angle between the liquid and solid approaches 3.____
   A. 0° B. 45° C. 90° D. 135°

4. Kneading of softened dental compound in water will 4.____
   A. cause the flow to increase because water acts as a plasticizing agent
   B. cause the flow to decrease because the water temperature weakens intermolecular bonds
   C. cause the flow to increase because the water temperature anneals the compound
   D. not affect the flow

5. The "setting" of plaster is a result of 5.____
   A. a difference in solubility between $CaSO_4 \cdot \frac{1}{2}H_2O$ and $CaSO_4 \cdot 2H_2O$
   B. a reaction between $CaSO_4 \cdot 2H_2O$ and water
   C. the nucleation and growth of $CaSO_4 \cdot \frac{1}{2}H_2O$ crystals
   D. a reaction between $CaSO_4 \cdot \frac{1}{2}H_2O$ and $CaSO_4 \cdot 2H_2O$

6. When porcelain is baked against metal, it should possess a 6.____
   A. high fusion temperature
   B. high setting expansion
   C. linear coefficient of thermal expansion less than that of the metal
   D. linear coefficient of thermal expansion greater than that of the metal

7. Placing a cast under tap water is to be avoided because 7.___
   A. water interferes with hygroscopic expansion
   B. water inhibits polymerization of the denture resin
   C. water interferes with crystallization of the dehydrate
   D. gypsum is slightly soluble in water and the surface of the cast will be eroded

8. The hysteresis of reversible hydrocolloids is exhibited by the fact that the temperature of gelation is _____ the temperature of liquefaction. 8.___
   A. higher than
   B. lower than
   C. about the same as
   D. not related to

9. In preparing a gold-alloy partial denture framework, the dentist would subject it to a hardening heat treatment in order to 9.___
   A. increase the proportional limit
   B. decrease the modulus of resilience
   C. decrease the modulus of elasticity
   D. increase the ultimate tensile strength

10. When alginate powder is mixed with water, the reactor FIRST reacts with the 10.___
   A. borac
   B. calcium sulfate
   C. potassium alginate
   D. trisodium phosphate

11. Localized porosity positioned sporadically on the surface of and/or within the structure of a cured acrylic denture results from 11.___
   A. the monomer not being diffused homogeneously throughout the resin dough prior to curing
   B. the use of acrylic resin of sticky consistency for packing the denture mold
   C. insufficient pressure on the acrylic resin in the denture mold
   D. the use of only a boiling water bath for curing purposes

12. When selecting a matrix for a cavity preparation in a primary tooth, a dentist should consider all of the following requirements EXCEPT that the matrix should 12.___
   A. allow the restoration to exceed the outline form of the cavity preparation
   B. have sufficient strength to permit proper condensation of the alloy
   C. provide a form to restore paper contour of the tooth
   D. be designed and constructed to protect the soft tissues

13. The MOST important mechanical property involved when a chromium cobalt partial denture clasp is adjusted is 13.___
   A. hardness
   B. elongation
   C. yield strength
   D. tensile strength

14. Listed below are four substances: 14.___
   I. Plaster II. Densite III. Hydrocal IV. Cristobalite
   Which of these substances have the SAME chemical formula?
   A. I, II, III
   B. I, II, IV
   C. I, III, IV
   D. II, II, IV

15. Listed below are five factors involved in surveying a cast: 15.____
    I. The path of insertion
    II. The height of the contour or guide line
    III. The tissue line or height
    IV. Marking retentive and bracing areas with colored pencils
    V. Orienting the case in a horizontal position

    Which of these factors are MOST important?
    A. I and II only B. I, II, III C. I, II, IV D. I, IV, V

16. Which of the following etiological factors in the development of distocclusion is generally considered to be conjectural? 16.____
    A. Heredity
    B. Developmental defects
    C. Premature loss of teeth
    D. Malnutrition

17. A 34-year-old patient has all maxillary teeth present except the third molars. Missing teeth in the mandibular arch include the right premolars and first molar, left premolars and molars. 17.____

    Should the right second molar be retained?
    A. Yes, because a noncarious well-supported tooth is not extracted when planning a mandibular partial denture.
    B. No, because the second molar would make attainment of bilateral balance difficult.
    C. No, because the second molar would trip distally with a partial denture.
    D. Yes, because the second molar would help maintain posterior vertical dimension of occlusion.

18. In treating a patient with a root fracture in a primary tooth, a dentist should take all of the following steps EXCEPT to 18.____
    A. examine the fracture roentgenographically
    B. remove all but the tip of the root
    C. construct a space maintainer if indicated
    D. take roentgenograms again within six weeks

19. A dentist may advocate complete crowns on partial denture abutments. Of the following, the BEST reason for this treatment is that 19.____
    A. the caries problem is eliminated
    B. periodontal problems can be controlled
    C. more adequate occlusion can be achieved
    D. abutment morphology can be controlled

20. Stability in partial dentures is BEST insured by 20.____
    A. using monoplane teeth
    B. incorporating harmonious occlusion
    C. incorporating all undercut areas available
    D. using tight clasping and indirect retention

21. In Class I occlusion, the mesiolingual cusp of the maxillary permanent first molar occludes with the 21.____
    A. central fossa of the first molar
    B. central fossa of the second molar
    C. embrasure between the first molar and the second molar
    D. embrasure between the second premolar and the first molar

22. To help insure the success of a mandibular distal extension partial denture, the denture base should cover the 22.____
    A. complete lingual area
    B. residual alveolar bone only
    C. same distal and buccal areas as a complete denture
    D. residual alveolar bone and the soft tissue of the lingual flange

23. The restoration of a tooth following vital pulp therapy would NOT include the use of 23.____
    A. zinc oxide-eugenol
    B. silver amalgam
    C. a chrome steel crown
    D. silicate cement

24. Thymol-phenol is the solution of choice in the desensitization of cavity preparations in primary teeth because it is all of the following EXCEPT a(n) 24.____
    A. sterilizing agent
    B. protein coagulant
    C. analgesic
    D. chemically inactive substance

25. Maxillary major connectors should be separated from the gingiva by 3-6 mm. of space in order to 25.____
    A. minimize food impaction
    B. prevent injury to paragingival tissues
    C. allow sufficient length for the minor connectors
    D. facilitate movements of the tongue and allow acceptable phonetics

KEY (CORRECT ANSWERS)

1. A
2. C
3. A
4. A
5. A

6. C
7. D
8. B
9. A
10. D

11. A
12. A
13. B
14. A
15. B

16. D
17. D
18. B
19. D
20. B

21. A
22. C
23. D
24. C
25. B

TEST 2

DIRECTIONS: Each question or incomplete statement is followed by several suggested answers or completions. Select the one that BEST answers the question or completes the statement. *PRINT THE LETTER OF THE CORRECT ANSWER IN THE SPACE AT THE RIGHT.*

1. The MOST useful radiographic observation which would suggest whether a patient's alveolar bone is capable of withstanding the occlusal forces of a removable partial denture is the 1.___
   A. contour of the alveolar crest
   B. condition of the cortical plate
   C. radiopacity of the medullary spaces
   D. bone level surrounding the abutment teeth

2. Which one of the following mechanisms of fluoride action is generally considered to be LEAST significant in the prevention of caries? 2.___
   A. Stabilizing the apatite lattice
   B. Reducing acid solubility of enamel
   C. Promoting recrystallization of carious lesions
   D. Lessening bacterial acid formation

3. Suppose that the marginal ridge on a patient's mandibular left second molar has been reduced approximately 2 mm. and the correct dimensions of the rest seat have been established. 3.___
   Next, the marginal ridge must be beveled or rounded again in order to
   A. reduce food trapping around the rest
   B. provide better retention by the clasp
   C. achieve better distribution of the vertical load
   D. reduce the possibility of fracture of the metal rest

4. A characteristic that alginate and agar hydrocolloid impression materials have in common is that 4.___
   A. both materials can be converted from gels to sols
   B. inaccuracies in the completed impressions made from both materials can be caused by fracture of the fibrils during gelation
   C. gelation of both materials is retarded by temperature increases
   D. both materials can be successfully stored in humidors without any significant dimensional change

5. Which of the following is NOT a type of space maintainer? 5.___
   A. Band and loop
   B. Pontic
   C. Cable balance
   D. Lingual arch

6. Of the following statements regarding indirect retainers on the mandibular arch, the one which is ACCURATE is that they 6.___
   A. are generally located on the cingulum of mandibular incisor teeth because this is as far away from the fulcrum line as possible
   B. most often take the form of a lingual plate where there is a low lingual attachment of the tongue

C. are not required with an all tooth-borne partial denture
D. are not necessary where there is a good base adaptation to the basal structures

7. If a patient has defective occlusal contacts between opposing natural teeth, the dentist should correct them 7.____
   A. prior to making the final impression
   B. with the guidance of the master casts
   C. during the first post-insertion adjustment appointment
   D. immediately prior to inserting the completed denture

8. In partial denture construction for a maxillary arch involving the replacement of anterior teeth, the relation of anterior teeth to the residual ridge is important because it determines all of the following EXCEPT the 8.____
   A. tongue space
   B. clarity of speech
   C. degree of vertical overlap
   D. thickness of the denture flange when needed

9. All of the following are advantages to the dentist of using a rubber dam in restorative procedures for children EXCEPT that the rubber dam 9.____
   A. aids in the management of the child
   B. prevents contamination of the filling material
   C. allows the dentist greater vision of the teeth that are being prepared
   D. allows the child full movement of his tongue

10. A patient who has worn a new denture for three months complains of a burning sensation in the palatal area of the maxillary denture. 10.____
    Which one of the following areas should the dentist relieve to solve the problem?
    A. Frenum area
    B. Post dam area
    C. Labial flanges
    D. Incisive foramen

11. The percentage of malocclusion which may be attributed to the early loss of a second primary molar has been estimated to be _____ percent. 11.____
    A. about 25
    B. at least 60
    C. between 80 and 90
    D. over 90

12. Which one of the following is the PRIMARY reason for a dentist to have full-mouth radiographs made for an edentulous patient? To 12.____
    A. aid in determining the denture foundation (bearing surface) available for the new dentures
    B. discover any general systemic debility that is affecting the tissues of the mouth
    C. reveal any retained roots or residual areas of infection
    D. reassure the patient that his previous dental care was adequate

13. The Pogonion is defined as 13.____
   A. an anterior point of the mandible on the midline
   B. the protuberance of the cheek bones
   C. the posterior point of the angle of the mandible
   D. a point in the lower arch

14. Which one of the following is a reason for the dentist to use a clear surgical tray when fitting an immediate denture? 14.____
   A. As an aid in placing sutures
   B. To prevent bleeding for the first 24 hours
   C. As an aid in trimming bone to fit the immediate denture
   D. To facilitate shortening the borders so the denture will fit securely

15. Which one of the following is the MAJOR reason why a dentist would not reduce the vertical overlap of anterior teeth in an attempt to reduce the incisal guidance? 15.____
   A. The advantage of duplicating the position of the natural teeth with artificial teeth in the immediate denture would be lost.
   B. The posterior cusp inclination would be increased and stability decreased.
   C. The interior contact necessary for balanced occlusion would be lost.
   D. The vertical dimension of occlusion would be changed.

16. Recording centric relation accurately with wall-constructed occlusion rims and on stabilized record bases will improve the accuracy of the immediate denture by 16.____
   A. aiding in the selection and setting of the artificial teeth
   B. reducing the number of processing errors
   C. contributing to accurate occlusal relations in the finished dentures
   D. eliminating the need for equilibrating the finished dentures

17. In a patient wearing complete dentures, a generalized soreness over the entire mandibular ridge is USUALLY caused by 17.____
   A. excessive increase in the vertical dimension
   B. impingement on the buccal frenum
   C. high muscle attachments
   D. undue border thickness

18. Perleche has long been considered a lesion caused PRIMARILY by 18.____
   A. bruxism and malnutrition
   B. vitamin deficiency and sialorrhoea
   C. vitamin B_2 deficiency associated with loss of vertical dimension
   D. an increased vertical dimension of occlusion and vitamin deficiency

19. Assume that a dentist examines a patient wearing complete dentures and determines that the vertical dimension of occlusion has been decreased. For this patient, the term *decreased vertical dimension of occlusion* refers to a(n) 19.____
   A. vertical dimension that leaves the teeth in a clenched, closed relation in normal positions
   B. occluding vertical dimension which results in an excessive interocclusal distance when the mandible is in rest position
   C. insufficient amount of interarch distance because of heavy, bony ridges
   D. condition in which the patient cannot open the mandible because of temporomandibular joint pathosis

20. In examining the edentulous mouth of an aged patient who has worn a complete maxillary denture for many years against six mandibular anterior teeth, dentist is MOST likely to find 20.____
   A. cystic degeneration of the formation of the anterior palatine nerve
   B. loss of osseous structure in the anterior maxillary arch
   C. flabby ridge tissue on the posterior maxillary arch
   D. insufficient interocclusal distance

21. The angle of convexity is 21.____
   A. imaginary
   B. the curved line formed by the occlusal surface of the lower teeth
   C. the distal angle of the mandible
   D. the line from the Pogonian to a point A and to the mesian

22. The gonion is defined as 22.____
   A. the posterior point of the angle of the lower jaw
   B. the mandible
   C. a point on the cheekbone
   D. a point in the upper jaw

23. Periodontal disease is a multifactorial disease and is predominantly inflammatory in origin. Which one of the following etiological agents may be considered to be the MAJOR cause of periodontal disease? 23.____
   A. Dental plaque
   B. Maculation
   C. Occlusal disharmonies
   D. Environmental factors

24. The esthetic results possible in a treatment plan involving malposed teeth and diatemata can be predetermined by 24.____
   A. the appearance and health of the gingival tissues
   B. the proper use of diagnostic casts
   C. the alveolar bone support
   D. an occlusal analysis

25. One should be mindful that restricting carbohydrate intake, in general, could result in serious problems.
Which one of the following statements regarding carbohydrate utilization is generally considered to be INCORRECT? 25.___
   A. Carbohydrates provide an inexpensive source of energy.
   B. Carbohydrates conserve water and electrolytes.
   C. Body fat is oxidized efficiently in the absence of carbohydrates.
   D. Acidosis can develop in the absence of enough dietary carbohydrates.

KEY (CORRECT ANSWERS)

1. D
2. D
3. D
4. B
5. C

6. A
7. A
8. C
9. D
10. D

11. B
12. C
13. A
14. C
15. A

16. C
17. A
18. C
19. B
20. B

21. B
22. A
23. A
24. B
25. B

TEST 3

DIRECTIONS: Each question or incomplete statement is followed by several suggested answers or completions. Select the one that BEST answers the question or completes the statement. *PRINT THE LETTER OF THE CORRECT ANSWER IN THE SPACE AT THE RIGHT.*

1. In cases in which complete maxillary dentures oppose distal extension mandibular partial dentures, resorption of the maxillary anterior ridge is frequently noted. 1.____
This condition is USUALLY attributed to
   A. excessive overjet
   B. improper curve of Spee
   C. faulty occlusal planes
   D. lack of protrusive balance

2. Topical fluoride applications have proven to be of some value in the percent reduction in D.M.F.S. Which of the following statements regarding fluoride applications is INCORRECT? 2.____
   A. A 0.05 percent sodium fluoride solution mouthwash every day decreases increments in D.M.F.S. by almost 50 percent.
   B. Self-application of an acidulated phosphate gel is the most effective topical fluoride.
   C. Sodium monofluorophosphate dentrifices increase the stains on silicate restorations.
   D. The prescription of fluoride lozenges is contraindicated when communal water is fluoridated.

3. In making a decision as to whether to extract the deciduous tooth of a patient, the dentist should consider all of the following factors EXCEPT 3.____
   A. occlusion, alignment, and arch development
   B. amount of root resorption of the tooth in question
   C. presence of infection
   D. degree of discoloration of the tooth

4. In the edentulous patient, the interarch distance measured when the occlusion rims or teeth are in uniform contact defines the 4.____
   A. freeway space
   B. rest vertical dimension
   C. occlusal vertical dimension
   D. centric relation at a given vertical dimension

5. The impression material which would record the tissues with the LEAST amount of pressure is a 5.____
   A. mouth flowable wax
   B. thin mix of plaster
   C. rubber base impression material
   D. zinc oxide-eugenol base material

6. When the dentist is making an impression of flabby or hypertrophic tissue, which one of the following applies? 6.____
   A. A close-fitting resin tray is desirable to help mold the tissue in a desired position.
   B. Intimate contact of the impression material with the tissue is not desirable.
   C. Wax is an ideal impression material to be used.
   D. A tray with a spacer should be used.

7. Following are five ways in which forces acting through a bridge may be directed: 7.____
   I. As far as possible at right angles to the long axes of the teeth
   II. Parallel to the long axes of the teeth
   III. By decreasing the buccolingual dimension of the pontic
   IV. By decreasing the mesiodistal
   V. In a mesial direction so that teeth nearer the midline will offer additional support

   In which of these ways should forces acting through a bridge on the abutment tooth may be directed?
   A. I, III, IV B. I, III, V C. I, IV, V D. II, III

8. Following are five ways in which a pontic may be constructed: So that the 8.____
   I. pontic contacts the mucosa, but does not impinge the mucosa
   II. pontic completely fills the edentulous space
   III. lingual embrasures of the pontic are widened
   IV. buccolingual width of the pontic is maintained the same size as that of the natural teeth lost
   V. buccolingual width of the pontic is reduced slightly

   In which of these ways should the pontic for a maxillary posterior bridge with normal alveolar resorption be constructed?
   A. I, II, IV B. I, II, V C. I, III, V D. I, III, IV

9. The choice and number of abutments for a fixed bridge would usually be influenced by all of the following factors EXCEPT the 9.____
   A. length of span of the bridge
   B. oral hygiene of the patient
   C. crown-root ratio of the abutments
   D. amount of periodontal support for the abutments

10. Following are four statements regarding the situation of a patient for whom fixed bridges are indicated and who also requires periodontal treatment: 10.____
    I. Normally, the bridges should be inserted before the treatment is started.
    II. The treatment should always be completed before the fixed bridges are started.
    III. The procedure can vary depending upon the stability of the teeth and the individual case.
    IV. Normally, periodontal disease should be treated before restorative procedures are undertaken.

    Which of these statements are ACCURATE?
    A. I, III B. II only C. III only D. III, IV

11. Following are five factors which influence the success of a fixed partial denture: 11.____
    I. Parallel vertical relation of abutment teeth
    II. Bilateral edentulous areas
    III. Good oral hygiene habits of the patient
    IV. Involving teeth of dissimilar function
    V. designing a bridge to permit slightly independent movement of abutment teeth

    Which of these factors are favorable influences?
    A. I, II B. I, II, V C. II, III, IV D. I, III

12. All of the following are frequent causes of fracture or separation of porcelain from metal in the porcelain-fused-to-gold technique when used as a crown and bridge restorative material EXCEPT 12.____
    A. poor design of the metal framework
    B. excessive thickness of the opaque layer
    C. contamination of metal before application of the opaque layer
    D. centric occlusal contacts at the junction of metal and porcelain

13. Which one of the following is NOT a requirement for the successful soldering of fixed partial dentures? 13.____
    A. The melting range of the solder must be at least 50°F to 100°F below that of the casting.
    B. The area to be soldered must be clean.
    C. The casting should be almost in contact.
    D. An oxidizing flame should be used.

14. The ADVANTAGE of using an annealed copper band rather than an unannealed band for a compound impression is that 14.____
    A. it is stronger
    B. the compound adheres more readily
    C. it adapts more readily to the form of the prepared tooth
    D. it retains the heat in the compound, thus maintaining the working consistency for a longer time

15. Which one of the following is NOT a criterion for the working qualities of silver amalgam as used in restorations? 15.____
    A. Time of amalgamation
    B. Compressive strength
    C. Consistency
    D. Carving characteristics

16. Suppose that a maxillary first molar has extruded 1.8 mm. into a mandibular first molar space. 16.____
    A. Construct the bridge to the existing occlusion.
    B. Extract the maxillary extruded tooth and bridge the maxillary and mandibular spaces.
    C. Restore the maxillary first molar to give a better plane of occlusion before constructing the bridge.
    D. Reduce the maxillary first molar on the cast, construct the bridge to this occlusion and adjust the maxillary molar after the bridge has been inserted.

17. The anterior three-quarter crown preparation is DIFFICULT to accomplish because it 17.____
    A. has the longest external margin
    B. is possible for the disk to slip and cut the lip
    C. must satisfy both esthetic and biomechanic demands
    D. must be modified in some cases to increase frictional retention

18. The PRIMARY reason or water quenching a gold alloy casting (in its investment) immediately after the dull redness disappears from the button is to 18.____
    A. produce a high degree of ductility in the casting
    B. facilitate removal of the casting from the mold
    C. obtain a desirable surface on the casting
    D. reduce corrosion

19. The objective of using a hinge axis face-bow is to record the 19.____
    A. centric relation
    B. lateral condylar inclination
    C. horizontal condylar inclination
    D. opening and closing axis of the mandible

20. The functional movements of the mandible are combinations of hinge and glide movements. With vertical limits, the mandible may take a pure hinge movement without a simultaneous glide.
    The one relation of the condyle to the fossae in which this pure hinge movement is possible is called the 20.____
    A. centric occlusion
    B. terminal hinge position
    C. retruded contact position
    D. postural position of the mandible

21. In selecting the color of cement for use in cementing a porcelain jacket crown, the dentist should mix the powder being tested with 21.____
    A. glycerin water solution
    B. cement liquid
    C. alcohol
    D. soap

22. If a patient experiences prolonged sensitivity to heat, cold, and pressure after cementation of a crown or bridge, it is USUALLY related to 22.____
    A. occlusal trauma
    B. improper cementation
    C. impingement on the marginal gingival sulcus
    D. failure to desensitize the abutment teeth

23. The MOST important procedure to be carried out by the dentist following cementation of a fixed bridge is to 23.____
    A. verify the occlusion again and adjust it if necessary
    B. thoroughly remove cement debris from embrasures and the gingival sulcus of abutment teeth
    C. take a radiograph of each abutment before dismissing the patient
    D. instruct the patient in specific oral hygiene procedures for this appliance

24. When changes occur in alveolar bone in the area around abutment teeth, these changes are adjustments to added function and load. Such adjustments are USUALLY shown by 24.____
    A. a widening of the periodontal ligament space and a lessening of density of the cribriform plates of the alveolar bone
    B. more definit4e and dense cribriform plates and increased trabeculation of the alveolar bone, with widening of the periodontal ligament space
    C. histologic thickening of the cementum and consequent decrease in the width of the periodontal ligament
    D. pronounced tooth mobility, sensitivity to masticatory pressure, and hyperemia of the soft tissues

25. Correct contour of a crown in maintaining and protecting the health of the gingival tissues is MOST important in the 25.____
    A. occlusal or incisal third
    B. infrabulge or gingival third
    C. height of contour of suprabulge
    D. interproximal gingival embrasure areas

KEY (CORRECT ANSWERS)

1.	D	11.	D
2.	C	12.	B
3.	D	13.	D
4.	C	14.	C
5.	B	15.	B
6.	D	16.	C
7.	D	17.	C
8.	C	18.	A
9.	B	19.	D
10.	D	20.	C

21. A
22. A
23. A
24. B
25. B

TEST 4

DIRECTIONS: Each question or incomplete statement is followed by several suggested answers or completions. Select the one that BEST answers the question or completes the statement. *PRINT THE LETTER OF THE CORRECT ANSWER IN THE SPACE AT THE RIGHT.*

1. The GREATEST cause of porosity in a porcelain jacket crown is usually 1.____
   A. excessively high firing temperature
   B. failure to anneal the platinum matrix
   C. excessive condensation of the porcelain
   D. inadequate condensation of the porcelain

2. In the case of a child who has had an injury resulting in a displaced primary tooth which is intruded, a dentist should take all of the following steps EXCEPT to 2.____
   A. examine the injury roentgenographically
   B. treat local lacerations
   C. administer penicillin or Aureomycin for 48 hours following the injury
   D. attempt to move the tooth into position

3. If a dentist wishes to open pits in occlusal cavities, it would usually be MOST efficient for him to use a 3.____
   A. small inverted cone bur
   B. tapered fissure bur
   C. straight fissure bur
   D. No. 2 round bur

4. Which one of the following is NOT a basic principle in the preparation of Class II cavities in deciduous teeth? 4.____
   A. There should be sufficient extension on the occlusal surface to include all pits and fissures.
   B. The cavity outline should include areas of carious involvement and, in addition, those that will retain food and plaque material.
   C. The width at the isthmus should be at least one-half or more of the intercuspal dimension of the tooth.
   D. The occlusal portion of the preparation should be established approximately 0.5 mm. pulpally from the dentinoenamel junction.

5. The type of pontic MOST commonly used in the posterior maxillary area is the _____ type. 5.____
   A. saddle
   B. ridge lap
   C. sanitary
   D. spheroidal

6. A clean, dry field is necessary prior to making an impression with a hydrocolloid type material because this type of material 6.____
   A. is unstable
   B. will not retract gingival tissue
   C. will not distort or tear if a dry field is maintained
   D. is capable of taking an impression of blood and saliva

7. Successful application of vital pulp therapy in the primary dentition depends upon all of the following EXCEPT 7.____
   A. correct diagnosis
   B. maintenance of a clean, uncontaminated field of operation
   C. proper cavity preparation that provides access to, and clear visibility of, all areas of the pulp chamber
   D. the presence of early root resorption

8. Of the following, the MOST important reason why patients wearing partial dentures should be re-examined periodically is that 8.____
   A. esthetics should be preserved
   B. a partial denture is considered a treatment service, not a cure
   C. the incidence of caries increases with partial dentures
   D. abutment teeth are subject to added stress and can become involved periodontally

9. Guidelines have been developed for the post-treatment evaluation of the quality of dental care given to patients in public health programs. 9.____
   On the basis of these guidelines, which of the following statements about evaluating the construction of a complete denture is INCORRECT?
   A. Generally, the lower first molar should be set two millimeters above the retro-molar pad.
   B. Dentures click when the occlusal plane is set too high.
   C. Increased overbite may result in general soreness.
   D. Frequent biting of the tongue may be the result of overclosure.

10. Failure of partial dentures, for reasons other than structural defects, usually can be attributed to 10.____
    A. inadequate diagnosis
    B. lack of patient adaptability
    C. improper handling of impression material
    D. incomplete advice to the patient at the time of delivery of the dentures

11. The following are some elements of a good treatment program. Which one of these elements BEST enables the senior dentist to evaluate adequacy and appropriateness of care? 11.____
    A. Examination
    B. Diagnosis
    C. Treatment Plan
    D. Prognosis

12. Quality has been described in terms of "level" of care. With which one of the following levels should public health dentists generally be MOST concerned? 12.____
    The _____ level
    A. individual service
    B. community
    C. individual
    D. mouth

13. Which one of the following statements regarding the auditing of publicly funded health-care services is generally considered to be ACCURATE? 13.___
   A. Monies spent in auditing would be better spent for more service.
   B. Practitioners in public health services are honest, prudent, and sensitive to the public welfare, making auditing unnecessary.
   C. There should be no auditing since there are no established norms of quality.
   D. Monies saved by auditing have justified auditing many times over.

14. Which one of the following is NOT an objective of auditing publicly funded health-care services? To 14.___
   A. assess the quality of health care in accordance with stipulated standards
   B. ascertain over- or under-utilization of services by the practitioner or by the patient
   C. identify fraud
   D. determine the penalty for misuse of funds

15. Which one of the following is generally NOT considered to be a pre-treatment quality control mechanism? 15.___
   A. Service benefit priorities
   B. Site evaluation
   C. Procedural limitations
   D. Continuing education

16. The overall objective of a dental health plan should be the achievement of an optimum oral health program for all persons eligible to participate in the program. 16.___
FIRST in order of priority among the following standards for such a program should usually be the
   A. correction of all defects
   B. maintenance of an optimum level of oral health, once achieved
   C. prevention of disease
   D. thorough diagnosis of such patient's oral, physical, and attitudinal status

17. Listed below are five procedures or tests: 17.___
I. Urinalysis
I. Complete blood count
III. Clotting time
IV. Radiographs of the chest
V. Complete physical examination
Which of these procedures or tests should make up the pre-operative examination of a handicapped or emotionally disturbed child who is about to undergo extensive restorative treatment and minor oral surgery under general anesthesia?
   A. All of the above
   B. I, II, III
   C. I, II, V
   D. V only

18. Which one of the following methods is generally considered to be LEAST effective in achieving the goal of modifying behavior regarding oral health? 18.___
   A. Use of mass media
   B. School units
   C. Individual counseling
   D. Organization in the community

19. Of the following statements relating to work simplification in dental practice, which statement is generally considered to be LEAST correct? 19.____
   A. Tools and materials should be pre-positioned wherever possible.
   B. The two hands should begin as well as complete their motions at the same time.
   C. A chair of the type of height to permit good posture should be provided for every worker.
   D. Work areas, cabinets, and trays should be at elbow level.

20. Suppose that several patients have complained to you that one of the dentists under your supervision has treated them in a condescending manner. Of the following, which is the course of action which would generally be the MOST desirable for you, as the senior dentist, to take FIRST? 20.____
   A. Ignore these complaints since patients may be inclined to be overly-sensitive.
   B. Inform the dentist that his manner is inappropriate and that he should improve it.
   C. Observe the dentist's behavior with patients.
   D. Ask the other dentists on staff for their opinion of the dentist's behavior with patients.

21. It has been said that one reason for the failure of many public health programs lies in the areas of communications. Which one of the following statements regarding communications between the dental examiner and the patient is LEAST likely to be considered accurate? 21.____
   A. Some patients receive inappropriate treatment because they do not understand the dental examiner and the dental examiner does not understand them.
   B. Sizeable groups in our city are limited in their ability to speak and understand English.
   C. Dental examiners readily admit to a handicap or failure in communication.
   D. Where the same language is ostensibly spoken, there may be differences in interpretation of what is said.

22. Suppose that a senior dentist who has recently assumed his position has reacted unfavorably to a highly-rated dentist now under his supervision. Which one of the following steps would it generally be MOST desirable for the senior dentist to take FIRST in this situation? 22.____
   A. Give the dentist a low rating if he, the senior dentist, feels it is deserved.
   B. Discuss his reservations about the dentist's performance with the dentist.
   C. Recommend that the dentist be transferred to a clinic under the supervision of another senior dentist.
   D. Refer the matter to the administration.

23. The arbitration of disputes between subordinates is one of the most difficult supervisory tasks. 23.____
If two dentists give widely differing versions of the nature of the dispute, which one of the following courses of action would generally be considered LEAST desirable for the senior dentist to take?
   A. Listen to both sides.
   B. Conduct his own investigation of the facts.
   C. Determine which of the dentists is actually at fault in the matter.
   D. Find out how to prevent a recurrence of the situation.

24. Suppose that a new directive has been promulgated by the central office. 24.____
When you inform your professional staff of this change at a meeting, you encounter heated resistance from a substantial number of them.
Of the following courses of action, the LEAST desirable for you as the senior dentist to take would be to
   A. listen to all sides.
   B. inform the staff that you are conveying the desires of administration and that the directive must be implemented.
   C. advise the staff that their objections and any suggestions will be brought to the attention of the administration
   D. reinterpret the directive to the staff

25. Suppose that a dentist has a patient who is resistant to the dentist's instructions regarding oral health and hygiene because of certain cultural reasons. 25.____
The one of the following courses of action which would be LEAST likely to help improve this patient's attitude would be for the dentist to
   A. show an interest in the patient
   B. relate instructions, as far as possible, to things which are familiar and acceptable to the patient
   C. attempt to eliminate any of the patient's customs or beliefs which seem to be erroneous
   D. recognize the patient's own ideas about his dental problem

KEY (CORRECT ANSWERS)

1. D
2. D
3. A
4. C
5. B

6. D
7. D
8. B
9. A
10. A

11. C
12. B
13. D
14. D
15. B

16. C
17. A
18. A
19. B
20. C

21. C
22. B
23. C
24. B
25. C

EXAMINATION SECTION
TEST 1

DIRECTIONS: Each question or incomplete statement is followed by several suggested answers or completions. Select the one the BEST answers the question or completes the statement. *PRINT THE LETTER OF THE CORRECT ANSWER IN THE SPACE AT THE RIGHT.*

1. Which of the following is an infrahyoid muscle involved in elevating the larynx? 1.____

   A. Sternothyroid
   B. Omohyoid
   C. Geniohyoid
   D. Thyrohyoid

2. The primary purpose of a facebow is to 2.____

   A. register the teeth's relationships to the rotational center of the jaw
   B. register the teeth's relationships to the features of the skull
   C. record centric occlusion
   D. force an eccentric registration of the jaw

3. A technician is boxing a cast with plaster of Paris and pumice. By volume, the ratio of plaster of Paris to pumice flour should be 3.____

   A. 2:1
   B. 1:1
   C. 1:2
   D. 1:3

4. In a ______ occlusion, the distal surface of the man- dibular canine is mesial to the mesial surface of a maxillary canine by a width of at least one premolar. 4.____

   A. Class I
   B. Class II, Division I
   C. Class II, Division II
   D. Class III

5. Which of the following is NOT an advantage associated with flasking dentures in a silicone mold? 5.____

   A. Rapid retrieval of cured denture from flask
   B. No application of tinfoil substitute required
   C. Excellent retention of denture teeth
   D. Reduced finishing time

6. A technician is constructing a baseplate out of autopolymerizing resin using the finger-adapted method. Potential disadvantages of this procedure include each of the following, EXCEPT 6.____

   A. variable polymer/monomer ratio
   B. greater risk of contamination than sprinkle-on method
   C. necessity of continuing to adapt until resin has completely polymerized
   D. difficulty in achieving uniform thickness

7. A technician is articulating a 20-degree maxillary first molar. In centric occlusion, the 7.
   I. mesiobuccal cusp rests in the anterior buccal groove of the mandibular first molar
   II. distal inclined plane touches the mesiolingual cusp of the mandibular second molar
   III. mesiolingual cusp fits in the central fossa of the mandibular second molar
   IV. distolingual cusp contacts the distal ridge of the lower second molar

   A. I only
   B. I and II
   C. II and III
   D. I, II, III and IV

8. In determining the forward position of the maxillary central incisor in a complete denture, a useful guide is the 8.

   A. existing ridge
   B. natural relationship between the upper central and the incisal papilla
   C. arch form
   D. position of the canine

9. A large ______ is a distinctive characteristic of the primary maxillary first molar. 9.

   A. mesiofacial
   B. mesiolingual
   C. distofacial
   D. distolingual

10. Crowding and lapping of teeth are most likely to occur in the ______ cusp configuration. 10.

   A. Square
   B. Square-tapering
   C. Tapering
   D. Ovoid

11. An alginate impression has torn. Which of the following.is the most likely explanation? 11.

   A. Impression removed too slowly
   B. Water temperature too high
   C. Too much powder in mix
   D. Impression removed too quickly

12. A technician is carving the gingival margin around the posterior teeth of a trial maxillary denture. The technician should use a carver or #7 spatula, held at an angle of approximately______degrees. 12.

   A. 30
   B. 45
   C. 60
   D. 90

13. From the incisal perspective, crowns of the anterior teeth are wider at the 13.____

   A. facial than the lingual
   B. mesial than the distal
   C. lingual than the facial
   D. distal than the mesial

14. Which of the following bones includes the posterior nasal spine? 14.____

   A. Maxilla
   B. Palatine
   C. Mandible
   D. Hyoid

15. The articulator method of relining a denture includes each of the following procedures, EXCEPT 15.____

   A. Blocking out palatal and lingual regions with modeling clay
   B. Curing in a pressure pot for 15 psi for 30 minutes
   C. Removing a thin layer of resin from the interior of the denture
   D. Leaving the borders of the denture intact

16. The tongue space on mandibular casts should 16.____

   A. be trimmed flat
   B. incline slightly posteriorly
   C. resemble the floor of the mouth as much as possible
   D. be removed

17. A technician observes that after tinting, the denture base has a gaudy red appearance. The technician has applied too much of pigment 17.____

   A. A
   B. B
   C. E
   D. F

18. During the construction of custom acrylic trays, the technician does NOT 18.____

   A. usually chemically cure the tray
   B. mix tray acrylic and adapt it directly to the cast
   C. use a wax spacer to develop a consistent thickness of impression material
   D. observer the material heat up as it polymerizes

19. A mandibular occlusion rim should be about ______ mm in width. 19.____

   A. 4
   B. 6
   C. 8
   D. 10

20. The most common location for a non-separated fracture of the denture base is the

    A. distobuccal end of a maxillary denture
    B. canine eminence of a mandibular denture
    C. midline of a maxillary denture
    D. midline of a mandibular denture

21. Synonyms for "centric occlusion" include each of the following, EXCEPT

    A. intercuspal position
    B. habitual occlusion
    C. neutroclusion
    D. convenience occlusion

22. When hand adapting an acrylic resin to a cast for the purpose of forming an impression tray, the technician should take special care to

    A. avoid overthinning the resin on the convex portions of the cast
    B. extend the resin well past the tuberosities
    C. avoid pressing the resin into undercuts
    D. be aware of the locations of tissue stops and add a little extra pressure at these points

23. A technician is flasking a mandibular denture. After the initial placement in stone, the technician will need to remove all stone undercuts that would prevent separation of the flask halves. In mandibular dentures, the most likely place for these undercuts to appear would be the ______ region.

    A. posterior lingual
    B. anterior lingual
    C. anterior labial
    D. posterior buccal

24. Which of the following materials has the lowest dimensional stability?

    A. Addition silicone
    B. Polysulfide
    C. Condensation silicone
    D. Alginate

25. Which of the following materials is LEAST appropriate as a material for a soft denture liner?

    A. Vinyl
    B. Silicone rubber
    C. Natural rubber
    D. Soft acrylics

KEY (CORRECT ANSWERS)

1. D
2. A
3. B
4. D
5. C

6. A
7. A
8. B
9. A
10. C

11. A
12. B
13. A
14. B
15. D

16. A
17. A
18. B
19. C
20. C

21. C
22. A
23. A
24. D
25. C

TEST 2

DIRECTIONS: Each question or incomplete statement is followed by several suggested answers or completions. Select the one the BEST answers the question or completes the statement. *PRINT THE LETTER OF THE CORRECT ANSWER IN THE SPACE AT THE RIGHT.*

1. "Anatomic teeth" are defined as denture teeth with a cusp angle of ______ degrees or more.

   A. 10
   B. 20
   C. 30
   D. 45

2. While the sprinkle-on method is preferred by many technicians for making an acrylic resin impression tray, it does have some problems. The main drawback is the difficulty in

   A. attaching a handle to the tray
   B. achieving the correct polymer/monomer ratio
   C. completing the tray before the resin has hardened
   D. controlling the thickness of the impression tray

3. After teeth have been removed, the loss of bone structure is usually

   A. greater on the buccolabial aspect of the maxillary ridge than on the palatal aspect
   B. greater on the palatal aspect of the maxillary ridge than on the buccolabial aspect
   C. uniform along the buccolabial and palatal aspects of the maxillary ridge
   D. dependent on the arch form of the individual

4. Which of the following occlusions is most often associated with a retrognathic profile?

   A. Class I
   B. Class II, Division I
   C. Class II, Division II
   D. Class III

5. A technician is articulating a 20-degree maxillary second molar. In centric occlusion, the

   I. mesiolingual cusp contacts ridges formed by the protrusive and retrusive lingual cusp planes of the mandibular second molar
   II. ridge of the mesiobuccal cusp rests in the buccal groove of the mandibular second molar
   III. mesiolingual cusp fits into the central fossa of the mandibular second molar
   IV. buccal cusps contact the buccal cusps of the mandibular second molar

   A. I and II
   B. I, II and IV
   C. II and III
   D. IV only

6. The mandibular occlusion rim should be approximately ______ mm from the incisal edge in the central incisor area to the deepest part of the labial vestibule.

   A. 18 B. 22 C. 32 D. 36

7. The mandibular anterior teeth of a complete denture should usually be arranged with 7.____

A. the lateral incisors tilted slightly labially from the horizontal plane.
B. the canines tilted slightly inward
C. their long axes projecting toward one common center
D. no axial rotation

8. A technician is preparing a nonseparated fracture line on a denture base for repair. Which of the following is NOT a guideline to be followed for this procedure? 8.____

A. Use a #558 bur to grind out the fracture line from beginning to end.
B. Bevel the widened fracture outward
C. In the palate of maxillary dentures, place shallow dovetails
D. In the lingual area of mandibular dentures, place a retaining wire

9. When settling a wax denture into a flask, the technician should be careful to 9.____

A. avoid tilting the occlusal plane
B. keep the denture from getting wet
C. submerge the gingival margin
D. push the cast base into contact with the flask interior

10. Which of the following statements is/are TRUE regarding the maxillary first molar and mandibular first molar? 10.____

I. The mandibular crowns are wider mesiodistally than faciolingually.
II. The mandibular first molar has only two facial cusps of similar size
III. The maxillary first molar crowns are wider mesiodistally than faciolingually
IV. The maxillary molars have two roots; the mandibular molars have three roots

A. I only
B. I and II
C. II only
D. II, III and IV

11. The most significant difference between replacing anterior and posterior teeth in a complete denture is that replacing posterior teeth involves 11.____

A. the removal of some of the resin denture base
B. remounting for occlusal correction
C. pressure curing
D. preserving the facial margin

12. Which of the following muscles does NOT play a role in pulling down on the hyoid bone? 12.____

A. Thyrohyoid
B. Sternothyroid
C. Stylohyoid
D. Omohyoid

13. A technician is constructing a baseplate out of autopolymerizing resin using the sprinkle-on method. The baseplate will be ready to be cured when the resin has reached a thickness of ______ mm. 13.____

A. 1 B. 2 C. 3 D. 4

14. A technician is arranging Anatoline posterior teeth in a bilateral balanced occlusion. The mandibular teeth should be occluded to the maxillary teeth with the articulator set at a(n) ______ -degree condylar inclination and a(n) ______ -degree incisal inclination.

    A. 30; 0
    B. 30; 10
    C. 10; 30
    D. 30; -10

15. After flasking a tinted resin denture base, a technician observes that the tinted surface is porous. This is most likely because

    A. there was no coating of tinfoil substitute provided
    B. the tinting resin monomer evaporated before the denture was packed
    C. too much monomer was added to the tint
    D. the resin did not sit long enough before packing

16. Acrylic resin teeth are best polished with a

    A. rubber prophy cup and pumice flour
    B. plain ragwheel
    C. pumice stone
    D. emery cloth

17. Compared to acrylic denture teeth, porcelain teeth

    A. form stronger chemical bonds to the denture base
    B. cause fewer scratches/abrasions to opposing ridges
    C. are more wear resistant
    D. are more easily ground and shaped

18. For fast-set alginate impression material, mixing should be completed within ______ seconds

    A. 30
    B. 45
    C. 60
    D. 75
    E.

19. A Class I occlusion, the

    I. maxillary first molar is slightly posterior to the mandibular first molar
    II. mesiobuccal cusp of the maxillary first molar is directly in line with the buccal groove of the mandibular first molar
    III. distal surface of the mandibular canine is within one premolar's width of the mesial surface of the maxillary canine.
    IV. incisal margins of the mandibular incisors lie behind the middle of the lingual surfaces of the maxillary incisors

    A. I and II
    B. I, II and III
    C. II and IV
    D. I, II, III and IV

20. A technician is mounting a cast on a semi-adjustable articulator with curved condylar pathways. The medial guiding surface of this instrument forms a fixed angle of _______ relative to the midsagittal plane of the skull. 20.____

A. 3
B. 7
C. 11
D. 15

21. Which of the following materials must be poured immediately after mixing? 21.____

A. Addition silicone
B. Condensation silicone
C. Polyether
D. Reversible hydrocolloid

22. In order to avoid porosity in the base, thick dentures should be 22.____

I. bench cured before being heated
II. heated slowly to 74° C (165° F)
III. packed as late in the polymerization process as possible
IV. flasked in silicone

A. I only
B. I and II
C. II, III and IV
D. I, II, III and IV

23. While boxing an impression with wax, beading wax should be applied around the periphery of the impression. This wax should be approximately ______ mm wide and ______ mm below the border of the impression. 23.____

A. 4; 3 to 4
B. 2; 3 to 4
C. 5; 1 to 2
D. 4; 1 to 2

24. A technician has made a denture base out of fluid resin. After deflasking, the denture base is porous. Which of the following is LEAST likely to have been the cause of this? 24.____

A. Accelerated polymerization
B. Denture placed in curing unit after polymerization began
C. Inadequate air pressure
D. Loose pieces of hydrocolloid left in the mold

25. Molars are each characterized by 25.____

I. at least two functional cusps and two afunctional cusps
II. the largest occlusal surfaces of any teeth
III. two to six major cusps
IV. two or three roots

A. I and III
B. I and II
C. II and IV
D. I, II, III and IV

KEY (CORRECT ANSWERS)

1. C
2. D
3. A
4. B
5. C

6. A
7. B
8. D
9. A
10. A

11. B
12. C
13. B
14. B
15. B

16. A
17. C
18. A
19. B
20. B

21. D
22. B
23. A
24. D
25. C

TEST 3

DIRECTIONS: Each question or incomplete statement is followed by several suggested answers or completions. Select the one the BEST answers the question or completes the statement. *PRINT THE LETTER OF THE CORRECT ANSWER IN THE SPACE AT THE RIGHT.*

1. Which of the following exists when mandibular molars are buccal to maxillary molars? 1.____

   A. Overbite
   B. Retrusion
   C. Crossbite
   D. Overjet

2. When dental impression compound sticks are used today, their uses typically include 2.____
   I. forming the palatal seal in impressions for complete dentures
   II. molding the peripheral borders of custom trays
   III. preliminary impressions of edentulous ridges for complete dentures
   IV. bite registration

   A. I only
   B. I and II
   C. II and III
   D. III and IV

3. A technician has just completed a set of acrylic resin impression trays for a patient. The trays should be stored ______ until they are needed. 3.____

   A. in a humidor
   B. in water
   C. on the casts
   D. slightly below room temperature

4. During the polymerization of a chemical-cured acrylic resin, a pressure pot may be used for each of the following, EXCEPT 4.____

   A. decreasing porosity
   B. decreasing shrinkage
   C. increasing wear resistance
   D. increasing strength

5. Which of the following is a disadvantage associated with porcelain denture teeth? 5.____

   A. Difficulty in restoring surface polish after grinding
   B. Difficulty in polishing denture base
   C. Unnatural appearance
   D. Poor wear resistance

6. The peripheral roll of a preliminary impression should be complete and no deeper than ______ mm. 6.____

   A. 1 to 2 B. B. 3 to 4
   C. 5 to 6 D. D. 7 to 8

7. A technician discovers a marked lack of interridge space in the tuberosity area. Esthetically and functionally, the best tooth to leave out of the setup is the

   A. first premolar
   B. second premolar
   C. second molar
   D. third molar

8. A malfunction of the ______ may cause a deviation to one side during protrusion of the mandible.

   A. lateral pterygoid
   B. medial pterygoid
   C. masseter
   D. sternocleidomastoid

9. A technician is constructing a baseplate out of autopolymerizing resin by confining the resin in a stone index. Other than the time involved in this procedure, the main disadvantage associated with it is the

   A. tendency to overlap impression boundaries
   B. creeping of resin into undercuts
   C. tendency to form voids in the baseplate
   D. poor thickness control

10. A technician is mounting a maxillary cast on a Whip-Mix articulator. Which of the following procedures would be performed LAST?

   A. Placing the plastic are projections over the pins of the condylar guides
   B. Placing a cast support between the undersurface of the transfer fork and the lower member of the articulator
   C. Adjusting the condylar guides
   D. Resting the anterior portion of the articulator on the crossbar of the face bow

11. After relining a denture, the technician observes a clear line between the denture base and the added resin. Which of the following is LEAST likely to have caused this?

   A. Added resin was too dry when placed in the denture
   B. Existing resin not freshened or cleaned prior to application of additional resin
   C. The relined denture was not cured in a pressure pot
   D. Aerosol of oil was used in the compressed air that was used to clean debris from base interior

12. What is the term used to describe the junction of the cementum of the root of the tooth and the enamel of the crown?

   A. dentinoenamel
   B. dentinocemental
   C. cementoenamel
   D. root and crown

13. When flasking a denture, a technician paints the first stone set with Super-Sep, a separating medium. When resin teeth are used, it is important not to allow such a separating medium to contact the occlusal surfaces or incisal edges of the teeth, because they may 13.____

   A. corrode
   B. separate from the flask
   C. become stained
   D. separate from the base

14. Each of the following maxillary teeth would be found near the floor of the maxillary sinus, EXCEPT the 14.____

   A. first molar
   B. third molar
   C. first premolar
   D. lateral incisor

15. The mandibular ridge is a fairly reliable guide to tooth arrangement for the edentulous patient, because it 15.____

   A. does not resorb to the extent that the maxillary ridge does
   B. resorbs more on the buccolabial aspect than on the lingual
   C. usually resorbs straight downward, retaining the lower arch outline
   D. resorbs more on the lingual aspect than the buccolabial

16. When repairing a small nonseparated fracture of the denture base, a repair cast is typically made incorporating the fracture and extending about ______ to either side of the fracture line. 16.____

   A. 2
   B. 5
   C. 7
   D. 10

17. Disinfectants appropriate for polysulfide impression materials include 17.____
   I. sodium hypochlorite
   II. complex phenolics
   III. glutaraldehydes
   IV. iodophors

   A. I only
   B. I and II
   C. III and IV
   D. I, II, III and IV

18. Each of the following is indicated by baseplates and occlusion rims, EXCEPT 18.____

   A. jaw relationships
   B. midline
   C. intercuspation
   D. cuspid line

19. When deflasking a denture, the first cut made into the investment is usually

    A. opposite the central incisors
    B. straight into the rear of the palatal or lingual area
    C. at either of the distobuccal ends
    D. opposite a canine

20. A patient's maxillary first molar is tipped forward so that its distal marginal ridge touches the mesial marginal ridge of the lower second molar and the middle of the mandibular first molar. This molar would be described as

    A. stolarized
    B. intercusped
    C. attritional
    D. crowded

21. If a technician chooses to stipple the waxed trial denture, it should be done

    A. with a soft-bristled brush
    B. over both lingual and buccofacial surfaces of the gingiva
    C. with a focus on root prominences
    D. primarily in the interproximal areas of the teeth

22. The hard tissue that completely surrounds the pulp is the

    A. enamel
    B. dentin
    C. cementum
    D. alveolar bone

23. A brown pigment, used to tint denture bases for patients with heavy gingival pigmentation, is distributed in bottles labeled

    A. B
    B. E
    C. F
    D. H

24. The largest and strongest root of the maxillary molar is the

    A. distofacial
    B. mesiofacial
    C. facial
    D. lingual

25. A technician is arranging 33-degree anatomic maxillary posterior teeth. Typically, the ______ of the maxillary first molar will touch the occlusal plane.

    I. mesiobuccal
    II. mesiolingual
    III. distobuccal
    IV. distolingual

    A. I only
    B. I and II
    C. III and IV
    D. I, II, III and IV

KEY (CORRECT ANSWERS)

1. C
2. B
3. C
4. C
5. A

6. B
7. C
8. A
9. C
10. B

11. C
12. C
13. C
14. D
15. C

16. D
17. D
18. C
19. A
20. A

21. D
22. B
23. A
24. D
25. B

TEST 4

DIRECTIONS: Each question or incomplete statement is followed by several suggested answers or completions. Select the one the BEST answers the question or completes the statement. *PRINT THE LETTER OF THE CORRECT ANSWER IN THE SPACE AT THE RIGHT.*

1. A technician is boxing an impression with wax. The tongue area of the mandibular impression should be waxed smooth and sealed ______ mm below the border of the impression.

   A. 0.5 to 1.0
   B. 1 to 2
   C. 3 to 4
   D. 5 to 6

2. Which of the following is NOT a step involved in the fabrication of a light-cured custom record base?

   A. Buffing the surface of the edentulous cast with a very fine-grained abrasive prior to fabrication
   B. Pressing the resin on the cast in a way that insures no air pockets exist between the cast and the resin
   C. Cutting a 2-cm-long slit in the back of the palate of the maxillary record base resin
   D. Inverting the record base after curing, and curing again

3. Because of its compressive strength, the favored medium for flasking a denture is

   A. alginate
   B. silicone
   C. dental stone
   D. dental plaster

4. A technician is articulating a 20-degree mandibular second premolar. In centric occlusion, which of the following is FALSE?

   A. The tip of the lower buccal cusp contacts the mesial marginal ridge of the maxillary second premolar.
   B. The tip of the lower buccal cusp contacts the distal marginal ridge of the maxillary first premolar.
   C. The lingual cusp is at the embrasure between the maxillary first and second premolars.
   D. The mesiolingual ridge contacts the mesial slope of the buccal cusp of the maxillary first premolar.

5. As a rule, incisal guide-table angulations of more than 20 degrees may indicate the use of

   I. 33-degree anatomic teeth
   II. Pilkington-Turner 30-degree posterior teeth
   III. 20-degree posterior teeth
   IV. 0-degree Rational posterior teeth

   A. I or II
   B. II only
   C. III only
   D. III or IV

6. In a ______ occlusion, the mesiobuccal cusp of the maxillary first molar is directly over the buccal groove of the mandibular first molar. 6.____

A. Class I
B. Class II, Division I
C. Class II, Division II
D. Class III

7. A technician has constructed a baseplate out of autopolymerizing resin. To strike the optimal balance between low porosity and good fit, the baseplate should be cured 7.____

A. in a pressure pot
B. at normal atmospheric pressure, under an inverted plaster bowl
C. on the bench
D. in a vacuum

8. When it is present, the cusp of Carabelli is located on the ______ of the maxillary first molar. 8.____

A. mesiofacial
B. mesiolingual
C. distolingual
D. distofacial

9. What is the term for a small elevation on some portions of a crown that is produced by the extra formation of enamel? 9.____

A. Calculus
B. Lamella
C. Cusp
D. Tubercle

10. When repairing an anterior denture tooth, resin should be removed from the ______ area. 10.____

I. lingual
II. labial
III. mesial
IV. distal

A. I only
B. I and II
C. III and IV
D. I, II, III and IV

11. Maxillary occlusion rims are usually made to measure ______ from the highest point on the labial flange to the occlusal surface in the central incisor region. 11.____

A. 18
B. 22
C. 32
D. 36

12. After constructing a set of gold occlusals, the technician observes that the occlusals don't function properly in the functional positions on an articulator. This is most likely because 1

    A. the articulator settings were disturbed after mounting
    B. the wax-up wasn't checked in the lateral and protrusive positions
    C. wax wasn't flowed onto the ridge laps and lingual surfaces of the resin teeth before flasking
    D. the investment index was overtrimmed occlusogingivally

13. Each of the following muscles elevates the mandible, EXCEPT the

    A. medial pterygoid
    B. lateral pterygoid
    C. temporal
    D. masseter

14. A technician is forming an acrylic resin impression tray using the sprinkle-on method. She has outlined the impression tray on the cast and blocked out the most severe undercuts with wax. Her next step would be to

    A. paint tinfoil substitute on the stone cast
    B. sift powdered polymer onto the cast
    C. adapt a layer of baseplate wax to the cast for relief
    D. make a resin handle

15. In a Class III occlusion, the incisal margins of the mandibular incisors lie _______ middle of the lingual surfaces of the maxillary incisors.

    A. in front of
    B. behind
    C. directly below
    D. to either side of

16. What is the term for the line in the soft palate that marks the junction between stationary tissue and tissue that moves?

    A. Vibrating line
    B. Frenum
    C. Vermilion border
    D. Philtrum

17. Which of the following is most likely to be the ultimate result of packing a denture too late?

    A. Increased processing error through tooth movement
    B. Curing shrinkage
    C. Excessive porosity
    D. Teeth coming loose from denture base

18. Which of the following impression materials is typically the most costly? 18.____

A. Alginate
B. Reversible hydrocolloid
C. Polyether
D. Polysulfide

19. Occasionally it may be necessary to add a posterior palatal seal to a maxillary denture. At the beginning of this procedure, the technician pours a stone cast to include all of the palatal seal and to extend ______ beyond it posteriorly. 19.____

A. 2 to 3
B. 4 to 6
C. 8 to 10
D. 13 to 15

20. Which of the following would be a secondary lymph node of involvement with infection of a maxillary premolar? 20.____

A. Submandibular
B. Upper deep cervical
C. Retropharyngeal
D. Submental

21. The purposes of stippling the resin base of a denture during the finishing and polishing process include 21.____

I. breaking up light reflections
II. correcting or hiding minor imperfections in the resin
III. increasing the surface area
IV. imitating the natural look of gingiva

A. I only
B. I and II
C. II and IV
D. II, III and IV

22. Which of the following is NOT typically caused by porosity in an acrylic denture? 22.____

A. Growth of microorganisms
B. Decreased thermal conductivity
C. Staining
D. Decreased strength

23. When adding a resilient liner to a denture base, it is important to maintain a denture base thickness of at least ______ over the crest of the alveolar ridge. 23.____

A. 1
B. 3
C. 5
D. 7

24. If a disposable plastic tray is used to make alginate impressions, the technician should make sure the tray is ______ before pouring. 24.___

A. perforated
B. rim-locked
C. treated with surfactant
D. rigid

25. When repairing an anterior denture tooth, resin should be removed from the ______ area. 25.___

I. lingual
II. labial
III. mesial
IV. distal

A. I only
B. I and II
C. III and IV
D. I, II, III and IV

KEY (CORRECT ANSWERS)

1. C
2. A
3. C
4. D
5. A
6. A
7. B
8. B
9. D
10. A
11. B
12. B
13. B
14. C
15. A
16. A
17. A
18. C
19. B
20. B
21. B
22. B
23. B
24. D
25. A

EXAMINATION SECTION
TEST 1

DIRECTIONS: Each question or incomplete statement is followed by several suggested answers or completions. Select the one the BEST answers the question or completes the statement. *PRINT THE LETTER OF THE CORRECT ANSWER IN THE SPACE AT THE RIGHT.*

1. Of the following, the most appropriate use for impression wax is 1.____

   A. making custom trays for wash injections
   B. making dies for temporary crowns
   C. preliminary impressions of edentulous ridges for complete dentures
   D. making direct wax pattern inlays

2. In the ideal centric occlusion, the ______ teeth occlude. 2.____

   A. posterior
   B. anterior
   C. canine
   D. incisor

3. The principal advantage associated with the construction of two-piece impression trays over stock or one-piece custom trays is their 3.____

   A. greater dimensional stability
   B. shorter time requirements
   C. ability to be disassembled and reassembled
   D. lack of bulk

4. A technician is arranging 33-degree anatomic maxillary posterior teeth. Typically, each of the following teeth will contact the occlusal plane at some point, EXCEPT the 4.____

   A. first premolar
   B. second premolar
   C. first molar
   D. second molar

5. During mastication, the ______ keeps food on occlusal surfaces. 5.____

   A. orbicularis oris
   B. orbicularis oculi
   C. zygomaticus minor
   D. depressor anguli oris

6. A technician is carving the gingival margin around the anterior teeth of a trial maxillary denture. The technician should use a carver or #7 spatula, held at an angle of approximately ______ degrees. 6.____

   A. 30
   B. 45
   C. 60
   D. 90

7. Before flasking a denture with artificial stone, the interior of the flask is best lubricated with 7

A. silicone lubricant
B. mineral oil
C. tinfoil substitute
D. powdered talc

8. Which of the roots in on the maxillary first molar is longest? 8

A. Mesiofacial
B. Distal
C. Lingual
D. Facial

9. The last step in deflasking is usually to 9

A. remove stone from the distobuccal corners
B. tap away the stone enclosing the cast
C. remove the denture base from the cast
D. remove the sectioned lingual or palatal area

10. Which of the following is NOT a purpose of a baseplate? 10

A. Carrying occlusal rims
B. Checking the accuracy of previous records
C. Holding the teeth for the try-in stage
D. Establishing the occlusal plane

11. Often, the ______ cusp of the maxillary third molar is missing. 11

A. distolingual
B. distofacial
C. mesiolingual
D. mesiofacial

12. The most significant advantage offered by resin denture teeth is that they 12

A. are chip-resistant
B. can bond to most heat-cured denture base resins
C. have great wear resistance
D. can be re-polished

13. Of the following muscles, the movement of the temporomandibular joint is most directly affected by the 13

A. masseter
B. trapezius
C. lateral pterygoid
D. medial pterygoid

14. Which of the following is NOT a typical characteristic in a tapering maxillary arch? 14.

A. Incisal tips of the canines are slightly below the incisal edges of the lateral incisors.
B. Lateral incisors are slightly above the occlusal plane.

C. Central incisors are farther forward of the canines than in other types of arches.
D. Central incisors are rotated inward at the distal aspect.

15. A patient has dental decay that has progressed into the tooth, exposing the dentin. Which is likely to happen as a result of this irritation? 15.____

A. The dentinal tubules will become sealed off.
B. The pulp will die as it is contacted by air.
C. Ameloblasts will attempt to cover the exposure with enamel.
D. Secondary dentin will form in an attempt to repair the tissue.

16. In a typical arrangement of Pilkington-Turner 30-degree posterior teeth, the 16.____

A. buccal cusps of the first and second premolars touch the occlusal plane
B. long axes of the premolars should be tilted slightly from vertical (in the buccal view)
C. lingual cusps of the first and second premolars touch the occlusal plane
D. long axes of the molars should be at right angles to the occlusal plane (in the buccal view)

17. The ______ muscle has two origins on the zygomatic arch. 17.____

A. sternocleidomastoid
B. masseter
C. lateral pterygoid
D. temporal

18. A technician is deflasking a denture. After the wax trial base and baseplate have been discarded, and no teeth are determined to have been dislodged, the next step is usually to. 18.____

A. flush each half-flask with boiling detergent water
B. scrub each half-flask with a brush and detergent
C. remove larger bits of remaining stone with a scalpel
D. paint tinfoil substitute on the exposed stone surfaces

19. Agar hydrocolloid impression materials 19.____

A. have high tear strength in narrow spaces
B. are hydrophobic
C. can be poured after several hours if kept in water
D. are compatible with a moist field

20. Usually, ______ g of dental stone is adequate for most impressions. 20.____

A. 50
B. 100
C. 200
D. 350

21. All other factors aside, the quickest and easiest method of making a usable baseplate is to 21.____

A. vacuum mold a sheet of thermoplastic resin to the cast
B. hand-adapt a rolled resin sheet

C. sprinkle on polymer and add monomer
D. confine resin in a stone index for curing

22. Heat-cured acrylic resin is packed into the denture flask to form the denture base during 22
the ______ stage of polymerization.

A. ropy
B. sandy
C. stringy
D. dough

23. Rebasing a denture is most often due to dissatisfaction with the ______ of the denture. 23

I. color
II. teeth
III. porosity
IV. fit

A. I only
B. I or III
C. I, III or IV
D. II, III or IV

24. A technician has received a transfer fork that registers the occlusal relationships of a 24
patient's teeth. The technician coats the indentations with a thin layer of zinc oxide/eugenol impression paste, for the purpose of

A. making the wax less porous
B. fastening the transfer fork to the articulator
C. preventing the wax from distorting
D. keeping the cast from sticking to the wax during articulation

25. Which of the following is NOT an advantage associated with the use of metal denture 25
bases?

A. Ease in relining
B. No warpage
C. Less tissue change under the base
D. Increased accuracy

KEY (CORRECT ANSWERS)

1. C
2. A
3. D
4. D
5. B

6. C
7. A
8. C
9. B
10. D

11. A
12. B
13. C
14. A
15. D

16. C
17. B
18. A
19. D
20. C

21. A
22. D
23. B
24. C
25. A

TEST 2

DIRECTIONS: Each question or incomplete statement is followed by several suggested answers or completions. Select the one the BEST answers the question or completes the statement. *PRINT THE LETTER OF THE CORRECT ANSWER IN THE SPACE AT THE RIGHT.*

1. A heat-processed denture is NOT _______ than a chemically cured denture. 1

   A. harder
   B. less dimensionally accurate
   C. more porous
   D. stronger

2. Which of the following impression materials is transformed from a liquid to a gel when set? 2

   A. Zinc oxide/eugenol
   B. Polysulfide
   C. Condensation silicone
   D. Alginate

3. A technician is constructing a baseplate out of autopolymerizing resin. He has used soft-curing resin to block out several undercuts. Occasionally, this soft-curing resin can flow out of the undercuts instead of remaining in place. The technician can prevent this problem by 3

   A. warming the cast in hot water, or with a chip blower
   B. using hard-curing resin
   C. chilling the cast slightly
   D. using baseplate wax

4. In recent years, many technicians have switched from reversible hydrocolloid impression material to newer elastomeric impression materials. Which of the following is NOT a reason for this? 4

   A. Elastomers are more accurate
   B. Impressions don't have to be poured immediately
   C. Surfactants are usually not required
   D. Elastomers don't require as much equipment

5. When arranging the maxillary anterior teeth, the cervical third of the canines should be tilted 5

   A. mesially
   B. lingually
   C. distally
   D. buccally

6. Which of the following premolars is commonly bifurcated? 6

   A. Maxillary first
   B. Maxillary second

C. Mandibular first
D. Mandibular second

7. Boxing final impressions before pouring 7.____

I. controls the form and thickness of the base of the cast
II. facilitates the placement of remounting plates
III. preserves the extension and thickness of borders
IV. conserves dental stone

A. I and III
B. I, II and III
C. II only
D. I, II, III and IV

8. When packing a denture, resin flash should be trimmed with a 8.____

A. sharp scalpel
B. dull spatula
C. carbide bur
D. PKT #2 tool

9. The suprahyoid muscles include each of the following, EXCEPT the 9.____

A. stylohyoid
B. thyrohyoid
C. digastric
D. geniohyoid

10. When repairing a plastic anterior denture tooth, which of the following is done FIRST? 10.____

A. Grinding the labial gingival margin
B. With a bur, placing shallow indentations in the denture-tooth ridge lap
C. Pouring a plaster index on the labial surface of the tooth to be replaced
D. Securing a replacement tooth in the base with sticky wax

11. In making a custom tray from chemical-cured resin, some technicians place three or four 2-mm holes in the anterior and posterior ridge regions of the wax spacer before adapting the tray material over it. Ultimately, this technique results in 11.____

A. the stabilization of wax rims during a try-in
B. insulating the patient from the heat of the exothermic reaction
C. blocking out tissue undercuts before the final construction
D. the prevention of large areas of tissue being compressed during the taking of an impression

12. The tint for a denture base's basic pink color is distributed in bottles labeled 12.____

A. A
B. B
C. E
D. H

13. Which of the following is NOT a guideline to be followed in constructing metal occlusals for denture teeth? 13

   A. When flasking the occlusals and teeth, the buccal surfaces should be depressed slightly toward the cervical aspect.
   B. Before forming the castings, maxillary and mandibular teeth should be reduced to provide about 4 mm of interocclusal space.
   C. Castings should be about 2 mm thick.
   D. Incisal shade resin should be sifted into the mold last when occlusals and resin teeth are cured in the flask.

14. Which of the following nerves innervates the lingual gingiva of the maxillary central incisor? 14

   A. Nasopalatine
   B. Posterior superior alveolar
   C. Inferior alveolar
   D. Trigeminal

15. A technician is articulating a 33-degree anatomic mandibular second premolar. In centric occlusion, the tip of the buccal cusp will typically contact the 15

   A. buccal groove of the maxillary first molar
   B. distal slope of the lingual cusp of the maxillary first premolar
   C. mesial marginal ridge of the maxillary second premolar
   D. the mesiobuccal slope of the maxillary second premolar

16. The main disadvantage associated with the use of thermoplastic shellac baseplate materials for making impression trays is their 16

   A. intense exothermic reaction
   B. dimensional instability
   C. difficulty in trimming
   D. complexity

17. Which of the following is NOT an advantage associated with heat-cured compression-molded resin baseplates? 17

   A. Bases can become part of the denture themselves
   B. Excellent preservation of master casts
   C. Minimal finishing and polishing requirements
   D. Thickness can be controlled during wax-up

18. Which of the following is associated with a Class III occlusion? 18

   A. Prognathic lower jaw
   B. Retrognathic lower jaw
   C. Enlarged lower jaw
   D. Lateral mandibular glide

19. Finished complete dentures should have a palate thickness of about ______. 19

   A. 1
   B. 2

C. 3
D. 4

20. Cracks in dental enamel are called 20.____

A. spindles
B. imbrications
C. lamellae
D. villi

21. When finishing and polishing a denture, the first area to receive attention is usually the 21.____

A. outer border
B. gingival margins
C. palate or lingual border
D. incisal or occlusal surfaces

22. In the ideal protrusive movement, the ______ teeth touch. 22.____

A. canine and posterior
B. anterior
C. canine
D. anterior and posterior

23. Each of the following is a typical procedure involved in the waxing of a trial maxillary denture, EXCEPT 23.____

A. forming a slight bulge over the maxillary premolars, from the canine eminence to the molar process
B. developing a slight root prominence over the maxillary central incisors
C. developing a gingival bulge that is approximately 5 to 6 mm wide over the second molar
D. carving a slight fossa between the root of the central incisor and the canine eminence

24. The superior aspect of the external auditory meatus, often used as a reference point in dental work, is known as the 24.____

A. porion
B. nasion
C. A-point
D. B-point

25. A technician plans to make a denture base out of fluid resin. The most important adjustment to make in this procedure is to 25.____

A. add more water to the flasking material
B. leave at least a 0.5 mm diastema between each canine and first premolar
C. increase the interocclusal distance about 0.5 mm in the incisal guide-pin area of the articulator
D. apply a coat of separating fluid to the incisal or occlusal surfaces of the teeth

---

KEY (CORRECT ANSWERS)

1. C
2. D
3. A
4. C
5. D

6. A
7. D
8. B
9. B
10. D

11. D
12. D
13. A
14. A
15. C

16. B
17. B
18. A
19. B
20. C

21. A
22. B
23. A
24. A
25. C

TEST 3

DIRECTIONS: Each question or incomplete statement is followed by several suggested answers or completions. Select the one the BEST answers the question or completes the statement. *PRINT THE LETTER OF THE CORRECT ANSWER IN THE SPACE AT THE RIGHT.*

1. On the facial surface of the anterior teeth, the greatest convexity will be found at the 1.____

   A. junction of the middle and incisal thirds
   B. incisal third
   C. middle third
   D. cervical third

2. A technician is trimming a diagnostic cast. The simplest and most effective way to align the back cuts of the maxillary and mandibular portions of the cast is to 2.____

   A. articulate the casts with pins and then trim them simultaneously
   B. articulate the casts with a wax bite and then trim them simultaneously
   C. trim the longer cast first and then articulate the casts with a wax bite
   D. trim the shorter cast first and then articulate the casts with a wax bite

3. Characteristics typical of a Class II, division II occlusion include 3.____

   I. mesioclusion
   II. crowded maxillary incisors
   III. a deep overbite
   IV. an abnormal overjet

   A. I and II
   B. II and III
   C. I, II and IV
   D. I, II, III and IV

4. Which of the following is NOT a significant problem associated with the flask method of rebasing a denture? 4.____

   A. Air inclusions in the flasking material producing nodules on the rebased denture
   B. Risk of dislodging a tooth from the flasking material when packing
   C. Breaking the cast while separating the denture
   D. Occlusal errors

5. Before making a wax baseplate, it is advisable to apply a separating layer of _______ on the cast surfaces. 5.____

   A. powdered talc
   B. Super-Sep fluid
   C. mineral oil
   D. slurry water

6. In centric occlusion, the lingual cusps of the maxillary molars strike their antagonists 6.____

   A. facial to the facial cusps of the mandibular teeth
   B. lingual to the lingual cusps of the mandibular teeth

C. on the facial portion of the facial cusps
D. on the central portion of the mandibular occlusal surface

7. A technician is boxing an impression with wax. The height of the wax should generally be adjusted so that it extends approximately _____ mm above the highest point on the impression. 7

A. 4
B. 7
C. 13
D. 22

8. The first step in removing a denture from a cast is to 8

A. direct a blast of air between the denture and the cast base
B. divide the cast base into several sections
C. make a saw cut opposite the central incisors
D. thin the cast base as much as possible with a cast trimmer

9. Which of the following is a term that denotes the dislocation of the temporomandibular joint? 9

A. Prognathicism
B. Malocclusion
C. Glide
D. Subluxation

10. What is the term for the area where the head of the mandible lies? 10

A. Glenoid fossa
B. Emenentia
C. External auditory meatus
D. Articular eminence

11. Metal occlusal surfaces for denture teeth may be indicated when 11
   I. their use is needed to reinforce and strengthen the denture
   II. constructing a denture that will be opposed by a reconstructed dentition with gold occlusal surfaces
   III. constructing a denture with a functionally generated path concept in which considerable modification of the teeth is necessary
   IV. special wax carving techniques are completed on a fully adjustable articulator

A. I and II
B. I and III
C. II, III and IV
D. I, II, III and IV

12. A technician discovers a lack of space for setting the mandibular first premolar in a complete denture. Each of the following is a possible solution, EXCEPT 12

A. leaving a 1 mm space between the mandibular canine and the first premolar
B. grinding the lower premolar carefully on mesial and distal surfaces

C. leaving out the lower central or lateral incisor
D. leaving out the mandibular second premolar

13. The most commonly used impression tray materials are 13.____

A. special autopolymerizing acrylic resins
B. thermoplastic resin sheets
C. hard thermoplastic waxes
D. thermoplastic shellac baseplate materials

14. A technician wants to add a plastic palate form to a trial denture before flasking. With a fissure bur, the existing palate should be cut at a distance of about ______ from the denture teeth. 14.____

A. 3 to 4
B. 5 to 6
C. 7 to 8
D. 9 to 10

15. Which of the following arteries supplies the muscles of mastication? 15.____

A. pterygoid plexus
B. superficial temporal
C. mental
D. maxillary

16. In the ______ arch configuration, the long axes of the anterior teeth generally deviate most noticeably from the sagittal plane, or midline. 16.____

A. Square
B. Square-tapering
C. Tapering
D. Ovoid

17. Gold alloys of Type(s) ______ are sufficiently rigid for use as cast metal denture bases. 17.____

A. I only
B. I and II
C. III and IV
D. V only

18. ______ exists where the premolars occlude during a lateral mandibular glide. 18.____

A. Group function
B. The balancing side
C. The working side
D. Posterior coupling

19. If a technician makes a denture base out of poured fluid resin, the denture will be flasked in 19.____

A. dental plaster
B. dental stone

C. silicone
D. hydrocolloid

20. Occlusal trauma is characterized by 20.

A. healing occurring with the inflammation
B. thinning of principal fibers due to tension
C. reparation after the inflammation is removed
D. bone resorption from obstruction of blood flow to principal fibers

21. A technician is constructing a baseplate out of autopolymerizing resin using the sprinkle-on method. When relief is applied to the cast, 21.

A. soft-curing resin should be used to block out only the severest undercuts
B. baseplate wax should be used to block out only the severest undercuts
C. soft-curing resin should be used to block out all the undercuts
D. baseplate wax should be used to block out all the undercuts

22. After deflasking, a technician is painting tinfoil substitute over the cast and stone. The technician should be careful to avoid applying tinfoil substitute to the 22.

A. ridgelaps of resin teeth
B. distolingual area
C. interproximal areas
D. peripheral roll

23. Which of the following gypsum products requires the highest water-to-powder ratio? 23.

A. High strength dental stone
B. High strength/high expansion dental stone
C. Dental stone
D. Model plaster

24. In centric occlusion, the mesiobuccal inclined plane of the mandibular second molar contacts the 24.

A. central fossa of the maxillary second molar
B. marginal ridge of the mesiolingual cusp of the maxillary first molar
C. mesiobuccal cusp of the maxillary second molar
D. marginal ridge of the distobuccal cusp of the maxillary first molar

25. Most dentists agree that for most patients, the average period of satisfactory service for a denture is about _______ years. 25.

A. 2
B. 5
C. 7
D. 10

KEY (CORRECT ANSWERS)

1. D
2. C
3. B
4. C
5. A
6. D
7. C
8. D
9. D
10. A
11. D
12. D
13. A
14. B
15. D
16. C
17. C
18. A
19. D
20. D
21. B
22. A
23. D
24. D
25. C

TEST 4

DIRECTION: Each question or incomplete statement is followed by several suggested answers or completions. Select the one the BEST answers the question or completes the statement. *PRINT THE LETTER OF THE CORRECT ANSWER IN THE SPACE AT THE RIGHT.*

1. A technician is using the double-pour method to make a working cast. Most often, this means that the anatomic portion 1

   A. and the art portion will be poured in stone, each separately
   B. and the art portion will be poured in plaster, each separately
   C. plaster; the base in dental stone
   D. dental stone; the base in plaster

2. Which of the following is MOST likely to have a transverse ridge? 2

   A. Maxillary first premolar
   B. Mandibular first premolar
   C. Maxillary second premolar
   D. Mandibular second premolar

3. Boxing with wax is usually most appropriate for impressions that are made from 3

   A. silicone
   B. alginate
   C. zinc oxide/eugenol impression paste
   D. rubber

4. A technician is placing the maxillary anterior teeth of a denture. Which of the following is typically FALSE? 4

   A. The central incisor is inclined slightly from the vertical.
   B. The incisal edge of the lateral incisor touches the occlusal plane.
   C. The canine is set at a right angle to the occlusal plane.
   D. The incisal edge of the central incisor touches the occlusal plane

5. Typically, _______ dental modeling compound softens at a higher temperature than other colors. 5

   A. white
   B. red
   C. green
   D. black

6. Flat tooth forms for a denture, such as Rational 0-degree posterior teeth, are appropriate for 6

   I. flat or heavily resorbed ridges
   II. crossbites
   III. patients with uncoordinated jaw movements
   IV. severe overbites

A. I and II
B. II and IV
C. I, II and III
D. I, II, III and IV

7. The mandible may be retruded or depressed by the _______ muscle. 7.____

A. thyrohyoid
B. masseter
C. medial pterygoid
D. digastric

8. A technician is rebasing a denture. If the teeth are porcelain, they will be removed by 8.____

A. heating them with a hot spatula
B. chilling with a cold spatula
C. grinding them down to near the margin
D. grinding them down to the retaining holes

9. A technician is mounting a mandibular cast on an articulator. The FIRST step in this process is usually to 9.____

A. fit the occlusal registration to the maxillary cast
B. invert the articulator with the maxillary cast in place
C. remove the maxillary cast from the articulator
D. set the incisal guide pin to the appropriate height

10. A technician is constructing a baseplate out of autopolymerizing resin using the sprinkle-on method. It is essential that the technician 10.____

A. adapt the resin by hand after it has been applied
B. have polymer and monomer ready in premeasured amounts
C. cure the baseplate in a pressure pot
D. perform the construction in a hood or well-ventilated area

11. Which of the following primary teeth has a lingual ridge on its lingual surface? 11.____

A. Mandibular central
B. Maxillary central
C. Mandibular canine
D. Maxillary canine

12. The most distinct feature of the maxillary first deciduous molar is its 12.____

A. mesial profile
B. transverse ridge
C. occlusion
D. buccal cervical ridge

13. Baseplate wax should NOT be used to block out undercuts in the construction of _______ baseplates. 13.____

A. vacuum-molded resin
B. sprinkle-on resin

C. hand-adapted resin
D. thermoplastic shellac

14. The starting point or "anchor" in the placement of mandibular posterior teeth is typically the 14

A. first premolar
B. second premolar
C. first molar
D. third molar

15. The soft palate is pulled into contact with the posterior pharyngeal wall by the ______ muscle. 15

A. uvula
B. styloglossus
C. levator veli palatini
D. procerus

16. Porcelain prosthetic teeth have retentive recesses known as ______ in the ridge laps that can retain the teeth in the denture base. 16

A. diastemas
B. pinholes
C. diatorics
D. obstinators

17. When waxing a mandibular trial denture, wax should be flowed onto the lingual surface and the gingival margins carved to produce a gingival marginal angle of about ______ below the horizontal. 17

A. 20
B. 35
C. 45
D. 60

18. A technician wants to make an acrylic resin soft and pliable. The technician should 18

A. use less monomer in the mix
B. use less powder in the mix
C. add benzoyl peroxide
D. add aromatic esters

19. Viewed from above, the narrowest part of the maxillary arch of a denture would typically be in the area of the 19

A. canines
B. first premolars
C. second premolars
D. first molar

20. What is the term used to denote carving of the denture base to simulate the contours of the natural tissues that are to be replaced by the denture? 20.____

A. Garnishment
B. Mimicry
C. Anatomizing
D. Festooning

21. ______ impression materials produce alcohol during setting and are subject to distortion as the alcohol evaporates. 21.____

A. Reversible hydrocolloid
B. Addition silicone
C. Zinc oxide/eugenol
D. Condensation silicone

22. A technician has remounted a denture on an articulator for adjustments. Which of the following is NOT a guideline to be followed in making these adjustments? 22.____

A. When adjusting the working position, adjust the buccal cusps of the upper teeth and the lingual cusps of the mandibular teeth to eliminate defective contacts.
B. In the working position, adjust maxillary buccal cusps and lingual cusps of mandibular teeth.
C. In the centric relation, grind the cusp tips rather than the fossae.
D. If possible, grind the inclines of the maxillary lingual cusps on the balancing side rather than the buccal cusps of mandibular dentures.

23. Another term for a Class II occlusion is 23.____

A. mesioclusion
B. distoclusion
C. neutroclusion
D. lateral excursion

24. The floor of the mouth is formed by the ______ muscle. 24.____

A. omohyoid
B. gastric
C. mylohyoid
D. stylohyoid

25. Cast metal denture bases should be each of the following, EXCEPT 25.____

A. dense
B. accurate enough to seat on the master cast without rocking
C. as thick as possible for maximum rigidity
D. of a biologically compatible alloy

KEY (CORRECT ANSWERS)

1. D
2. B
3. C
4. B
5. D
6. C
7. D
8. A
9. D
10. D
11. D
12. D
13. A
14. C
15. C
16. C
17. A
18. D
19. B
20. D
21. D
22. C
23. B
24. C
25. C

EXAMINATION SECTION
TEST 1

DIRECTIONS: Each question or incomplete statement is followed by several suggested answers or completions. Select the one the BEST answers the question or completes the statement. *PRINT THE LETTER OF THE CORRECT ANSWER IN THE SPACE AT THE RIGHT.*

1. Which of the following is a direct retainer? 1.____

   A. Y-bar
   B. Incisal hook
   C. Occlusal rest
   D. Lingual plate

2. A lingual bar should be rigid, with an upper border located at least ______ mm form a line connecting the gingival margins. 2.____

   A. 1 to 1.5
   B. 1.5 to 2
   C. 3 to 4
   D. 4 to 5

3. The principal advantage associated with acrylic resin as a denture base material is that it 3.____

   A. maintains its form without distortion
   B. conforms over time to fit the edentulous ridge
   C. has a high thermal conductivity that increases patient comfort
   D. can be re based or relined

4. What is the term for prepared, flattened surfaces on restored abutment teeth that are parallel to the selected path of insertion for a removable partial denture? 4.____

   A. Occlusal planes
   B. Guiding planes
   C. Subcoronals
   D. Surveying lines

5. The retentive arm of a clasp is so named because it 5.____

   A. maintains the clasp assembly in its proper position on the tooth
   B. resists the forces that tend to displace the denture occlusally
   C. protects the soft tissues
   D. counteracts lateral forces exerted on the abutment tooth

6. Semi-adjustable arcon articulators with preformed condylar controls that permit immediate sideshift can be adjusted by using eccentric wax interocclusal records. For optimal accuracy, they may be used with simplified mandibular motion analyzers. These analyzers 6.____

   I. begin in a position where incisal edges meet
   II. can be used to program a fully adjustable articulator
   III. measure the amount of immediate sideshift
   IV. trace the form of the protrusive condylar pathways

A. I only
B. I and II
C. III and IV
D. IV only

7. After a custom tray has set completely, a technician makes a number of perforating retention holes. These holes should typically be spaced about ______ mm apart. 7.

A. 2
B. 4
C. 6
D. 8

8. If a double palatal bar is used as a major connector for a removable partial denture, the anterior bar should be at least ______ mm from the anterior teeth. 8.

A. 3 to 4
B. 5 to 6
C. 7 to 8
D. 10 to 12

9. ______ is a material that is broken into pieces to remove it from the mouth and then reassembled in the laboratory for making an impression. 9.

A. Plaster
B. Wax
C. Dental compound
D. Zinc oxide/eugenol

10. A patient is missing all of his maxillary incisors, along with a canine. This patient is a candidate for a Kennedy Class ______ removable partial denture. 10.

A. I
B. II
C. III
D. IV

11. Of the following, the tool most likely to be used to bead a maxillary cast would be the 11.

A. spoon excavator
B. long beavertail
C. PKT #3 tool
D. Roach carver

12. With all other factors remaining equal, doubling the length of a clasp arm will 12.

A. reduce its flexibility by half
B. have no effect on its flexibility
C. double its flexibility
D. increase its flexibility by a factor of 5

13. After rebasing a removable partial denture, a technician observes an orange discoloration of the resin base that extends to one of the artificial teeth. The most likely cause of this was 13.

A. too much monomer in the resin when processed
B. the intrusion of stone separating fluid onto the waxed-up base and the tooth
C. movement or distortion of the framework during resin packing
D. contaminated tinfoil substitute

14. After a cast has been separated from an impression, it should not be washed or trimmed for a minimum of ______ hours. 14.____

A. 8
B. 12
C. 24
D. 48

15. Which of the following is NOT an advantage associated with the simple circlet (Akers) clasp? 15.____

A. Ease of design and construction
B. Excellent support
C. Minimal coverage of tooth surface
D. Reduced tendency to collect food

16. A wrought wire clasp can be used on terminal abutments of distal extension partial dentures, and is usually placed in a ______ undercut. 16.____

A. mesiofacial
B. mesiolingual/mesiopalatal
C. distofacial
D. distolingual/distopalatal

17. When used with alginate material, a properly selected impression tray should be deep enough to provide at least ______ mm of space beyond the incisal and occlusal surfaces of the teeth. 17.____

A. 1
B. 2
C. 3
D. 4

18. The term "desirable undercuts," in relation to removable partial dentures, concerns 18.____

A. the clasping of abutment teeth
B. buccal or labial portions of the residual ridge
C. a lack of interference with the nonflexible portions of the framework
D. esthetics

19. A technician has made a corrected cast impression by boxing it with a plaster and pumice mixture, but has trouble removing it from the corrected cast. Which of the following is LEAST likely to have been the cause? 19.____

A. Undercuts in impression tray
B. Impression tray locked into dental stone because too much of it was exposed during boxing
C. Original cast was dry when new stone was poured into ridge areas
D. Failure to heat modeling plastic used for border molding

20. After a refractory cast has been removed from a mold, the best way to remove debris from the cast is with 20

A. a soft-bristled brush
B. tap water
C. clear slurry water
D. gentle blasts of air

21. Each step of the "lost wax" procedure for making castings can cause inaccuracies in the final product. The most significant property-common to the impression material, the die stone, wax, investment material, and the cast metal-that must all be controlled by the technician to achieve the best possible final casting is 21

A. vaporization
B. condensation
C. strength and durability
D. expansion and contraction

22. Which of the following is NOT a purpose of an occlusion rim? 22

A. determining high and low lip lines
B. recording the maxillomandibular relationship
C. determining the path of insertion for a denture
D. determining the length and width of replacement teeth

23. Cobalt-chromium alloys should be cleaned and have oxides removed after devestment by 23

A. pickling and sandblasting
B. pickling and shellblasting
C. sandblasting only
D. pickling only

24. If no framework is attached to a record base, the usual means of separating it from a cast after fabrication is 24

A. directing a blast of air under the periphery and then gently lifting
B. turning the cast upside down and shaking the record loose
C. prying slightly on the side with the undercuts
D. prying slightly on the side opposite the undercuts

25. The wax-up for a removable partial denture framework is usually best smoothed and finished by 25

A. flaming with a torch
B. polishing with a soft cloth
C. dipping in warm water
D. smoothing with the fingertips

KEY (CORRECT ANSWERS)

1. A
2. C
3. D
4. B
5. B
6. C
7. C
8. B
9. A
10. D
11. A
12. D
13. B
14. B
15. C
16. A
17. B
18. A
19. C
20. D
21. D
22. C
23. C
24. A
25. B

TEST 2

DIRECTIONS: Each question or incomplete statement is followed by several suggested answers or completions. Select the one the BEST answers the question or completes the statement. *PRINT THE LETTER OF THE CORRECT ANSWER IN THE SPACE AT THE RIGHT.*

1. "Tripod marks" are used on a surveyed cast to 1.

   A. determine the gingival extent of a retentive clasp tip
   B. evaluate the buccolingual inclination
   C. determine the most desirable undercut for the abutment teeth
   D. re-establish the selected path of insertion if the cast is removed and replaced

2. Before an acrylic resin tray material sets completely, it is often a good idea to 2.
   I. add some of the material to the front of the tray to form a handle
   II. hold the plastic to the cast with one's fingers
   III. remove it and check for undercuts
   IV. perforate it with a No. 6 or 8 round bur

   A. I and II
   B. II only
   C. II and IV
   D. I, II, III and IV

3. The arms of extra-coronal retainers should encircle the abutment tooth at least _______ degrees. 3.

   A. 120
   B. 180
   C. 220
   D. 270

4. A patient is missing the first, second, and third molars on the left mandibular side only. This patient is a candidate for a Kennedy Class _______ removable partial denture. 4.

   A. I
   B. II
   C. III
   D. IV

5. Which of the following is NOT an advantage associated with the double palatal bar? 5.

   A. Bracing of anterior teeth with weakened periodontal support
   B. Excellent strength
   C. Provision of access to palatal tissues for the tongue
   D. Usefulness for long spans

6. After relining, the rests of a removable partial denture don't seat completely into the rest seats of the abutments. Of the following, which is LEAST likely to have caused this? 6

   A. Resin was too dry when packed
   B. Reline was processed in a flask with incomplete closure

C. Reline jig was not completely closed
D. Rests were not seated when impression was made

7. Cast extensions should include an area ______ mm beyond the hamular notches on the maxillary cast, and the same distance beyond the retromolar pad on the mandibular cast. 7.____

A. 1 to 2
B. 3 to 4
C. 5 to 6
D. 8 to 10

8. A left lateral tilt of a cast on a surveyor will increase the undercuts on the 8.____

A. lingual or palatal surfaces of the left side
B. buccal surfaces of the left side
C. mesial side
D. distal side

9. Simple circlet cast clasps are used primarily in 9.____

A. tooth-supported partial dentures
B. Kennedy Class I dentures
C. Kennedy Class II dentures
D. posterior teeth only

10. Which of the following connectors is most rarely used for partial dentures? 10.____

A. Lingual bar
B. Labial bar
C. Lingual plate
D. Palatal strap

11. A technician is making a resin record base, without incorporating a framework, using the sprinkle-on method. Of the following, which would be performed FIRST in this procedure? 11.____

A. Adapting a reinforcing wire
B. Placing the cast in a slurry solution
C. Blocking out interproximal undercuts
D. Beading the border with wax

12. Gold-alloy castings should be bench-cooled for a period of about ______ minutes before quenching in water. 12.____

A. 6
B. 12
C. 30
D. 60

13. Of the following elastomers, ______ must be poured with gypsum material within a few hours after the impression is made. 13

I. polysulfide
II. polyether
III. condensation silicone
IV. addition silicone

A. I only
B. II only
C. II and IV
D. III and IV

14. After a stone cast has set, but while it is still warm from crystallization, it is often helpful to place the poured impression in ______ for 3 to 5 minutes. 14

A. denatured alcohol
B. tap water
C. distilled water
D. slurry water

15. If the base of a refractory cast is too large to fit into a casting ring, it must be trimmed 15

A. immediately after removal from the hydrocolloid
B. after setting for at least an hour
C. after soaking in clear slurry water for 3 to 5 minutes
D. before it is coated with model spray

16. The use of infrabulge clasps should generally be avoided when 16

I. a "push" type of retention is desirable
II. the abutment tooth has a severe buccal or lingual inclination
III. there are significant aesthetic concerns
IV. there is a large soft tissue undercut in the gingival area of the abutment tooth

A. I only
B. I and II
C. II and IV
D. I, II, III and IV

17. The multiple circlet clasp is most often used to provide additional support for weakened 17

A. incisors
B. canines
C. premolars
D. molars

18. In general, the width of an abutment's guiding plane should extend from the buccal to the lingual lien angle of the abutment, and the height should be approximately ______ mm from the marginal ridge. 18

A. 0.5 to 1.0
B. 1.0 to 2.0
C. 1.5 to 3
D. 2 to 4

19. For nailhead retention, 19.____

A. 18-gauge round wax is attached to the ridge sheet, cut to about a 2-mm length, and flattened
B. nailheads are typically soldered after casting
C. pre-formed resin nailheads are attached to the ridge sheet
D. nailheads should be conical in shape, no matter what material is used

20. In alginate impression materials, potassium sulfate is added to 20.____

A. delay the set
B. increase stiffness and strength
C. prevent the alginate from interfering with the set of a gypsum cast
D. keep the impression surface from becoming sticky

21. A technician is mounting a maxillary cast on a Whip-Mix articulator. 21.____
In this type of articulator, _______ is/are substituted for the condylar spheres.

A. a universal clutch
B. a mounting bracket
C. jackscrews
D. adjustable axis indicators

22. A lingual rest is a metallic extension that is prepared on the ______ area of an anterior tooth. 22.____

A. cervical
B. proximal
C. cingulum
D. incisal

23. Relief blockout on a cast is used 23.____

I. to create a space between the framework and the cast or soft tissue
II. beneath lingual bars
III. in edentulous areas to provide for attachment of denture bases
IV. to form internal finish lines

A. I and II
B. I, III and IV
C. II and III
D. I, II, III and IV

24. A technician is trimming a diagnostic cast. The heels of the cast should be trimmed 24.____

A. at a 30° angle to the mid-sagittal line
B. parallel to the side cut
C. at a 90° angle to a line formed connecting the canine eminence to the opposite side/back cut
D. parallel to the anterior cut

25. Of the following, the fastest method of forming a record base is to use 25.

A. baseplate wax
B. visible light-cured resin sheets
C. shellac
D. thermoplastic vinyl sheets

KEY (CORRECT ANSWERS)

1. D
2. A
3. B
4. B
5. A

6. A
7. B
8. B
9. A
10. B

11. C
12. B
13. C
14. D
15. A

16. C
17. C
18. D
19. A
20. C

21. B
22. C
23. D
24. C
25. B

TEST 3

DIRECTIONS: Each question or incomplete statement is followed by several suggested answers or completions. Select the one the BEST answers the question or completes the statement. *PRINT THE LETTER OF THE CORRECT ANSWER IN THE SPACE AT THE RIGHT.*

1. The first step in pouring a corrected impression is typically to 1.____

   A. remove the residual ridge areas from the master cast
   B. box the impression
   C. lute the framework onto the master cast
   D. soak the cast in clear slurry water

2. A technician is surveying a diagnostic cast. The abutment teeth do not have the required amount of undercut for a removable partial denture. Which of the following is the LEAST appropriate option? 2.____

   A. Altering the contour of the abutment
   B. Using non-clasp-type retainers
   C. Restoring the abutment tooth with a retainer that has the appropriate contours
   D. Using a clasp made of flexible wire

3. Addition silicones 3.____

   A. do not require disinfection
   B. have a high dimensional stability
   C. require custom acrylic trays
   D. cost about the same as reversible hydrocolloids

4. During the second phase of prosthodontic treatment, a record base is typically used to 4.____
   I. obtain an accurate mounting of the diagnostic casts
   II. determine the maxillomandibular relationship of the master casts
   III. aid in fabricating the metal framework
   IV. determine an accurate occlusal relationship of the casts

   A. I and II
   B. II and III
   C. II, III and IV
   D. I, II, III and IV

5. The I clasp is a short, stiff clasp that is usually used on ______ for esthetics. 5.____

   A. incisors
   B. canines
   C. premolars
   D. molars

6. The junction of a rest and a clasp body must be approximately ______ thick for adequate strength. 6.____

   A. 0.5 to 1.0
   B. 1.0 to 1.5

C. 1.5 to 2.0
D. 2.0 to 2.5

7. Which of the following is NOT a step involved in pouring the anatomical portion of a double-poured cast?

    A. Vibrate the anatomical after pouring for 2-3 seconds
    B. Smooth the surface of the anatomical portion that will contact the base
    C. Let the anatomical portion set for at least 10 minutes before mixing the base portion
    D. After bringing the portions together, use the spatula to fill the heels and sides of the impression

8. What type of blockout is used on buccal or lingual surfaces of a cast to facilitate accurate ledging of plastic or wax patterns for clasp arms?

    A. Relief
    B. Parallel
    C. Arbitrary
    D. Shaped or ledging

9. Which of the following is NOT a guideline to be used in removing a refractory cast from a mold?

    A. do not touch the anatomic portion of the cast
    B. remove the hydrocolloid and the cast from the body of the flask in one piece
    C. cut the hydrocolloid carefully in four or five places
    D. pry the cast gently from the mold

10. What is the term for the portion of the crown of a tooth gingival to the survey line?

    A. Infrabulge
    B. Suprabulge
    C. Cingulum
    D. Collar

11. Clasps must NOT

    A. be passive, exerting no force on the tooth whatsoever
    B. have reciprocity provided by the reciprocal arm
    C. have a high degree of frictional retention
    D. have a design that involves encirclement of the tooth

12. A technician is using a transverse bar to cast multiple units. If the horizontal bar is formed with a 10-gauge sprue pin, the sprue formers for the individual units will generally be made with ______ -gauge pins.

    A. 8
    B. 10
    C. 12
    D. 14

13. When using a gypsum-bound investment, the temperature of a burnout furnace should not rise above _______ °F. 13._____

A. 1000
B. 1150
C. 1300
D. 1450

14. Which of the following is NOT a function of a partial denture retainer? 14._____

A. Support
B. Guiding insertion
C. Base retention
D. Bracing

15. A palatal bar is indicated for each of the following, EXCEPT 15._____

A. Class II partial dentures where the denture base is relatively short
B. a removable partial denture where anterior teeth must be replaced
C. posterior dentures where the force of opposing occlusion is less than if it were opposed by another removable partial denture
D. Class III dentures where the number of teeth to be replaced is not extensive

16. On a removable partial denture, the most common point of fracture in the connecting apparatus is the 16._____

A. junction of the rest and the clasp body
B. junction of the clasp body and the minor connector
C. face of the rest
D. junction of the major and minor connectors

17. A rule of thumb for designing custom trays is to provide about _______ mm relief for alginate impression materials and _______ mm relief for elastomeric materials. 17._____

A. 6; 3
B. 4; 2
C. 2; 4
D. 3; 6

18. Wax record bases 18._____

A. usually must be readapted before each application
B. should not be reinforced with wire
C. are potentially harmful to cast teeth
D. often interfere with the placement of occlusion rims

19. An impression material that has two different temperatures for melting and solidifying is described as 19._____

A. syneretic
B. colloidal
C. semisolid
D. hysteretic

20. On the master cast, the outer strut of open retention is most often made from ______ wax. 20.

A. 16-or 18-gauge pear-shaped
B. 16-or 18-gauge round
C. 12- or 14-gauge half-round
D. 12- or 14-gauge round

21. Compared to the infrabulge clasp, a suprabulge clasp generally 21.

A. requires less alteration to the coronal contour
B. has better retention
C. has better aesthetics
D. provides better stabilization and bracing

22. If a cast on a surveyor is tilted anteriorly, the 22.

I. mesial undercuts on abutment teeth and residual ridges will be increased
II. distal undercuts will be decreased
III. undercuts on the buccal surfaces of the right side will be increased
IV. undercuts on the lingual palatal surface of the left side with be increased

A. I and II
B. II and III
C. II and IV
D. I, II, III and IV

23. After flasking a denture, a technician should wait at least ______ after the fourth pour of investment before beginning wax elimination. 23

A. 30 minutes
B. 1 hour
C. 4 hours
D. 8 hours

24. In Kennedy Class III removable partial dentures, 24

A. there is a distal extension base (free-end saddle) on one side only
B. edentulous areas are bounded anteriorly and posteriorly by abutments
C. the abutment teeth are situated anterior to edentulous areas
D. the anterior area is edentulous

25. A technician is mounting a maxillary cast on a Hanau articulator. He is attempting to align the orbital pointer of the facebow with the axis-orbital plane indicator on the articulator. This adjustment can be made simpler by 25

A. using the mounting pin, rather than the incisal guide pin
B. using a stone index to guide the placement of the cast
C. springing the facebow
D. placing the cast on the transfer fork before initiating

KEY (CORRECT ANSWERS)

1. A
2. D
3. B
4. B
5. B
6. B
7. B
8. D
9. D
10. A
11. C
12. C
13. C
14. B
15. B
16. A
17. A
18. A
19. D
20. C
21. D
22. A
23. B
24. B
25. A

TEST 4

DIRECTIONS: Each question or incomplete statement is followed by several suggested answers or completions. Select the one the BEST answers the question or completes the statement. *PRINT THE LETTER OF THE CORRECT ANSWER IN THE SPACE AT THE RIGHT.*

1. In the polymerization of acrylic resins, hydroquinone functions 1

   A. as a cross-linking agent
   B. to activate chemical-cured resins
   C. to inhibit the polymerization of monomer during storage
   D. to reduce translucency

2. The function of the reciprocal arm of a clasp is to 2

   A. hold the denture base tightly to the edentulous ridge
   B. resist the vertical components of masticatory forces
   C. protect the soft tissues
   D. counteract lateral forces

3. Which of the following is an inelastic impression material? 3

   A. Agar hydrocolloid
   B. Alginate
   C. Dental compound
   D. Polyether

4. Which of the following components of a surveyor is used for the initial determination of undercuts on abutment teeth? 4

   A. Analyzing rod
   B. Wax knife
   C. Carbon rod
   D. Tripod

5. Each of the following is an indication for a lingual plate, EXCEPT when 5

   A. anterior teeth have a severe lingual inclination
   B. teeth are periodontally compromised
   C. there is a space problem between the gingival tissues and the floor of the mouth
   D. anterior tooth placement is anticipated

6. A technician has made a corrected cast impression by boxing it with wax. Later, the completed denture rocks in the patient's mouth. Potential causes include the possibility that the framework was 6

   I. improperly oriented to the teeth when the impression was made
   II. not completely seated when the impression was made
   III. too thick
   IV. moved when the cast was poured

   A. I and II
   B. I, II and IV

C. II, III and IV
D. I, II, III and IV

7. In general, a cast gold alloy clasp is designed for an undercut of ______ mm. 7.____

A. 0.25
B. 0.38
C. 0.5
D. 0.87

8. Soft tissue undercuts frequently affect the design of a removable partial denture, especially when considering the use of a(n) ______ clasp. 8.____

A. onlay
B. bar-type
C. circlet
D. embrasure

9. The most reliable way of accelerating the setting of dental stone is to 9.____

A. mix it with slurry concentrate, rather than water
B. use heat lamps
C. use less water in the mix
D. use an acrylic admixture

10. Before pouring a reversible hydrocolloid impression, it is often helpful to soak it in a solution of 10.____

A. denatured alcohol
B. hydrogen peroxide
C. green soap
D. potassium sulfate

11. As a rule of thumb, a sprue hole in the base of a refractory cast should be ______ mm in diameter and as near as possible to the center of the casting. It is inserted into a hole that extends ______ mm onto the pattern side. 11.____

A. 3; 5
B. 5; 7
C. 7; 10
D. 10;13

12. The PKT #1 instrument is designed for 12.____

A. refining triangular ridges and occlusal grooves
B. applying small drops of melted wax
C. remove loose particles of wax from a pattern
D. applying large drops of melted wax

13. The depth of beading on a maxillary cast should be no more than ______ mm, and should fade out as is approaches the gingival margin. 13.____

A. 0.5
B. 1

C. 2
D. 2.5

14. Which of the following is an elastomeric impression material that is considered to have poor "rebound"? 14.

A. Addition silicone
B. Condensation silicone
C. Polyether
D. Polysulfide

15. If a resin record base does not fit the master cast, possible reasons include each of the following, EXCEPT 15.

A. record base was removed from cast before adequate polymerization
B. storage of record base in damp environment
C. excessive grinding or polishing of the base
D. warpage of the record base from forceful prying from the cast

16. A circlet C clasp is indicated for 16.

I. tilted molars where space is not available for clasp shoulders
II. molars where tissue undercuts contraindicate an infrabulge clasp
III. abutments with compromised periodontal support
IV. mesially tilted molars with mesial undercuts

A. I and II
B. I, III and IV
C. II and IV
D. I, II, III and IV

17. The most significant function of a rest is to 17.

A. prevent food impaction between the clasp assembly and the abutment tooth
B. transfer occlusal forces from the prosthesis to the abutment tooth
C. protect the occlusal surface of the prosthesis
D. protect the mucosa

18. Before a refractory cast is poured, the agar hydrocolloid should be cooled to a temperature of approximately 18.

A. 45° C (113° F)
B. 60° C (140° F)
C. 85° C (185° F)
D. 120° C (248° F

19. If the teeth on a cast break when a custom impression tray is removed, the most likely reason is that 19

A. there was insufficient blockout of undercuts
B. the tray was too thick
C. tinfoil substitute was contaminated or not used
D. the tray was insufficiently perforated

20. In a Kennedy Class I denture, 20.____

A. support is received primarily from remaining teeth
B. lingual retention is often indicated
C. two clasps are used on the dentulous side
D. 0.010 inch of retention is usually sufficient for cast cobalt-chromium clasps

21. Which of the following tools would be LEAST appropriate for removing flash from the clasp arms, minor connectors, rests, and retention areas of a casting? 21.____

A. Knife-edge wheel
B. Carbide bur
C. Barrel-shaped mounted stone
D. Disk

22. Which of the following gypsum products has the lowest abrasion resistance? 22.____

A. High strength dental stone
B. High strength/high expansion dental stone
C. Dental stone
D. Model plaster

23. The major connector most often used for mandibular removable partial dentures is the 23.____

A. lingual bar
B. lingual plate
C. labial bar
D. double lingual bar

24. Final refinement of the guide planes on the wax patterns of abutments should be performed with a(n) 24.____

A. cylindrical bur
B. pumice slurry
C. surveyor-mounted wax knife
D. scalpel

25. Which of the following is NOT a disadvantage associated with the use of facings in a removable partial denture? 25.____

A. Poor esthetics
B. Difficulty in using on a resorbed ridge
C. Larger space requirements
D. Difficulty in relining

KEY (CORRECT ANSWERS)

1. C
2. D
3. C
4. A
5. A

6. B
7. B
8. B
9. A
10. D

11. C
12. D
13. B
14. D
15. B

16. C
17. B
18. B
19. A
20. D

21. A
22. D
23. A
24. A
25. C

EXAMINATION SECTION
TEST 1

DIRECTIONS: Each question or incomplete statement is followed by several suggested answers or completions. Select the one the BEST answers the question or completes the statement. *PRINT THE LETTER OF THE CORRECT ANSWER IN THE SPACE AT THE RIGHT.*

1. Which of the following procedures is NOT performed in the repair of a denture using a chemical-cured acrylic resin? 1.____

   A. Removing a layer of the old resin from around the fracture site
   B. Applying repair acrylic at the fracture site and allowing it to cure at room temperature in the laboratory
   C. Reassembling the broken pieces and holding them together with wax while a cast is poured
   D. Wetting the resin around the fracture with monomer before applying the repair acrylic

2. For distal extension denture bases, a tissue stop is often used to 2.____

   A. prevent distortion of the metal minor connector during flasking
   B. protect the edentulous ridge
   C. allow for normal intraoral thermal expansion of the resin
   D. create a void for the insertion of retaining wires

3. Perforated and solid metal rimlock trays are most often used with ______ impression materials. 3.____

   A. reversible hydrocolloid
   B. alginate
   C. polysulfide
   D. plaster

4. A technician has a cast mounted on a surveyor and is making a wax pattern for an abutment to a removable partial denture. The prosthesis is a tooth-borne denture that receives only vertical force. Which of the following is true? 4.____

   A. Retention can be gained by the use of a positive nodule above the clasp tip
   B. Retention can be gained by the use of a negative dimple above the clasp tip
   C. Either a dimple or a nodule can be used, because little rotation is anticipated
   D. Neither a dimple nor a nodule should be used

5. The T clasp should NOT be used when 5.____

   A. soft tissue contours would require placement of the approach arm in an undercut
   B. the mesial arm must be relied upon for bracing
   C. retention is needed in the maxillary arch
   D. there is no abutment on the opposite end of the denture

6. Which of the following are adjustable on a "semi-adjustable" articulator? 6.____
   I. angle of the eminentia
   II. amount of immediate sideshift

III. progressive sideshift
IV. intercondylar distance

E. I only
F. I and II
G. II and III
H. II, III and IV

7. When pouring a refractory cast into a mold, the investment material should FIRST be applied to the 7

A. peripheral roll
B. residual ridges
C. most posterior corner
D. tooth or teeth that will be clasped

8. Which of the following is NOT a factor the affects the setting expansion of dental investment? 8

A. Thermal expansion of the wax pattern
B. Thickness of ring liner
C. Configuration of the pattern
D. Rate of investment hardening

9. The stability of a record base can be enhanced by lining it with each of the following, EXCEPT 9

A. alginate impression materials
B. elastomeric impression materials
C. autopolymerizing resin
D. zinc oxide/eugenol impression paste

10. A hydrocolloid impression material is described as "irreversible" when it cannot 10

A. reverse from a gel to a sol
B. be altered in form
C. transform from a sol to a gel
D. be used in a wet field

11. In Kennedy Class I removable partial dentures, 11

A. the abutment teeth are situated anterior to edentulous areas
B. there is a distal extension base (free-end saddle) on one side only
C. edentulous areas are bounded anteriorly and posteriorly by abutments
D. the anterior area is edentulous

12. The shoulder of a clasp must be kept 12

A. near the gingival margin
B. below the survey line
C. in the undercut
D. on or above the survey line

13. Which of the following is NOT a type of suprabulge clasp? 13.____

A. Circlet (Akers)
B. Fishhook
C. I-bar
D. Back-action

14. Parallel blockout 14.____

I. is used in less critical areas to prevent the encroachment of metal on the soft tissues
II. is usually used beneath lingual bars
III. is made by using different styli to establish differing degrees of taper
IV. extends from the survey line to the gingiva

A. I and III
B. II, III and IV
C. III and IV
D. IV only

15. When a cast has been poured into an elastomeric impression, it is advisable to separate the cast from the impression in 15.____

A. 30 minutes
B. 1 hour
C. 3 hours
D. 6 hours

16. The borders of a maxillary framework are typically made by 16.____

A. laying a sheet of wax or plastic and trimming it directly on the outline
B. laying a sheet of wax or plastic and trimming it just short of the outline
C. pressing the edges of a wax or plastic layer into the beading, trimming them outside, and thinning the edges with a modified pencil eraser
D. flowing blue casting wax into the beading where it should be about 1 mm thick and then fading out toward the gingiva

17. A technician is making a custom tray from chemical-cured resin. Before applying a wax spacer to the cast, the cast may be treated in each of the following ways, EXCEPT 17.____

A. treated with a separating material
B. soaked in cold water
C. lightly coated with petroleum jelly
D. abraded with a fine-grained pumice rag

18. The burnout period for a removable partial denture typically involves a period of ______ during which the furnace is set at 538 °C (1000 °F). 18.____

A. 30-minute
B. 2-hour
C. 3-hour
D. 4-hour

19. According to the standards for describing a cast on a surveyor, each of the following statements is true, EXCEPT 19

A. if a clasp is described as "low" on a maxillary cast, it means that the clasp is toward the gingiva
B. if a clasp is described as "high" on a mandibular cast, it means that the clasp is toward the occlusal or incisal surface
C. The "right side" of the mandibular cast is the actual right side of the lower arch
D. The "left side" of the maxillary cast is the actual maxillary left quadrant

20. To function properly, the angle formed by the base of a rest and the proximal tooth surface face must be at least 20

A. 45° or less
B. 90° or less
C. 90° or more
D. 135° or more

21. The "survey line" on a cast identifies the 21

A. amount of undercut below the greatest convexity of the tooth
B. occlusal plane
C. edentulous ridge
D. greatest convexity of the abutment teeth and supporting tissues

22. Which of the following is NOT a type of mandibular major connector? 22

A. Double lingual plate
B. Double lingual bar
C. Labial bar
D. Lingual bar

23. When trimming the base of a mandibular cast, the technician should trim the anterior portion 23

A. to a point extending from the midline of the floor of the mouth
B. in a straight line that spans the canine-to-canine width
C. in a curved line from canine to canine
D. using the base of the maxillary cast as a guide

24. Which of the following is NOT an advantage associated with the use of shellac as a material for record bases? 24

A. Excellent dimensional stability
B. Low cost
C. Ease of handling
D. Readaptability

25. When flasking a removable partial denture, there should be at least ______ mm of clearance between the top of the second mix and the top of the upper half of the flask. 25.____

A. 7
B. 11
C. 16
D. 22

KEY (CORRECT ANSWERS)

1. B
2. A
3. B
4. C
5. A
6. B
7. D
8. B
9. A
10. A
11. A
12. D
13. C
14. C
15. B
16. D
17. D
18. B
19. D
20. B
21. D
22. A
23. C
24. A
25. A

TEST 2

DIRECTIONS: Each question or incomplete statement is followed by several suggested answers or completions. Select the one the BEST answers the question or completes the statement. *PRINT THE LETTER OF THE CORRECT ANSWER IN THE SPACE AT THE RIGHT.*

1. The use of a wrought wire clasp is indicated for 1

   A. situations that require both retentive and reciprocal arms to be made of wire
   B. an abutment tooth where the only usable undercut is on the mesiolingual surface
   C. the incisal edge of an abutment tooth
   D. an abutment tooth where the only usable undercut is on the mesiofacial surface

2. The refractory agent most often used to produce thermal expansion of an investment is some form of 2

   A. silica
   B. gypsum
   C. phosphate
   D. alumina

3. Functional impressions are usually made for 3

   A. Class IV partial dentures
   B. tooth-supported edentulous spaces
   C. anterior spans
   D. distal extension bases

4. The first stage in the addition polymerization reaction is known as 4

   A. sol stage
   B. initiation
   C. wet stage
   D. polymerization

5. Ideally, the tooth in a removable partial denture that is adjacent to a rest should be 5

   A. porcelain
   B. a metal pontic
   C. resin
   D. porcelain with a metal occlusal

6. The mesiodistal length of an open latticework connector should encompass the entire length of the maxillary ridge and ______ the length of the mandibular ridge. 6

   A. one-third
   B. one-half
   C. two-thirds
   D. all

7. Generally, record bases should have 7
   I. dimensional stability
   II. the same adaptation to the basal seat area as the finished denture base

III. a border form slightly larger than the finished denture base 7.____
IV. construction that permits use as a base for tooth arrangement

A. I and III
B. I, II and IV
C. II, III and IV
D. I, II, III and IV

8. The first step in obtaining any facebow recording is to 8.____

A. tighten the setscrews
B. position the nosepiece
C. prepare the wax transfer fork
D. fit the plastic projections into the patient's ears

9. Which of the following methods for pouring a corrected cast impression is LEAST appropriate when the dental arch is small? 9.____

A. North Carolina
B. Beading with wax and the two-stage pour
C. Beading and boxing with wax
D. Boxing with a plaster/pumice mix and wax

10. The water-powder ratio for christobalite investment for refractory casts is usually ______ parts water to 100 parts powder by weight. 10.____

A. 31
B. 65
C. 94
D. 124

11. The buccal cusps of the mandibular teeth and the palatal cusps of the maxillary teeth are called ______ cusps. 11.____

A. stamp
B. Stuart
C. shear
D. eccentric

12. Which of the following major connectors is indicated if the anterior mandibular teeth have a severe lingual inclination? 12.____

A. lingual bar
B. labial bar
C. lingual plate
D. double lingual bar

13. A technician has a cast mounted on a surveyor and is waxing a removable partial denture. The denture uses an I-bar connector with a distal extension base. Which of the following is true? 13.____

A. Retention can be gained by the use of a positive nodule above the clasp tip
B. Retention can be gained by the use of a negative dimple above the clasp tip

C. Either a dimple or a nodule can be used to prevent release of the clasp
D. Neither a dimple nor a nodule should be used

14. In a Kennedy Class I arch, the preferred method for clasping posterior teeth is 14

A. mesiobuccal retention using a reverse circumferential clasp
B. mesiobuccal retention using an 18-gauge wrought-wire clasp
C. distobuccal retention using an 18-gauge wrought-wire clasp
D. distobuccal retention using a vertical projection clasp

15. In the marginal ridge area of a molar, the width of a rest should be about ______ mm. 15

A. 0.5
B. 1.0
C. 1.5
D. 2.0

16. Which of the following types of clasps would typically involves the greatest risk of caries? 16

A. Multiple circlet
B. Onlay
C. T clasp
D. I-bar

17. Alginate impression material can be immersed in a disinfectant for up to ______ without the risk of distortion. 17

A. 10 minutes
B. 30 minutes
C. 1 hour
D. 3 hours

18. For removable partial dentures, probably the most frequent cause of incomplete castings, particularly of palatal connectors, is that 18

A. sprues were placed too far apart
B. the means of retention was too complex
C. the wax or plastic sheet was stretched too thin
D. localized shrinkage occurred

19. A shellac resin base is usually heated to a temperature of ______ before it is adapted to the cast. 19

A. 40° to 50° C (104° to 122° F)
B. 60° to 70° C (140° to 158° F)
C. 80° to 90° C (176° to 194° F)
D. 100° to 120° C (212° to 248° F)

20. When a maxillary wax-up is sprued from above, ______ -gauge round leads are typically used, and the height of the leads should be adjusted so that the base of the cast will be about ______ mm from one end of the investing ring when the crucible former is flush with the other end. 20

A. 18; 12
B. 16; 6
C. 12; 14
D. 10; 8

21. A rule of thumb used by technicians in boxing a cast with wax is that the wax should extend at least ______ higher than the highest point of the impression. 21.____

A. 5 mm
B. 1 cm
C. 0.5 inch
D. 1 inch

22. The first step in the transfer of a design from a diagnostic cast to a master cast is to 22.____

A. choose new tripod marks for the diagnostic casts
B. remount the diagnostic casts on a surveyor
C. mark survey lines on the master cast
D. mark rests on the master cast

23. Which of the following is NOT typically inserted directly into the spindle of a surveyor, but requires the use of a reinforcing rod? 23.____

A. Wax knife
B. Undercut gauge
C. Carbon rod
D. Analyzing rod

24. Parts of the infrabulge clasp arm include the 24.____

I. flexible tip
II. shoulder
III. approach arm
IV. retentive tip

A. I and IV
B. I and II
C. III and IV
D. IV only

25. Each of the following is an esthetic guideline for the arrangement of artificial denture teeth, EXCEPT 25.____

A. overlapping centrals with laterals slightly
B. reshaping the facial and incisal surfaces of the teeth for a more "natural" appearance
C. maintaining the same long axis for all the anterior teeth
D. setting one central incisor slightly facial to the other

KEY (CORRECT ANSWERS)

1. D
2. A
3. D
4. B
5. C

6. C
7. B
8. C
9. A
10. A

11. A
12. B
13. A
14. D
15. D

16. B
17. B
18. C
19. B
20. D

21. C
22. B
23. C
24. C
25. C

TEST 3

DIRECTIONS: Each question or incomplete statement is followed by several suggested answers or completions. Select the one the BEST answers the question or completes the statement. *PRINT THE LETTER OF THE CORRECT ANSWER IN THE SPACE AT THE RIGHT.*

1. Which of the following is an advantage associated with using a wrought wire clasp, rather than one that is cast? 1.____

   A. Excellent support and stability
   B. Ease of design and fabrication
   C. Simpler repair
   D. High resiliency

2. Which of the following steps in the survey of a cast would be performed FIRST? 2.____

   A. Evaluating the buccolingual inclination
   B. Establishing the survey line on the abutment teeth
   C. Inclining the cast so that the analyzing rod is perpendicular to the occlusal plane
   D. Determining the path of insertion for the partial denture

3. Custom trays or record bases can be made of light-cured acrylic resin. This material 3.____

   A. is more difficult to use than chemical-cured resins
   B. does not generate as much heat during polymerization as chemical-cured acrylic
   C. poses the risk of inhaling and handling monomer
   D. is typically dispensed in mixing powder-and-liquid form

4. Most of the vertical support for a partial denture is provided by 4.____

   A. retentive arms
   B. reciprocal arms
   C. major connectors
   D. rests

5. The maximum drying temperature for a refractory cast should be about 5.____

   A. 93° C (200° F)
   B. 121° C (250° F)
   C. 176° C (350° F)
   D. 260° C (500° F)

6. Typically, the strongest connector for retaining the denture base is 6.____

   A. beads
   B. twisted wire
   C. open latticework
   D. mesh

7. Each of the following is an advantage associated with the lingual plate, EXCEPT 7.____

   A. reduced likelihood of food impaction
   B. accommodation of lower vertical space

C. some splinting effect for anterior teeth with poor periodontal support
D. ability to add an anterior tooth to the denture

8. The borders of a cast should be trimmed to form a vestibular sulcus that is ______ mm deep. 8

A. 0.5 to 1.0
B. 1.5 to 3
C. 3 to 4
D. 5 to 6

9. Typically, the ______ stage in the polymerization of acrylic resins is longer for heat-cured resins due to the absence of a tertiary amine. 9

A. polymerization
B. stringy
C. dough
D. initial

10. When a wire is used to stabilize a record base, it typically spans the anterior space between 10

A. canines
B. first premolars
C. second premolars
D. first molars

11. Water-cooled metal impression trays are typically used with ______ impression materials. 11

A. silicone
B. polyether
C. reversible hydrocolloid
D. alginate

12. A technician receives a cast from a dentist that has the design for a removable partial denture drawn on it. Typically, areas that are drawn on the cast in red represent the location of 12

A. areas to be ground, prepared, or recontoured
B. the metal framework or denture base
C. the acrylic resin denture base
D. the survey line and tissue undercut areas

13. Disadvantages associated with condensation silicone impression materials include 13

I. poor wetting characteristics
II. unpleasant taste
III. long set time
IV. relatively rapid dimensional change

A. I only
B. I and IV
C. II and III
D. II, III and IV

14. When it is placed in a duplicating flask, a cast should have at least ______ mm of clearance on all sides in order to make a proper impression. 14.____

    A. 2
    B. 4
    C. 6
    D. 10

15. A technician has a cast mounted on a surveyor and is making a wax pattern for an abutment to a removable partial denture. Which of the following is typically FALSE? 15.____

    A. dislodgement of the denture can be prevented by making a dimple on the abutment
    B. the amount of undercut can be controlled by altering the wax pattern
    C. gauges should be used to determine the undercut
    D. the anatomical contours should not be altered

16. Which of the following steps in investing a sprued wax-up for a removable partial denture is usually performed FIRST? 16.____

    A. painting investment on the cast and sprues with a brush
    B. sealing the crucible former to the casting ring
    C. attaching the pattern to a crucible former
    D. placing the crucible former ring on a vibrator

17. For premolars, the proper width of a rest is approximately ______ the distance between the buccal and lingual cusps. 17.____

    A. one-quarter
    B. half
    C. three-quarters
    D. all

18. Which of the following types of clasps is NEVER indicated for a Kennedy Class I arch? 18.____

    A. Wrought-wire clasp engaging a mesiobuccal undercut
    B. Wrought-wire clasp engaging the distobuccal undercut
    C. Cast circumferential clasp engaging a mesiobuccal undercut
    D. Circlet clasp engaging a distobuccal undercuts

19. Before flasking, the wax base of a removable partial denture should be 19.____

    A. free of any gingival bulges
    B. slightly smaller than the finished resin base, to allow for investment expansion
    C. painted with Super-Sep or similar medium
    D. overwaxed slightly beyond finish lines

20. Which of the following impression materials CANNOT be repoured? 20.____

    A. Alginate
    B. Polyether
    C. Polysulfide
    D. Addition silicone

21. The major problem associated with thermoplastic vinyl impression trays is their 21

A. flexibility
B. difficulty in fabrication
C. brittleness
D. irregular thickness

22. Each of the following is a type of infrabulge clasp, EXCEPT 22

A. Roach
B. push-type
C. bar
D. onlay

23. A technician is forming wax patterns for abutments to a removable partial denture. The junction between the rest seat and the proximal guiding plane should be 23

A. angular
B. perpendicular
C. rounded
D. below the cusp of the abutment

24. Metal pontics are indicated for a removable partial denture if 24

I. there is severe ridge resorption
II. space is too narrow mesiodistally for a single denture tooth
III. relining is likely
IV. there is insufficient interarch space

A. I only
B. II and IV
C. I, III and IV
D. III and IV

25. Prior to investment, a technician attaches an 18-gauge sprue wire to a pattern, directly opposite the larger sprue pin. The technician terminates the wire close to the edge of the investment. The reason for this addition is that the technician believes 25

A. the pattern is too thick and the alloy may harden in the sprue during casting
B. the pattern has a long axial length that will require more "pull"
C. a transverse bar is indicated
D. the thin portion of the pattern, where the wire is attached, may harden too quickly during casting

KEY (CORRECT ANSWERS)

1. D
2. D
3. B
4. D
5. A
6. C
7. A
8. C
9. C
10. C
11. C
12. A
13. B
14. C
15. D
16. A
17. B
18. C
19. D
20. A
21. A
22. D
23. C
24. B
25. A

TEST 4

DIRECTIONS: Each question or incomplete statement is followed by several suggested answers or completions. Select the one the BEST answers the question or completes the statement. *PRINT THE LETTER OF THE CORRECT ANSWER IN THE SPACE AT THE RIGHT.*

1. When outlining the lingual plating on a master cast, whether it is on anterior or posterior teeth, it is crucial to draw the superior margin of the plate 1

   A. cervical to the survey line
   B. occlusal to the survey line
   C. to reflect the forms of the interdental papillae
   D. in blue

2. An embrasure clasp is most often used on 2

   A. incisors
   B. canines
   C. premolars
   D. molars

3. Generally, a sprue pin should be 3

   A. at least 5 mm in length
   B. slightly thinner than the thickest portion of the wax pattern
   C. thicker than the thickest portion of the wax pattern
   D. placed perpendicular to a flat portion of the pattern

4. When mixing alginate impression material, the technician uses a wide-bladed spatula and presses the material against the sides of the bowl. Which of the following will NOT be achieved by this procedure? 4

   A. Improving surface detail
   B. Preventing voids
   C. Preventing graininess
   D. Slowing set

5. Most natural posterior teeth are ______ than denture teeth. 5

   A. more inclined buccolingually
   B. larger buccolingually
   C. larger occlusogingivally
   D. less intercuspated

6. The choice of the undercut used in fabricating a partial denture is influenced by the 6

   I. type of clasp used
   II. relative height of the survey line
   III. metal alloy used
   IV. amount of blockout wax remaining

   A. I only
   B. I and II

C. I and III
D. III and IV

7. Ridge bases are NOT 7.____

A. preliminary structures analogous to pontics
B. used to establish the dimension between the upper and lower arches
C. constructed from the same material as trays
D. used in the construction stage of the denture

8. On a mandibular pattern, auxiliary sprues on a molar clasp that is separated from the lingual bar by a thin section are mostly likely formed with ______ -gauge round wax. 8.____

A. 18
B. 16
C. 14
D. 12

9. Advantages associated with the wax-confined dough method of fabricating a record base include each of the following, EXCEPT 9.____

A. increased stability of the record base
B. no damage to the cast upon removal
C. ease of fabrication
D. controlled record base thickness

10. In partial denture fabrication, a "rest" is a(n) 10.____

A. tissue stop
B. portion of a plate or bar that contacts the mucosa near the gingival margins
C. extension from the clasp body onto the occlusal surface
D. part of the denture base that contacts the edentulous ridge

11. In the ______ technique of pouring a corrected cast impression, the residual ridges of the original cast are ground out with a carborundum wheel. 11.____

A. boxing with a plaster/pumice mix and wax
B. beading and boxing with wax
C. beading with wax and the two-stage pour
D. North Carolina

12. A patient has a Kennedy Class III arch. One of the posterior abutment teeth is weak due to bone loss. It is advisable for the technician to 12.____

A. fabricate a retentive clasp for the abutment
B. use a labial bar
C. use a circlet (Akers) clasp on the abutment and the tooth immediately in front of it
D. use an occlusal rest and a nonretentive clasp arm

13. On a surveyor-mounted cast, a technician is forming a wax pattern for an abutment that will receive a lingual rest. Which of the following is NOT a guideline to be used in this procedure? 13.____

A. The pattern should be waxed to full contour.
B. A straight line should be marked mesiodistally.
C. The reduced portion of the wax pattern should be at least 0.5 mm thick.
D. The rest seat should be inclined toward the center of the abutment tooth.

14. A technician receives a cast from a dentist that has the design for a removable partial denture drawn on it. Typically, areas that are drawn on the cast in brown represent the location of 14.

A. the survey line and tissue undercut areas
B. the acrylic resin denture base
C. the metal framework or denture base
D. areas to be ground, prepared, or recontoured

15. In order to blend into the interproximal embrasure, a minor connector should be ______ in cross section 15.

A. circular or oblate
B. triangular
C. square or rectangular
D. trapezoidal

16. The main disadvantage associated with the use of denture teeth in a removable partial denture is that they 16.

A. require a relatively large space
B. cannot be used where ridge resorption is severe
C. have poor esthetics
D. have poor retention

17. In general, a wrought wire clasp is designed for an undercut of ______ mm. 17

A. 0.25
B. 0.38
C. 0.5
D. 0.87

18. Which of the following steps in forming an occlusion rim for a partial denture is performed FIRST? 18

A. Adapting wax to the edentulous area
B. Adapting tinfoil to the edentulous area
C. Grinding down the edentulous area
D. Flowing baseplate wax under and around the retention struts of the framework

19. If a partial denture is soaked in a cleaner that contains sodium hypochlorite, the metal framework will 19

A. effervesce and become shiny
B. corrode and darken
C. dissolve
D. not be cleaned

19. According to the standards for describing a cast on a surveyor, each of the following statements is true, EXCEPT 19.____

A. if a clasp is described as "low" on a maxillary cast, it means that the clasp is toward the gingiva
B. if a clasp is described as "high" on a mandibular cast, it means that the clasp is toward the occlusal or incisal surface
C. The "right side" of the mandibular cast is the actual right side of the lower arch
D. The "left side" of the maxillary cast is the actual maxillary left quadrant

20. To function properly, the angle formed by the base of a rest and the proximal tooth surface face must be at least 20.____

A. 45° or less
B. 90° or less
C. 90° or more
D. 135° or more

21. The "survey line" on a cast identifies the 21.____

A. amount of undercut below the greatest convexity of the tooth
B. occlusal plane
C. edentulous ridge
D. greatest convexity of the abutment teeth and supporting tissues

22. Which of the following is NOT a type of mandibular major connector? 22.____

A. Double lingual plate
B. Double lingual bar
C. Labial bar
D. Lingual bar

23. When trimming the base of a mandibular cast, the technician should trim the anterior portion 23.____

A. to a point extending from the midline of the floor of the mouth
B. in a straight line that spans the canine-to-canine width
C. in a curved line from canine to canine
D. using the base of the maxillary cast as a guide

24. Which of the following is NOT an advantage associated with the use of shellac as a material for record bases? 24.____

A. Excellent dimensional stability
B. Low cost
C. Ease of handling
D. Readaptability

KEY (CORRECT ANSWERS)

1.	B	11.	D
2.	C	12.	D
3.	C	13.	B
4.	D	14.	C
5.	B	15.	B
6.	C	16.	A
7.	A	17.	C
8.	C	18.	B
9.	C	19.	B
10.	C	20.	C

21. D
22. C
23. C
24. B
25. B

EXAMINATION SECTION
TEST 1

DIRECTIONS: Each question or incomplete statement is followed by several suggested answers or completions. Select the one the BEST answers the question or completes the statement. *PRINT THE LETTER OF THE CORRECT ANSWER IN THE SPACE AT THE RIGHT.*

1. Liquid plastic stains are usually not very effective in modifying the shading of resinous provisional pontics because of the 1.____

   A. tendency of resins to absorb fluids
   B. increased thickness of the resin
   C. high frequency of food impaction
   D. relative darkness of most pontic environments

2. When a gas/air torch is used to melt a dental alloy prior to casting, the tip of the _______ zone of the flame should be used. 2.____

   A. reducing
   B. mixing
   C. oxidizing
   D. combustion

3. A technician is preparing the veneer area of an incisal wax pattern for an acrylic resin crown. To create a peripheral undercut, the technician will 3.____

   A. scribe a ring with a scalpel blade around the gingival margin
   B. reduce labial wax to the depth of the guiding groove
   C. make small pinholes in the incisal edge
   D. extend the mesial and distal wings into the lingual surface

4. A removable die is rotating in a working cast. Of the following, the most likely cause is 4.____

   A. dowel pin too short in base of cast
   B. die ditched too deeply
   C. stone not vacuum-mixed
   D. debris in pinhole

5. Which of the following attachments is considered ideal for anterior nonparallel abutments? 5.____

   A. Mini-Rest
   B. McCollum
   C. Stern
   D. Interlock

6. A technician is adjusting a Hanau articulator to the protrusive record. The FIRST step in this procedure is to 6.____

   A. rotate the condylar post until the shoulder on the axle of the articulator makes contact with the medial aspect of the condylar sphere
   B. adjust the condylar inclination so that the teeth on the cast interdigitate fully into the indentations on the wax record

C. rotate the condylar posts inward 15 degrees
D. place the protrusive record between the maxillary and mandibular casts

7. Disinfectants appropriate for zinc oxide/eugenol impression materials include 7

I. sodium hypochlorite
II. complex phenolics
III. glutaraldehydes
IV. iodophors

A. I only
B. I and II
C. II, III and IV
D. III and IV

8. Which of the following is a type of porosity in dental castings that is caused by shrinkage during solidification? 8

A. Subsurface porosity
B. Gas inclusions
C. Pinhole porosity
D. Microporosity

9. Which of the following may be used to reduce the surface tension of a wax pattern prior to investment? 9

A. Slurry water
B. Separating solution
C. Pickling acid
D. Debubblizer

10. Prior to investment, the sprue pin should generally be attached to 10

A. the thickest portion of the wax pattern.
B. a marginal area
C. an axial contour
D. the thinnest portion of the pattern

11. A partial veneer crown is most likely to be used as a retainer for a fixed partial denture when 11

A. cast connectors are used
B. the abutment teeth have tipped toward the edentulous area
C. excessive forces are anticipated for the denture
D. the edentulous area is a long span

12. The teeth which tend to vary most in their appearance are the 12

A. molars
B. premolars
C. canines
D. incisors

13. Before fabricating a(n) ______ restoration, a technician must consult a preparation template of the tooth. 13.____

A. intracoronal
B. custom
C. polycarbonate
D. aluminum

14. The split cast technique for mounting a cast on an articulator 14.____
I. allows separation of the master cast and its base
II. is useful only with fully adjustable articulators
III. allows the technician to check the upper member with the mounted base as it closes into the maxillary cast
IV. is most often used to observe soft tissues

A. I and III
B. I, III and IV
C. II and IV
D. I, II, III and IV

15. When an individual die impression is poured, the die stone should be built ______ above the cervical area to facilitate handling of the die. 15.____

A. 0.3 to 0.5
B. 0.8 to 1.2
C. 1.0 to 1.5
D. 2.0 to 2.5

16. Which of the following is NOT a circumstance that would indicate a cast full veneer crown? 16.____

A. Existing large defective restorations
B. Extensive caries
C. Greater than average crown length
D. Fracture of the tooth

17. In a(n) ______, one or more of the anterior teeth discludes with the posterior teeth in working and nonworking movements. 17.____

A. anterior balanced posterior
B. unilateral balanced posterior
C. bilateral balanced posterior
D. anterior guided posterior

18. The best way to increase the tear strength of alginate impression material is to 18.____

A. leave the impression in the mouth for 1-2 minutes beyond the set point
B. increase the amount of water in the mixture
C. add diatomaceous earth
D. decrease the ambient temperature

19. A technician is using a vacuum investor. Vibration of the investment should be avoided if 19

A. the investment is gypsum-bonded
B. a wetting agent is applied to the pattern
C. the casting will be base metal
D. the investment has been spatulated by hand

20. After a brush has been used to apply opaque resin to a casting, it should be cleaned with 20

A. warm, soapy water
B. hydrogen peroxide
C. acetone
D. mineral oil

21. What is the term for the shape given to a restoration to enable it and the remaining tooth 21
structure to withstand masticatory stress?

A. Retentive form
B. Stabilization
C. Resistance form
D. Elastic form

22. A technician is trimming a diagnostic cast. Each anterior cut of the maxillary cast should 22
be made on a line 3mm out from, and parallel to, a line running

A. the midline between central incisors to the canine eminence
B. from each retromolar pad
C. from the buccal bone at the widest portion of the arch to the canine eminence
D. the canine eminence to the opposing side/back cut

23. Which of the following steps in soldering castings is typically performed FIRST? 23

A. sealing the joint area with sticky wax
B. sealing the connector area with sprue wax facially and lingually
C. making an occlusal stone index
D. filling the crowns with soldering investment

24. A technician is making a die using a dowel pin system. After the die stone has set, the 24
technician makes V-shaped grooves buccolingually on each side of the dowels. The purpose of these grooves is to

A. facilitate separation of the dies from the cast
B. guide the depth of the wax patterns
C. expose the ends of the dowel pins
D. prevent misplacement of individual dies in the working cast

25. The occlusal view of a mandibular second molar reveals 25

I. a central pit in the middle of the occlusal table
II. facial and lingual halves about equal in width
III. an occlusal table in the lingual two-thirds of the crown
IV. a crown with a wider mesial half than distal half

A. I only
B. I and IV
C. II, III and IV
D. I, II, III and IV

KEY (CORRECT ANSWERS)

1. B
2. A
3. D
4. A
5. D
6. C
7. D
8. D
9. D
10. A
11. B
12. A
13. B
14. A
15. D
16. C
17. D
18. A
19. B
20. C
21. C
22. A
23. A
24. D
25. D

TEST 2

DIRECTIONS: Each question or incomplete statement is followed by several suggested answers or completions. Select the one the BEST answers the question or completes the statement. *PRINT THE LETTER OF THE CORRECT ANSWER IN THE SPACE AT THE RIGHT.*

1. A technician is placing removal knobs on a wax pattern prior to investment. Appropriate locations for these knobs include the 1.

   I. mesial angle of the buccal surface
   II. mesial angle of the lingual surface
   III. mesial angle of the palatal surface
   IV. distal angle of the buccal surface

   A. I and IV
   B. II and III
   C. II, III and IV
   D. I, II, III and IV

2. Which of the following is NOT a good choice for extracoronal provisional coverage? 2.

   A. Provisional acrylic
   B. Provisional composite
   C. Polycarbonate crown
   D. Zinc oxide/eugenol

3. Resin can be used to reline temporary crowns that are made of 3.

   I. stainless steel
   II. polymer
   III. ceramic
   IV. base metal

   A. I only
   B. II only
   C. II and III
   D. III and IV

4. "Tipping" forces are occlusal forces that move a restoration 4

   A. circumferentially around the prepared tooth
   B. in buccolingual or mesiodistal directions
   C. occlusally
   D. apically

5. The cone-waxing technique is appropriate for ______ crowns. 5

   I. posterior partial veneer
   II. anterior full-veneer
   III. anterior partial-veneer
   IV. pinledge

   A. I only
   B. I and II

C. II and III
D. III and IV

6. A technician is mounting a mandibular cast on an articulator in a position of maximal occlusion. The incisal guide pin should be set 6.____

A. to increase the opening to compensate for the thickness of the recording material
B. at the appropriate level below zero, to compensate for the penetration of incisal edges beyond the occlusal plane
C. to allow for the placement of an anterior jig
D. at zero

7. After it is removed from the investment, a dental casting reveals a network of raised fins along its surface. The most likely cause of this was 7.____

A. underheating the investment
B. foreign substance intrusion into the mold
C. heating the investment too quickly
D. separation of the investment from the wax pattern

8. The root portion of a sectioned die should be at least ______ cm in length, to permit proper handling. 8.____

A. 1.0 to 1.5
B. 1.5 to 2.0
C. 2.0 to 2.5
D. 2.5 to 3.0

9. To position castings in an impression accurately, it is important to position them against a positive material. Which of the following, by itself, would NOT be suitable? 9.____

A. Plaster
B. Alginate
C. Compound
D. Acrylic

10. A technician has outlined the veneer area on a die. Zinc stearate powder is then dusted on the wax pattern and adjacent areas in order to 10.____

A. harden the wax
B. prevent the adhesion of wax particles to the pattern during veneer development
C. indicate the presence of pits and grooves on the pattern surface
D. lubricate the action of wax burs and other developmental tools

11. The purpose of a T-support in mounting a cast on an articulator is to ______ the mounting procedure is completed. 11.____

A. maintain intercondylar width
B. hold up the facebow fork and maxillary cast
C. orient the casts along two dimensions
D. maintain intercuspation

12. A technician has applied opaque resin to the casting. Typically, at room temperature, this 1
material will dry in about

A. 60 seconds
B. 5 minutes
C. 30-45 minutes
D. 1-2 hours

13. The facial view of a mandibular second premolar reveals 1

A. a grossly asymmetrical outline
B. a crown that is wider mesiodistally than occclusocervically
C. a cusp sloping at about a 20-degree angle from the tip
D. proximal contracts in the cervical third

14. After completing an investment, a technician places the invested casting ring into a 100° 1
F water bath for 30 minutes while the investment sets. This is to insure that the investment

A. expands to allow for the shrinkage of the metal casting as it cools
B. does not crack during heating
C. does not set too quickly
D. establishes a smooth, non-porous surface around the wax pattern

15. A technician can control the expansion of dental investment material in a number of 1
ways. Which of the following statements is FALSE?

A. A full cast crown generally calls for more investment than a partial-coverage crown.
B. Greater expansion can be achieved by attaching the sprue pin so that the pattern is oriented along the long axis of the casting ring.
C. A resilient liner will help offset the more-rapid contraction of the cooling ring after burnout.
D. Decreasing the powder-to-water ratio during mixing increases expansion slightly.

16. Irreversible hydrocolloid impression material is considered accurate enough for each of 1
the following, EXCEPT

A. diagnostic casts
B. final impressions for crown preparations
C. opposing casts for crown and bridge treatments
D. custom trays

17. Travel in the posterior direction of the dental arches reveals mandibular teeth that gradu- 1
ally incline more lingually, while maxillary teeth incline more buccally. This trend is represented by the

A. cross-bite
B. curve of Wilson
C. fovea palatinae
D. curve of Spee

18. A technician is pouring the base portion of a diagnostic cast. The mixture that is placed on the tile or in the base former should be at least ______ thick and slightly larger than the dimension of the filled impression and the tray. 18.____

A. 5 mm B. 1 cm C. 0.5 inch D. 1 inch

19. The PKT #5 instrument is designed for 19.____

A. refining triangular ridges and occlusal grooves
B. applying large drops of melted wax
C. carving grooves on the occlusal surfaces of posterior teeth
D. smoothing rough areas

20. All-ceramic crowns are considered preferable to porcelain-bonded-to-metal crowns in terms of their 20.____

A. workability
B. strength
C. ease of tinting
D. aesthetics

21. When soldering castings, the investment block is usually heated to approximately ______ before being placed on the soldering stand. 21.____

A. 200° C (392° F)
B. 350° C (662° F)
C. 550° C(1002° F)
D. 800° C(1472° F)

22. Cast posts 22.____

I. usually have the core attached
II. are used more frequently than preformed posts
III. can be cast using high noble, noble or base metal alloys
IV. are formed from a wax or acrylic resin pattern

A. I only
B. I, III and IV
C. II only
D. III and IV

23. Partial veneer crowns are generally NOT suitable for 23.____

I. teeth with extensive cervical caries
II. upper canines with long cusps
III. teeth with a poor long-axis relationship with the path of insertion
IV. short teeth

A. I and IV
B. I, II and III
C. III and IV
D. I, II, III and IV

24. Of the following, the type of crown that provides the best retention as an abutment for a fixed partial denture is the 24.

A. full veneer
B. three-quarter
C. pinlay
D. partial veneer

25. When an electrical resistance melting furnace is used to make dental castings, the 25.

A. piston should allow a small amount of blow-by
B. alloy is usually melted with a gas/air torch
C. button only remains molten for a brief moment
D. alloy is usually melted in a graphite crucible

KEY (CORRECT ANSWERS)

1. C
2. D
3. C
4. B
5. B

6. D
7. C
8. C
9. B
10. B

11. B
12. B
13. C
14. A
15. D

16. B
17. B
18. C
19. A
20. D

21. C
22. B
23. D
24. A
25. D

TEST 3

DIRECTIONS: Each question or incomplete statement is followed by several suggested answers or completions. Select the one the BEST answers the question or completes the statement. *PRINT THE LETTER OF THE CORRECT ANSWER IN THE SPACE AT THE RIGHT.*

1. A technician has just poured dental stone into an alginate impression. Ideally, the stone should set for a period of _______ before removal 1.____

   A. 30 minutes
   B. 60 minutes
   C. 4 hours
   D. 8-12 hours

2. As a rule of thumb, a cast should be trimmed so that the base accounts for about _______ of the total depth, or height, of the cast. 2.____

   A. one-fourth
   B. one-third
   C. two-thirds
   D. one-half

3. In developing spurs and pickups in an incisal wax pattern, each of the following is a recommended procedure, EXCEPT 3.____

   A. loops should be placed in the medial and distal edges of the veneer
   B. loops should bridge across the depression separating the facial surface and the flange of the wax pattern
   C. scalpel cuts should all be made at the same angle
   D. margins should be refined prior to retention development

4. What is the term for the lowermost point on the bony rim of the orbit? 4.____

   A. Zygion
   B. Gnathion
   C. Level of orbitale
   D. Foramen

5. Which of the following impression materials can be poured up to a week after it has been mixed? 5.____

   A. Reversible hydrocolloid
   B. Condensation silicone
   C. Polysulfide
   D. Polyether

6. The refractory material used in dental investment is often either quartz or cristobalite. Which of the following is/are true? 6.____

   I. quartz investment continues to expand uniformly until a temperature of about 566° C (1050° F) is reached

II. the maximum expansion of cristobalite occurs over a narrow temperature range, and then reaches a plateau
III. when a quartz investment is removed from the furnace, cooling contraction is generally slower and less pronounced
IV. the ultimate thermal expansion of cristobalite is greater than that of quartz

A. I only
B. I, II and IV
C. III and IV
D. I, II, III and IV

7. A technician is waxing a die for reverse pin facing. The technician should be careful to AVOID adding wax

A. to the cervical portion of the lingual surface
B. over the seated plastic pins
C. over the area of the edentulous ridge that will contact the casting
D. on the occlusal portion

8. Electroplating impressions produces dies that have more surface hardness and better surface detail than other dies. This procedure involves each of the following, EXCEPT

A. submersion in an electrolytic solution such as copper sulfate
B. copper anodes for wax or compound impressions
C. silver anodes for polysulfide impressions
D. metalization of the area to be plated with a fine gold powder

9. A technician is using a broken-arm centrifugal casting machine. To load the spring, _______ are usually sufficient to provide enough force for dental castings.

A. 1 to 2
B. 3 to 4
C. 5 to 7
D. 7 to 10

10. When a cast is mounted on a semiadjustable articulator, vertical separation of the casts is maintained by the

A. incisal guide pin
B. condylar heads
C. T support
D. vertical stop

11. The type of soft dental wax used for most indirect techniques is Type

A. A
B. B
C. C
D. D

12. From the incisal view, the mandibular lateral incisor has

I. a crown wider mesiodistally than faciolingually
II. a distal contact slightly more lingual than mesial

III. the prominence of the cingulum slightly mesial of center
IV. an incisal edge slightly facial of center

A. I and II
B. II only
C. II, III and IV
D. I, II, III and IV

13. A technician is using a prefabricated plastic key and keyway to form a nonrigid connector. The direction of insertion of the key and the line of draw of the bridge are determined with the key and keyway secured to a(n) 13.____

A. surveyor
B. Stuart articulator
C. Simplex articulator
D. die

14. Which of the following types of occlusion are suitable for fixed partial dentures? 14.____

I. Bilateral balanced posterior
II. Unilateral balanced posterior
III. Anterior guided posterior

A. I only
B. I and II
C. II and III
D. I, II and III

15. Typically, a ______ -mm gingival collar of metal is preserved in the formation of acrylic veneer crowns. 15.____

A. 0.5
B. 1.0
C. 1.5
D. 2.5

16. After it is removed from the investment, a dental casting reveals a series of minute ridges and veins on its surface. Of the following, the most likely cause of this was 16.____

A. underheating during burnout
B. air bubbles in the casting
C. too high a casting pressure
D. the formation of a water film over the pattern of the surface

17. In the fabrication of a crown, a die provides 17.____

I. access for finishing the marginal area of the wax pattern
II. the prepared crown's occlusal relationship to adjacent teeth
III. the prepared crown's proximal contours

A. I only
B. I and II
C. II and III
D. I, II and III

18. After a working cast has been trimmed, sectioned dies are typically trimmed to present a 18.
_______ section.

A. circular or oblate
B. square or rectangular
C. hexagonal or octagonal
D. triangular

19. Relief for resilient partial dentures must provide for both vertical and angular displacement. The relief should start at _______ gauge occlusally and increase as a wedge to _______ gauge gingivally. 19.

A. 18; 12
B. 22; 16
C. 28; 18
D. 36; 20

20. Possible consequences of improper provisional coverage of a tooth include 20.

I. periodontal irritation
II. tooth migration
III. tooth hypersensitivity
IV. food impaction

A. I and II
B. II and III
C. II, III and IV
D. I, II, III and IV

21. A technician is preparing to solder the connector areas of to castings. The technician 21
should be sure to do each of the following, EXCEPT

A. make an investment block that is at least an inch thick
B. make sure the connector areas are free of oxides
C. maintain the relationship of the castings with a stone index
D. prepare the joint surface with an abrasive

22. The third chamber of a hydrocolloid conditioner is used to 22

A. liquefy the impression material
B. solidify the impression material
C. maintain the impression material in a liquid state
D. temper the impression material before application

23. In _______ side-shift, the greatest rate of side-shift occurs throughout the first 4 mm of for- 23
ward movement of the orbiting condyle as it leaves centric relation.

A. distributed
B. progressive
C. early
D. immediate

24. The most appropriate area for attaching a sprue pin is the 24.____

    A. inner slope of the nonfunctional cusps
    B. outer slope of the nonfunctional cusps
    C. inner slope of the functional cusps
    D. outer slope of the functional cusps

25. Of the following types of resins used to make provisional crowns, splints, or fixed partial dentures, which have the lowest shrinkage upon polymerization? 25.____

    A. Epimines
    B. Hybrids
    C. Polymethyl methacrylates
    D. Polyethyl methacrylates

KEY (CORRECT ANSWERS)

1.	B	11.	C
2.	B	12.	B
3.	C	13.	A
4.	C	14.	C
5.	D	15.	B
6.	B	16.	D
7.	A	17.	A
8.	D	18.	C
9.	B	19.	D
10.	A	20.	D

21. A
22. D
23. A
24. B
25. A

TEST 4

DIRECTIONS: Each question or incomplete statement is followed by several suggested answers or completions. Select the one the BEST answers the question or completes the statement. *PRINT THE LETTER OF THE CORRECT ANSWER IN THE SPACE AT THE RIGHT.*

1. Which of the following impression materials has the highest dimensional stability? 1.

   A. Alginate
   B. Condensation silicone
   C. Addition silicone
   D. Polysulfide

2. A hinge-axis facebow relationship 2.

   A. is ideally recorded for all restorations
   B. does not require a clutch for measurement
   C. is most easily transferred from facebow to articulator
   D. is required to mount the maxillary cast in a fully adjustable articulator

3. The best method for pickling a dental casting is to place it in a solution 3.

   A. with stainless steel tongs
   B. that is slightly below room temperature
   C. that is heated, but not boiling
   D. that is boiling

4. Which of the following surfaces of the tooth is NOT covered by a three-quarter crown? 4.

   A. Labial
   B. Mesial
   C. Distal
   D. Lingual

5. Study of a diagnostic cast reveals too much space in the edentulous area. If a "supernumerary" tooth is required in a fixed partial denture, it is most likely to be a(n) 5

   A. maxillary lateral incisor
   B. mandibular central incisor
   C. mandibular first molar
   D. maxillary first premolar

6. In the centrifugal casting technique, factors which significantly affect the casting accuracy include the 6

   I. melting of the alloy
   II. time lapse between the removal of the investment ring from the furnace and the filling with molten alloy
   III. amount of centrifugal force used on the mold
   IV. length of the horizontal arm of the casting machine

   A. I only
   B. I and II

C. II and III
D. I, II, III and IV

7. A technician wants to make a provisional crown using tooth-colored acrylic resin, but a custom tray is not available. To provide the ideal thickness of impression material in a stock tray with polyvinyl siloxane material, the technician could use the ______. 7.____

A. abutment
B. twin viscosity, single-stage
C. two-step putty/wash
D. closed-tray impression post

8. Type I alloys are typically used for 8.____

A. small inlays that are easily burnished and subject to light stress
B. inlays subject to very high stress
C. veneering with dental porcelain
D. average thickness partial veneer crowns

9. Which of the following is NOT a situation that would necessitate the use of nonrigid connectors between retainers and pontics? 9.____

A. One abutment tooth has an edentulous area both anterior and posterior to it.
B. One abutment tooth has begun to incline toward the edentulous area.
C. The anterior and posterior definitions are joined
D. The path of insertion of a bridge cannot be paralleled, as one abutment tooth is tipped mesially or distally.

10. For a final check of occlusal contact on articulated casts that have been waxed, the technician applies a light coating of zinc stearate powder to the occlusal surface. One of the reasons zinc stearate is used is because it will 10.____

A. burn out easily during casting
B. help in fastening the sprue
C. double as a wetting agent during investment
D. helps to harden the wax during investment

11. The base of a cast should be thick enough to give strength to the cast, but not too thick to allow attachment to an articulator. Typically, this means a thickness of 11.____

A. 7 to 10 mm
B. 10 to 15 mm
C. 2 to 3 cm
D. 4 to 5 cm

12. Before mounting a face-bow on a semiadjustable articulator, several preparatory steps must be performed. The first of these preparatory steps is typically to 12.____

A. trim the face-bow fork
B. zero the incisal guide pin
C. confirm the intercondylar width
D. lock the maxillary and mandibular casts together in centric relation

13. In terms of fabrication, the most significant difference between resin veneer crowns and porcelain-fused-to-metal crowns is that 13.

A. resin veneer requires mechanical retention
B. porcelain is more likely to absorb fluids
C. resin veneer bonding produces an exothermic reaction
D. different metal substructures are required for each

14. Which of the following is NOT an extracoronal combined attachment? 14.

A. Bival
B. Schatzmann
C. Dalbo
D. ASC-52

15. Crowns made of polycarbonate material are used primarily on 15.

A. inlays
B. multiunit bridges
C. posterior teeth
D. anterior teeth

16. A stone cast that was poured into an elastomeric impression is distorted. Which of the following is LEAST likely to have been the cause? 16.

A. Incomplete polymerization
B. Lack of tray rigidity
C. Impression not poured immediately
D. Powder-water ratio too high

17. After pouring a cast beyond the marginal areas of an impression, a technician places three stone nodules on the base of the working cast. The purpose of these nodules is to 17.

A. apply more mass to hold the stone in the impression
B. help retain the second pour
C. aid in removing the working cast from the impression
D. aid in positioning individual dies

18. Hygroscopic expansion of dental investment is typically accomplished in each of the following ways, EXCEPT 18

A. applying a wetting agent to the was pattern before investment
B. submerging the ring in a water bath immediately after investment
C. adding a small amount of water to the investment as it sets
D. increasing the water-to-powder ratio during the mixing of the investment

19. Of the following methods of retention for an acrylic veneer, the one that involves the greatest risk for the percolation of fluids between resin and metal is 19

A. spurs and pickups
B. undercuts
C. wax bars
D. plastic beads

20. Generally, the cusp-to-fossa waxing technique is more widely used than the cusp-to-marginal-ridge technique for each of the following reasons, EXCEPT that it 20.____

A. avoids the "wedging" effect of a cusp articulated over the occlusal embrasure
B. allows occlusal forces to be axially diverted
C. provides the most stable tooth contact in the position of maximum intercuspation
D. represents the most prevalent kind of natural occlusal relationship

21. Which type of pontic is usually most suitable for any kind of maxillary and mandibular fixed partial denture? 21.____

A. Modified ridge-lap
B. Saddle
C. Hygienic
D. Spheroid

22. Which of the following is MOST likely to be a last step in setting up mounted models on an articulator? 22.____

A. Establishing the centric relationship
B. Fabricating a custom incisal guide table
C. Measuring a protrusive record
D. Recording sideshift

23. When the wax pattern for a fixed partial denture with an all-metal pontic is completed, gross excess is removed from the gingival surface to provide clearance between the pontic and the crest of the residual ridge. Ideally, this clearance should be ______. 23.____

A. 1
B. 2
C. 3
D. 5

24. In a(n) ______, the posterior teeth on the working side disclude the teeth on the non-working side. 24.____

A. anterior guided posterior
B. bilateral balanced posterior
C. anterior balanced posterior
D. unilateral balanced posterior

25. Solvents used with resinous bonding agents typically include 25.____

I. butyl alcohol
II. ethyl alcohol
III. ethyl acetate
IV. acetone

A. I and II
B. II and III
C. II and IV
D. I, II, III and IV

KEY (CORRECT ANSWERS)

1. C
2. D
3. C
4. A
5. A

6. B
7. C
8. A
9. B
10. A

11. B
12. C
13. A
14. B
15. D

16. D
17. B
18. A
19. B
20. D

21. A
22. B
23. C
24. D
25. C

EXAMINATION SECTION
TEST 1

DIRECTIONS: Each question or incomplete statement is followed by several suggested answers or completions. Select the one the BEST answers the question or completes the statement. *PRINT THE LETTER OF THE CORRECT ANSWER IN THE SPACE AT THE RIGHT.*

1. Which of the following is NOT an advantage associated with one-piece casting of retainers and pontics? 1.____

   A. It reduces the likelihood of distortion.
   B. It produces the ideal joint form.
   C. It creates a strong union between retainers and pontics.
   D. The cast metal has high corrosion resistance because solder is not used.

2. Which of the following steps is performed LAST in the formation of an acrylic resin-faced pontic? 2.____

   A. The pattern is sectioned with a saw
   B. Retentive tabs are developed in the periphery of the pontic window
   C. The gingival surface is removed lingually to the alveolar crest
   D. Interproximal embrasures are recontoured

3. A technician is developing a wax pattern for a full-veneer crown. In most posterior teeth, the contact areas should be located in the 3.____

   A. middle third
   B. central third
   C. occlusal third
   D. buccolingual center

4. The purpose of die spacers is to 4.____

   A. create an index for replacing the dies in a working cast
   B. make an allowance for the width of the saw blade used to cut the die from the working cast
   C. help compensate for the casting shrinkage of the alloy
   D. prevent a layer of cement from interfering with the complete seating of a casting

5. During sprue formation, the technician places a spherical mass of wax that surrounds the sprue pin near the point of attachment. The reason for this placement of this "reservoir" is that the technician believes the sprue is too 5.____

   A. short
   B. long
   C. wide
   D. perpendicular

6. A technician is mounting a maxillary cast on a Whip-Mix articulator. Which of the following procedures would be performed FIRST? 6.____

   A. Opening the facebow
   B. Adjustment of condylar guide pins by adding or removing spacers

C. Placing the maxillary cast into the depressions of the transfer fork
D. Removal of the incisal guide pin from the upper member of the articulator

7. In the hygroscopic technique of casting, the ring is heated to a temperature no greater than ______, because an appreciable thermal expansion of the investment is not desired. 7

A. 200° C (400° F)
B. 480° C (900° F)
C. 550° C (l002° F)
D. 685° C (1250° F)

8. A solid working cast may be tapered from the ______ to the base. 8

A. buccal fold
B. lingual fold
C. maxillary palatal portion
D. cervical areas

9. The principle advantage associated with the use of sulfuric acid as a pickling agent in the dental laboratory, as opposed to hydrochloric acid, is that sulfuric acid 9

A. does a more thorough job of removing investment and oxide coatings
B. has a lower boiling point
C. does not need to be renewed as often
D. has less corrosive fumes

10. In mounting a cast on an articulator, a technician observes an obvious error in the plane of occlusion. Of the following, the most likely cause is a failure to 10

A. support the face-bow fork properly
B. hold the cast together by cast stabilization
C. close the articulator completely
D. allow the plaster to set long enough

11. Which of the following is NOT a material used to make preformed metal posts? 11

A. Titanium
B. Titanium alloy
C. Stainless steel
D. Gold

12. Due to the phenomenon of ______, inlays are not generally acceptable retainers for fixed partial dentures. 12

A. retention
B. resistance
C. pitting
D. deflection

13. Which of the following types of crowns is used exclusively for the restoration of anterior teeth? 13.____

A. MOD onlay
B. Three-quarter
C. Four-fifths
D. Seven-eighths

14. The retentive design of connectors using frictional attachments, or frictional attachments aided by a mechanical lock, limits their application to crowns that are no shorter than ______ mm occlusogingivally. 14.____

A. 2
B. 3
C. 4
D. 5

15. Which of the following gypsum products has the highest porosity? 15.____

A. High strength dental stone
B. High strength/high expansion dental stone
C. Dental stone
D. Model plaster

16. Which of the following types of pontics is considered least hygienic? 16.____

A. Saddle
B. Spheroid
C. Ridge-lap
D. Modified ridge-lap

17. A reversible hydrocolloid impression has produced a chalky stone cast. Which of the following is LEAST likely to have been the cause? 17.____

A. Poor stone mixing
B. Contaminants in impression
C. Movement of tray during setting
D. Removal of cast before stone has set completely

18. When a resin bonding agent polymerizes, it creates resin tags that lock onto the tooth. The bond created is called a 18.____

A. hybrid layer
B. micromechanical retention
C. primary bond
D. secondary bond

19. A technician is making a wax pattern for a fixed partial denture. With cusp-to-marginal ridge occlusion, locations for occlusal contacts around each working cusp include 19.____

I. in a fossa
II. mesial to the cusp tip
III. distal to the cusp tip
IV. buccal to the cusp tip

A. I only
B. I, II and III
C. II and III
D. I, II, III and IV

20. Which of the following materials is most appropriate for imparting the final luster to a cast crown?

A. Cut-down fissure bur
B. Green silicon point
C. Soft bristle brush with tripoli and rouge
D. Chamois wheel and rouge

21. A removable die has broken at the neck. Of the following, the most likely cause is

A. base of die lacking positive seat
B. dowel pin seated too deeply in impression
C. saw cuts not tapered
D. die ditched to shallowly

22. A technician is mounting an anatomic cast on a nonadjustable articula-tor. After the casts have been intercuspated, the technician applies sticky wax directly on the teeth to maintain the relationship throughout the mounting procedure. Possible drawbacks to this method include

I. distorting the relationship
II. preventing the technician from observing any slippage or changes
III. surface alterations upon removal
IV. cast fracture upon removal

A. I and II
B. II only
C. II and III
D. I, II, III and IV

23. To ensure a complete casting for an acrylic veneer substrate, the wax remaining between the die and the veneer area should be no less than ______ mm in thickness.

A. 0.1
B. 0.4
C. 1.0
D. 1.3

24. A technician is determining how to reduce the vertical stress on a fixed partial denture. Each of the following factors should be incorporated in this devices occlusion, EXCEPT

A. a proportionate area of the food table relative to the periodontal support
B. shortening cusp height as much as possible within aesthetic requirements
C. incorporating supplemental grooves
D. simultaneous, even contact of teeth in the most intercusped position

25. For crown and bridge procedures, alginate impression material is sometimes used in combination with reversible (agar) hydrocolloid material. The advantages of this combination include 25.____

I. greater accuracy
II. easier tray preparation
III. reduced need for equipment
IV. extended pour time

A. I and II
B. I and III
C. II, III and IV
D. III and IV

KEY (CORRECT ANSWERS)

1.	A	11.	D
2.	A	12.	D
3.	C	13.	B
4.	D	14.	B
5.	B	15.	D
6.	D	16.	A
7.	B	17.	C
8.	A	18.	B
9.	D	19.	B
10.	A	20.	D

21. B
22. D
23. B
24. B
25. B

TEST 2

DIRECTIONS: Each question or incomplete statement is followed by several suggested answers or completions. Select the one the BEST answers the question or completes the statement. *PRINT THE LETTER OF THE CORRECT ANSWER IN THE SPACE AT THE RIGHT.*

1. Of the following methods of retention for an acrylic veneer, the weakest are typically

   A. wax bars
   B. undercuts
   C. plastic beads
   D. retentive loops

2. When a technician is using a gypsum-bound investment during a wax elimination procedure, the casting ring should be heated

   A. as quickly as possible
   B. slowly, with the heat concentrated at the sprue-pin end
   C. slowly and uniformly
   D. rapidly to about 1200°F and then cooled to the maximum expansion point

3. As a rule, during the casting of dental alloys, the amount of metal contained in the sprue and crucible button should be ______ than the amount in the casting.

   A. less
   B. about equal to
   C. about 2 to 3 grams more
   D. about 5 to 6 grams more

4. The vertical anatomic plane that extends mediolaterally and superoinferiorly is known as the ______ plane.

   A. coronal
   B. mandibular
   C. sagittal
   D. horizontal

5. Copings are effectively used

   I. in extensive treatment cases with multiple abutments and splinting
   II. to provide firm restoration foundations, in combination with dowels
   III. to support removable superstructures
   IV. to rebuild grossly defective teeth

   A. I and III
   B. I, II and IV
   C. II and III
   D. I, II, III and IV

6. A technician, preparing to solder a rigid connector for a fixed partial denture, makes a stone occlusal index. This index is used to register the

   I. cusp tips

II. linguofacial inclinations
III. mesiodistal inclinations
IV. undercuts

A. I only
B. I and II
C. II and III
D. I, II, III and IV

7. Which of the following statements about hydrophilic impression materials is TRUE? 7.____

A. The resist the uptake of water during gypsum curing
B. They require a dry field for best results
C. They repel saliva and blood
D. They will only absorb moisture after their final set

8. In developing patterns for crowns, a general guideline for contouring is ______ mm from the cementoenamel junction for the mandibular second premolars. 8.____

A. 0.5
B. 0.75
C. 1.0
D. 1.25

9. Drawbacks or risks associated with the use of a short sprue during investment and casting include 9.____

I. entrapment of gases during burnout
II. casting shrinkage
III. cracks or fins on the casting
IV. porosity at the sprue attachment point

A. I only
B. I and IV
C. III only
D. II and IV

10. A ridge-lap pontic 10.____

I. has a small total area of tissue contact
II. is usually used when there is extensive loss of the maxillary anterior or posterior alveolar bone
III. is contoured to contact the facial aspect of the ridge
IV. is usually made entirely of metal

A. I and II
B. I, II and III
C. III only
D. I, II, III and IV

11. The Stern JMS attachment 11.____

A. makes use of color-coded plastic jackets for different types of connections
B. usually requires the addition of a milled substructure bar
C. is an intracoronal-extracoronal combined attachment
D. is an intracoronal precious-metal attachment

12. The main disadvantage to the conventional (hand-placed) dowel pin system for preparing dies is that it requires 12

    A. two pins for most teeth
    B. full-arch impressions
    C. two pours
    D. the use of retention nodules

13. A technician has overpolished a dental casting to the point where there will be no proximal contact. This condition should be corrected by 13

    A. repeating the casting
    B. adding solder to the deficient area on the casting
    C. enlarging the castings of the abutments
    D. shaping one or two vertical spillways on the proximal contour of the casting

14. Which of the following steps is performed FIRST in the formation of an acrylic resin-faced pontic? 14

    A. The faciogingival surface is corrected on the working cast
    B. A facial window is developed
    C. The wax pattern segments are transferred to individual dies
    D. Interproximal embrasures are corrected on the working cast

15. The axial contour of a fixed restoration should represent an interpretation of protective versus stimulating features. This interpretation is relative to each of the following, EXCEPT 15

    A. statistical averages
    B. clinical crown length
    C. contour of adjacent teeth
    D. tissue architecture

16. A hydrocolloid impression has just been filled with wet stone. While the stone sets, the impression should be 16

    A. placed in a cool, dry place
    B. heated slightly
    C. stored in a covered humidor that contains a saturated sponge
    D. immersed in clear slurry water

17. Faciolingually, the base of a triangular ridge is located 17

    A. occlusally
    B. cervically
    C. toward the center of the tooth
    D. apically

18. Which of the following cements is generally most difficult to manipulate? 18

    A. Glass ionomer
    B. Zinc oxide/eugenol
    C. Resin
    D. Zinc polycarboxylate

19. Which of the following types of articulators is nonadjustable? 19.____

A. Whip-Mix
B. Hinge-axis facebow
C. Hinge with fixed condylar guidance controls
D. Gnathological

20. In mounting a diagnostic cast, the articulator does not seat together firmly. Of the following, the most likely cause of this is 20.____

A. slippage of the facebow during mounting of upper cast
B. a failure to set the intercondylar distance for upper and lower members at the same time
C. an inaccurate cast
D. distortion of the face-bow fork

21. Zinc oxide/eugenol impression material may be 21.____

A. used to make impressions of a crown preparation in the presence of inflamed gingiva
B. used by itself in a custom acrylic resin tray as a wash material
C. mixed to the same consistency as a provisional filling material
D. used as a temporary restorative

22. The abrasion resistance of the gypsum die can often be enhanced by treating the set surface with any of the following, EXCEPT 22.____

A. epoxy
B. styrene
C. colloidal silica
D. acrylic

23. One of the most effective hardening treatments for dental alloys is to "heat soak" castings at a specific temperature for about ______ before water-quenching. 23.____

A. 15 to 30 minutes
B. 30 to 60 minutes
C. 1 to 2 hours
D. 3 to 6 hours

24. Factors effecting the set time of polysulfide impression materials include 24.____

I. moisture
II. temperature
III. base/catalyst ratio
IV. amount of material used

A. I and II
B. I, II and III
C. III only
D. I, II, III and IV

25. The Schatzmann attachment is typically used as a major connector for each of the following, EXCEPT 25.

A. provisional fixed partial dentures
B. distal extension partial dentures
C. removable bridgework
D. removable partial dentures

KEY (CORRECT ANSWERS)

1. D
2. C
3. B
4. A
5. D
6. A
7. B
8. B
9. B
10. B
11. A
12. C
13. B
14. D
15. A
16. C
17. C
18. C
19. C
20. B
21. B
22. C
23. A
24. B
25. A

TEST 3

DIRECTIONS: Each question or incomplete statement is followed by several suggested answers or completions. Select the one the BEST answers the question or completes the statement. *PRINT THE LETTER OF THE CORRECT ANSWER IN THE SPACE AT THE RIGHT.*

1. Which of the following types of crowns is typically used on maxillary molars–and occasionally on maxillary premolars–that have extensive distal involvement by caries or a previous restoration? 1.____

   A. Full-veneer
   B. Three-quarter
   C. Four-fifths
   D. Seven-eighths

2. A technician is developing an acrylic veneer crown using a buildup. With tooth-colored powder, the ratio of powder to liquid is typically 2.____

   A. irrelevant, since the powder does not absorb additional liquid after it is mixed
   B. 1:2
   C. 1:1
   D. 2:1

3. The principle hardener in most dental alloys is 3.____

   A. palladium
   B. zinc
   C. copper
   D. iron

4. From a proximal viewpoint, the maxillary lateral incisor has 4.____

   A. a gently concave facial outline
   B. relatively high facial and lingual heights of contour
   C. an incisal edge centered in the middle of the crown
   D. a faciolingual width greater than its incisocervical length

5. After setting, addition silicone impression materials exhibit less deformation when poured than condensation silicones. In other words, they have 5.____

   A. lower flow
   B. higher flow
   C. lower viscosity
   D. higher viscosity

6. Mandibular side-shift in which the orbiting condyle moves essentially straight medially as it leaves centric relation is known as ______ side-shift. 6.____

   A. progressive
   B. early
   C. immediate
   D. distributed

7. A technician has just applied soft wax coping to a die. The technician applies finger pressure to the wax as it hardens, in order to 7.

A. control shrinkage
B. leave a depression for the central fossa of the crown
C. leave dermal ridges that will permit a firmer bond with the hard wax cap
D. flatten the soft wax layer

8. With extremely thick wax patterns, the gauge of sprue pin most often used is 8.

A. 6
B. 8
C. 10
D. 12

9. Nonadjustable articulators are considered appropriate for 9.

I. prostheses with complicated occlusal disharmonies
II. single restorations
III. small prostheses that are not involved in controlling anterior tooth guidance
IV. long-span partial dentures

A. I only
B. II and III
C. III only
D. IV only

10. About ______ of the proximal contacts of posterior teeth are in the located in the occlusal third of the crown. 10.

A. a fourth
B. half
C. three-quarters
D. seven-eighths

11. Before mounting a cast on the articulator, a technician carves three transverse notches in the bottom of each base. The purpose of this is to 11.

A. provide a positive index for accurately remounting the casts
B. expose the dowel-pin area
C. improve the mechanical bond between the cast and the mounting material
D. outline the wax fork registration

12. Which of the following is an advantage associated with polycarboxylate cements? 12.

A. Good tensile strength
B. High resiliency under load
C. Good compressive strength
D. Acid resistance

13. Establishing an occlusal relationship with three-point contacts is most applicable when it is desirable to 13

A. use both additive and subtractive techniques
B. have the mandible move from one position to another without interference

C. maintain a long centric relationship
D. have the teeth establish the condylar position at one point

14. In preparing dies, cyanoacrylate glue may be used to 14.____
    I. protect the surface of the die from abrasion
    II. cement the completed die to the working cast
    III. cement dowel pins into pinholes
    IV. reveal surface imperfections

A. I and II
B. I and III
C. II, III and IV
D. I, II, III and IV

15. A technician may sometimes develop spillways running from the mesial and lingual fossae of pontics to the embrasure lingually across the marginal ridge. The ultimate purpose for these spillways is to 15.____

A. provide rest seats
B. improve hygiene
C. hold the pontics in position
D. reduce the occlusal load

16. Which of the following devices is required for any nonretentive attachment that has little or no adjustment capability? 16.____

A. Interlock
B. Egg contour
C. Milled lingual retentive arm
D. Milled substructure bar

17. Which of the following elastic impression materials has the highest rigidity? 17.____

A. Compound
B. Polyether
C. Polysulfide
D. Alginate

18. Which of the following is NOT a facial margin design typically used with a full-veneer crown? 18.____

A. Chamfer
B. 75-degree shoulder
C. Shoulder
D. Shoulder with bevel

19. Casting procedures for gold alloys assume a casting temperature that is ______ ^{o}F higher than the melting point of gold. 19.____

A. 50
B. 150
C. 250
D. 400

20. A technician wants a dental casting to remain somewhat soft after the casting procedure, so that it can be easily burnished. The casting should

   A. be heat soaked for 30 minutes at a medium-high temperature before quenching
   B. have a high copper content
   C. be quenched immediately after casting
   D. be quenched as soon as the crucible button stops emitting a dull red glow

21. Of the following methods of retention for an acrylic veneer, the strongest are typically

   A. wax bars
   B. undercuts
   C. spurs or pickups
   D. plastic beads

22. A technician has placed a wax pattern on a working cast to begin preparations for an acrylic veneer. Which of the following is NOT a guideline that should be followed in forming the "resin window"?

   A. vertical and horizontal bars are recessed in the pontic cavity for mechanical retention
   B. the pontic tip and the buccal cusp should be left in metal
   C. the window is developed with a scalpel
   D. the occlusal contact should be verified on an articulator

23. An impression tray has been filled with dental stone. The impression tray may be vibrated or moved

   A. before the stone begins to lose its gloss
   B. as soon as the stone begins to lose its gloss
   C. using the tray handle
   D. only after the initial setting of the stone

24. In finishing and polishing a dental casting, a garnet disc

   A. will probably be needed only where the sprue was removed
   B. is a good general-purpose burnisher
   C. is too abrasive for use on noble alloys
   D. should be used to define the margins

25. Which of the following materials may be used to customize the internal fit of a preformed crown?

   I. Polycarbonate
   II. Zinc phosphate
   III. Acrylic provisional
   IV. Composite provisional

   A. I and II
   B. II, III and IV
   C. III only
   D. III and IV

KEY (CORRECT ANSWERS)

1. D
2. D
3. C
4. C
5. A

6. C
7. A
8. B
9. B
10. B

11. A
12. C
13. D
14. B
15. D

16. C
17. C
18. B
19. B
20. D

21. D
22. C
23. D
24. A
25. D

TEST 4

DIRECTIONS: Each question or incomplete statement is followed by several suggested answers or completions. Select the one the BEST answers the question or completes the statement. *PRINT THE LETTER OF THE CORRECT ANSWER IN THE SPACE AT THE RIGHT.*

1. After the die stone has set, the technician removes the cast from the impression. Which of the following procedures would be appropriate before trimming the cast on a cast trimmer? 1

    A. Defining the margins
    B. Soaking the cast in clear slurry water
    C. Sectioning the dies
    D. Stapling the second pour to the first

2. Nonrigid connectors are appropriate for uniting a retainer with a pontic when 2

    I. connectors must be soldered
    II. the edentulous area is a short span, with normal conditions
    III. two abutment teeth cannot be made parallel
    IV. an abutment tooth has an edentulous area on both sides

    A. I and III
    B. II and III
    C. III and IV
    D. IV only

3. Which of the following is an advantage associated with the partial veneer crown over the full-veneer crown? 3

    A. Better retention
    B. Usually no visible metal
    C. Increased rigidity
    D. More favorable periodontal response

4. In developing a wax pattern, the ______ of the artificial tooth are the most important in terms of the patient's periodontal health. 4

    A. axial contours
    B. cusp cones
    C. marginal and cusp ridges
    D. triangular ridges

5. For pinledge wax patterns, sprue pins are generally 5

    I. placed toward the cervical aspect of the lingual surface
    II. placed toward the incisal aspect of the lingual surface
    III. angled toward the surface of the pattern
    IV. perpendicular to the surface of the pattern

    A. I and III
    B. II and III
    C. I and IV
    D. II and IV

6. A technician has mixed and hand spatulated dental stone for a cast. Of the following procedures, the one that should be performed next is to 6.____

A. place the mix in small increments in one corner of the impression
B. fill the impression with stone up to the cervical area
C. place the mix in a vacuum spatulator for 15 seconds
D. vibrate the mix for several seconds

7. A post is used for the purpose of 7.____

A. permanent sealing of the root canal filling material
B. core material retention
C. root strengthening
D. core material strengthening

8. A technician is casting a dental alloy. As the metal becomes fluid, the technician sprinkles it with borax. Each of the following is a possible benefit of this procedure, EXCEPT 8.____

A. minimizing the porosity of the metal
B. preventing oxidation
C. hardening the metal
D. increasing the fluidity of the metal

9. An impression made from _______ will swell when immersed in water. 9.____

A. addition silicone
B. condensation silicone
C. polysulfide
D. polyether

10. The vertical anatomic plane that extends anteroposteriorly and superoinferiorly is known as the _______ plane. 10.____

A. horizontal
B. sagittal
C. coronal
D. maxillary

11. From the occlusal view, the maxillary second premolar has 11.____

I. proximal contacts facial to the middle of the crown
II. supplemental grooves and ridges radiating from the pits
III. a facial cusp tip slightly mesial of center
IV. a facial half that is wider lingually than mesiodistally

A. I and II
B. I, II and IV
C. III only
D. III and IV

12. When fabricating a stainless steel crown, a technician FIRST determines the 12.____

A. contour of the finish line
B. occlusal height

C. mesial/distal dimensions
D. occlusal/incisal to gingival dimensions

13. A technician wants fast, accurate, and inexpensive attachment of a cast to an articulator. The most appropriate material for this purpose is 13.

A. dental stone
B. baseplate wax
C. dental plaster
D. dental compound

14. When an acrylic resin-faced pontic is employed in a fixed partial denture, 14.

A. wax caps for the retainers are made directly on the working cast
B. the retainers and the pontic may be waxed at the same time
C. the pontic is contoured along the entire coronal length
D. the final form of the pontic should be slightly concave

15. A technician has removed casts from the impression. The floor of the mouth and the palatal area are best trimmed with a 15.

A. coping saw
B. set of plaster nippers
C. cast trimmer
D. scalpel

16. Type IV alloys are typically used for each of the following, EXCEPT 16

A. inlays subject to very high stress
B. average thickness partial veneer crowns
C. long-span fixed prostheses
D. removable partial denture components

17. To insure a strong enough substrate, the thickness of a resin veneer should be a maximum of ______ mm. 17

A. 0.5 to 1.0
B. 1.0 to 1.5
C. 1.5 to 2.0
D. 2.0 to 2.5

18. Teeth can be waxed in relation to the temporomandibular joint in one of three positions. Which of the following is NOT one of these? 18

A. Centric relation-occlusion (CR-O)
B. Long centric (LC)
C. Long axial (LA)
D. Intercuspal position (ICP)

19. A technician, preparing an impression tray with regular-set alginate, mixes the material for 45 seconds. How much time remains to load the tray, wipe on the alginate, and seat the tray? 19

A. 45 seconds
B. 75 seconds
C. 3 minutes
D. Indefinitely, as long as a catalyst has not been applied

20. The main disadvantage to the use of gypsum as a die material is its 20.____

A. susceptibility to abrasion
B. incompatibility with several impression materials
C. poor dimensional accuracy
D. complexity of use

21. The ______ attachment is an intracoronal precious metal attachment widely used in fixed restorations. 21.____

A. Stern
B. McCollum
C. Interlock
D. Schatzmann

22. Which of the following layers in a resin buildup should be slightly enlarged to allow for postpolymerization correction? 22.____

A. Opaque
B. Tooth-colored
C. Dentin
D. Enamel

23. "Localized shrinkage" in a dental casting 23.____

A. is a result of trying to force too much metal into the casting
B. generally occurs at the portion of the casting that is farthest from the sprue
C. generally occurs near the sprue-casting junction
D. can be alleviated with investment venting rods

24. Pickling agents commonly used with gold alloys include 24.____

I. hydrochloric acid
II. sulfuric acid
III. hydrogen peroxide
IV. sodium cyanide

A. I and II
B. I and III
C. III only
D. I, II, III and IV

25. Design guidelines for full veneer crowns include each of the following, EXCEPT 25.____

A. maintenance of cingulum as low as possible
B. parallel proximal walls
C. maintenance of cingulum parallel with the facial surface
D. rounding all sharp angles

KEY (CORRECT ANSWERS)

1. B
2. C
3. D
4. A
5. B

6. B
7. B
8. C
9. D
10. B

11. A
12. C
13. C
14. B
15. A

16. B
17. B
18. C
19. B
20. A

21. B
22. C
23. C
24. A
25. A

EXAMINATION SECTION
TEST 1

DIRECTIONS: Each question or incomplete statement is followed by several suggested answers or completions. Select the one the BEST answers the question or completes the statement. *PRINT THE LETTER OF THE CORRECT ANSWER IN THE SPACE AT THE RIGHT.*

1. If the porcelain used for a crown fuses at 980°C (1760°F), the melting temperature of the alloy used must be higher than 1.____

   A. 1080° C (1976° F)
   B. 1240° C (2264° F)
   C. 1460° C (2660° F)
   D. 1600° C (2912° F)

2. The most significant advantage of hydrocolloid impression materials is that they 2.____

   A. have a high degree of dimensional accuracy
   B. can be used in a wet field
   C. may be poured multiple times over an extended period
   D. come in premixed units

3. Which of the following molars has four almost equally divided cusps? 3.____

   A. mandibular first
   B. mandibular second
   C. maxillary first
   D. maxillary third

4. Technicians who make porcelain-fused-to-metal crowns typically use larger sprues during wax elimination because 4.____

   A. porcelain is difficult to force through a sprue
   B. ceramic noble alloys have a higher melting point and flow slowly
   C. castings for metal copings tend to be smaller than full-crown castings
   D. most porcelain-fused-to-metal crowns are used on anterior teeth

5. The occlusal surface of a stock porcelain facing should not be reduced, because reduction 5.____

   A. will shorten the pinholes and compromise retention
   B. may expose the porcelain to fracture forces
   C. may compromise the shape of the gingival margin
   D. will expose an unsightly amount of metal

6. The solder joint between a pontic and a retainer should be extended at least ______ mm over the gingival margin on the working cast to insure an adequate interdental embrasure. 6.____

   A. 0.5
   B. 1.0

C. 1.5
D. 2.0

7. Each of the following is a type of dental depression, EXCEPT the 7.

A. fossa
B. pit
C. transverse ridge
D. groove

8. The most common problem associated with the addition of porcelain to restorations that have already been fired is that 8.

A. the added porcelain is too dry
B. a thinner mix is used, resulting in greater porosity
C. a different shade is used, resulting in a color mismatch
D. dentin and enamel portions are grossly overbuilt

9. Alumina is sometimes added to porcelain powder in order to 9

A. increase translucency
B. simulate natural tooth colors
C. facilitate condensation
D. increase strength

10. Sectioned dies are typically trimmed to allow an extension of ______ mm beyond the margin of the die, with a tapered root form. 10

A. 0.4 to 0.8
B. 1.0 to 1.5
C. 1.7 to 2.0
D. 2.0 to 2.5

11. After a metal substructure is cast, it may be cleaning either by pickling or abrasive blasting. Advantages of pickling include 11

A. surface decontamination
B. fewer safety risks
C. establishing micropores
D. preservation of thin margins

12. An aluminous porcelain jacket crown has cracked after the first bake. Which of the following is the LEAST likely cause? 12

A. No allowance for shrinkage
B. Too-rapid firing cycle
C. Not enough drying time
D. Outside layer dried without condensing the inner layer

13. In the preporcelain veneer method of fabricating a partial denture, 13

I. the relationship of castings is recorded by a stone index
II. the metal framework is cast into two segments
III. uses castings made of two different metals
IV. castings can be fitted to individual dies

A. I and II
B. I, II and IV
C. II and IV
D. I, II, III and IV

14. The most common way to eliminate bubbles or voids in a porcelain restoration is to 14.____

A. fire the porcelain in a partial vacuum
B. cool the fused porcelain under pressure
C. substitute a diffusible gas for the ordinary furnace atmosphere
D. induce self-glazing by reheating

15. A technician is pouring the anatomic portion of a diagnostic cast. After beginning by picking up a small increment of gypsum with a spatula, the technician begins by placing the increment at ______ of the impression. 15.____

A. the anterior portion
B. one posterior corner
C. both posterior corners
D. both canines

16. What is the term for the angle formed between the axis-orbital plane and the superior wall of the glenoid fossa? 16.____

A. Suprameatal triangle
B. Eminentia
C. Parietal notch
D. Styloid process

17. From the incisal view of a mandibular central incisor, the 17.____

I. crown is wider faciolingually than mesiodistally
II. lingual outline tapers toward the cingulum
III. mesial and distal halves are nearly identical
IV. incisal edge is slightly facial of center

A. I and II
B. I, II and III
C. III only
D. I, II, III and IV

18. The ______ molars have only one antagonist. 18.____

A. mandibular first
B. mandibular third
C. maxillary second
D. maxillary third

19. After a casting is seated on a die, the technician observes a black shadow at the porcelain-gold junction. If the cause is determined to be over-glaze lapping over the margins, the technician should 19.____

A. redo the casting
B. grind off excess porcelain until porcelain and gold are ground together, and then refire

C. grind the porcelain down near the opaque layer and then build up again
D. use a rubber wheel to remove the overglaze from the metal, and then polish

20. With a thin scalpel, a technician makes interproximal cuts in the porcelain powder down to the opaque layer before firing. The purpose of these cuts is to 20

A. distribute the shrinkage associated with firing
B. increase the translucency of the final layer
C. prepare the area for contour correction
D. accelerate condensation

21. A gypsum-bonded investment material that is mixed with a colloidal silica liquid- such as Divestment-is most appropriate for 21

A. porcelain-fused-to-metal crowns
B. all-porcelain full-veneer crowns
C. conventional gold alloys
D. porcelain jacket crowns

22. The distal contact area of the maxillary canine is located 22

A. in the incisal third
B. near the incisal ridge
C. apical to the middle
D. in the middle

23. In the wax-added technique of developing a pattern, the ______ developed last. 23

A. triangular ridges
B. facial and lingual contours
C. cusp cones
D. marginal and cusp ridges

24. A technician is adding translucent powder to the incisal area of a restoration. The buildup should be about ______ percent larger in all directions than the final dimensions in order to allow for shrinkage during firing. 24

A. 1-3
B. 5-10
C. 15-20
D. 25-33

25. Methods for eliminating localized shrinkage in dental castings include. 25

I. increasing the water-to-powder ratio of the investment
II. extending the period of burnout by a minute or two
III. flaring the point of the sprue attachment
IV. lowering the casting temperature by about 30° C

A. I and II
B. II, III and IV
C. III and IV
D. I, II, III and IV

KEY (CORRECT ANSWERS)

1. B
2. B
3. B
4. B
5. A

6. B
7. C
8. B
9. D
10. B

11. D
12. A
13. B
14. A
15. B

16. B
17. B
18. D
19. D
20. A

21. C
22. D
23. A
24. C
25. C

TEST 2

DIRECTIONS: Each question or incomplete statement is followed by several suggested answers or completions. Select the one the BEST answers the question or completes the statement. *PRINT THE LETTER OF THE CORRECT ANSWER IN THE SPACE AT THE RIGHT.*

1. A technician is adding incisal powder over dentin powder in a fixed partial denture. If the incisal powder is too wet, it may result in 1

   A. a loss of translucency
   B. the separation of the buildup
   C. gross surface distortion
   D. hindered condensation

2. A working cast for crown preparation should first be trimmed 2

   A. buccolingually
   B. marginally
   C. mesiodistally
   D. facially

3. For what reason would a technician add lithium carbonate to porcelain prior to fusion with the metal coping? 3

   A. To remove oxidizing materials from the metal interface
   B. To make the porcelain less likely to deform when fired
   C. To increase the porcelain's coefficient of thermal expansion
   D. To decrease the porosity of the porcelain

4. Which of the following is NOT an advantage associated with porcelain jacket crowns? 4

   A. Low abrasion
   B. Excellent simulation of natural colors and forms
   C. Well tolerated by surrounding tissues
   D. Excellent marginal adaptation

5. After it is removed from the investment, a dental casting is covered with a carbon coating that proves nearly impossible to remove by pickling. The most likely cause of this was 5

   A. too low a water-powder ration in the investment
   B. underheating during burnout
   C. improper orientation of the pattern in the investment
   D. insufficient casting pressure

6. Which of the following premolars often has three cusps? 6

   A. maxillary first
   B. maxillary second
   C. mandibular first
   D. mandibular second

7. A technician has just completed torch soldering a pair of dental castings. Some of the solder has flowed outside of the joint. Which of the following was LEAST likely a cause? 7.____

A. Excess flux
B. Heat improperly applied
C. Contamination or oxidation of solder
D. No antiflux adjacent to joint gap

8. For most porcelain systems, firing is done at a pressure range roughly between ______ in. Hg. 8.____

A. 10-15
B. 18-22
C. 25-30
D. 35-45

9. If porcelain is fired in a vacuum, the vacuum should be applied 9.____

A. while the restoration is still at a low temperature
B. at a temperature no lower than 400°C (752°F)
C. just before the restoration has reached fusion temperature
D. just after the restoration has reached fusion temperature

10. Which of the following gypsum products gives the best dimensional accuracy? 10.____

A. High strength dental stone
B. High strength/high expansion dental stone
C. Dental stone
D. Model plaster

11. The most common type of die spacer is made by coating a gypsum die to within about ______ mm of the margin. 11.____

A. 0.1
B. 0.5
C. 1.0
D. 1.3

12. Methods for condensing wet porcelain powder include 12.____

I. vibration
II. brushing
III. tapping
IV. gravitation

A. I only
B. I, III and IV
C. II and III
D. I, II, III and IV

13. Nonarcon articulators

    A. have condyles attached to the upper member and the guiding surfaces attached to the lower member
    B. have condyles attached to the lower member and the guiding elements attached to the upper member
    C. are fully adjustable
    D. are a good choice for articulating casts of patients who have temporo-mandibular joint disturbances

14. A technician has fashioned a full veneer crown using the porcelain facial margin technique. After firing, the technician observes that the porcelain lifts at the mental juncture. This is most likely due to

    A. firing the crown too rapidly
    B. failing to wet the opaque surface with dentin slurry before building up the crown
    C. failing to moisten the dentin porcelain before applying the enamel porcelain
    D. applying the porcelain too thinly over the opaque layer

15. After a technician has formed a stone index for a glazed stock facing, she removes the facing from the cast and uses a porcelain stone to define the bevel and remove any glaze. The next step is to

    A. begin construction of the occlusal anatomy of the pontic
    B. flow wax into the pinholes
    C. place the facing and the backing pattern back on the cast
    D. add wax to the occlusal surface of the backing pattern

16. After scribing the outline of a veneer, a technician takes a wax bur and creates a single longitudinal groove on the facial surface of the crown. The purpose of the groove will be to

    A. embrace the sprue
    B. guide the development of a uniform depth for the veneer
    C. create bonding embrasures on the surface of the metal coping
    D. make the casting easier to remove from the investment

17. From the facial view of a maxillary central incisor, the

    A. surface is smoothly convex, with labial lobe grooves
    B. mesial outline is more convex than the distal, with proximal contact more cervical
    C. the crown is longer mesiodistally than incisocervically
    D. mesioincisal angle forms a 45-degree distoincisal angle more rounded in form

18. Of the following, the longest longitudinal groove exists in the ______ surface of the ______.

    A. distal; maxillary first premolar
    B. mesial; mandibular first premolar
    C. mesial; maxillary first premolar
    D. mesial; maxillary second premolar

19. A porcelain facing, after being contoured, is placed on a cast with utility wax. An opposing working cast is seated on an articulator. The facing should be seated on the edentulous ridge to insure that there is at least ______ mm clearance between the occlusal surface of the facing and the opposing functional cusp. 19.____

A. 0.5
B. 1.0
C. 2.0
D. 3.0

20. To make them easier to trim, cast bases made of dental stone should be 20.____

A. soaked in water for 5 to 10 minutes prior to trimming
B. mixed with a higher water content than the anatomical portion
C. fabricated without mechanical vibration
D. heated to at least 130°F before trimming

21. Technically, the fusion of porcelain particles to form a restoration is known as 21.____

A. fritting
B. sintering
C. muffing
D. vitrification

22. The PKT #3 instrument is designed for 22.____

A. applying small drops of melted wax
B. all-purpose wax carving
C. carving grooves on the occlusal surface of posterior pattern teeth
D. refining wax pattern margins

23. An impression material, in its gel state, tends to contract and exude liquid. This property is known as 23.____

A. syneresis
B. reversibility
C. hysteresis
D. imbibition

24. In order to be properly supported by the substructure, the porcelain from the incisal edge to the facial surface of a pontic in a porcelain-fused-to-metal fixed partial denture should not exceed ______ mm in thick-ness. 24.____

A. 0.3 to 0.5
B. 0.5 to 0.8
C. 1.0 to 1.5
D. 1.7 to 2.0

25. After the opaque layer of a porcelain jacket crown has been fired, the platinum apron is most appropriately removed with a(n) 25

A. beavertail instrument
B. flexible diamond disk
C. silicon bur
D. scalpel

KEY (CORRECT ANSWERS)

1. A
2. A
3. C
4. D
5. B

6. D
7. C
8. C
9. A
10. A

11. B
12. D
13. A
14. B
15. B

16. B
17. A
18. C
19. C
20. A

21. B
22. C
23. A
24. C
25. B

TEST 3

DIRECTIONS: Each question or incomplete statement is followed by several suggested answers or completions. Select the one the BEST answers the question or completes the statement. *PRINT THE LETTER OF THE CORRECT ANSWER IN THE SPACE AT THE RIGHT.*

1. When recontouring a porcelain restoration of an anterior tooth after firing, the technician should FIRST correct the 1.____

   A. interproximal surfaces
   B. coronal length
   C. facial surface
   D. incisail thickness

2. The greatest potential for failure of a porcelain-fused-to-metal crown lies in the possibility of 2.____

   A. thermal expansion of the porcelain
   B. breaking of porcelain under occlusal forces
   C. distortion of the metal coping
   D. thermal constriction of the porcelain resulting in cracks and eventual fractures

3. A politic backing and retainers have just been cast, devested, and pickled. The next step would be to 3.____

   A. adjust the occlusion
   B. fit the cast backing to the porcelain facing
   C. remove shiny exposed spots on the metal with a bur
   D. separate the sprues

4. Which of the following is an anterior tooth point angle? 4.____

   A. Mesiolingual
   B. Distolabioincisal
   C. Linguoincisal
   D. Distolinguoocclusal

5. The porcelain and metal components of a restoration should meet in a ______ . 5.____

   A. tenon
   B. lap
   C. slot
   D. butt

6. A technician is trimming a diagnostic cast. To remove excess gypsum distal to the retro-molar pads (maxillary) and tuberosities (mandibular), the technician should use 6.____

   A. plaster nippers
   B. an acrylic bur
   C. a cast trimmer
   D. a ragwheel

7. The postporcelain veneer method is typically used to fabricate 7

    I. long-span fixed partial dentures
    II. fixed partial dentures in the posterior region that are composed of two different metals
    III. dentures that span from incisors to canines or canines to premolars
    IV. porcelain-fused-to-metal crowns

    A. I only
    B. I and II
    C. II and III
    D. I, II, III and IV

8. Describing an impression material as "hydrophilic" means that it 8

    A. repels water
    B. can be immersed in water without losing its structure
    C. has good surface-wetting characteristics
    D. needs water to set

9. In preparing dies with a dowel pin system, staples are sometimes used to 9

    A. fasten the cast securely to an articulator
    B. mark pinhole locations
    C. prevent separation of the base cast from the impression cast
    D. prevent a die from being separated from an abutment

10. Low-fusing porcelains are MOST likely to be used in the construction of 10

    A. artificial denture teeth
    B. partial veneer crowns
    C. porcelain jacket crowns
    D. rigid connectors

11. A technician is preparing a fast-set alginate impression. For this material, the ADA recommends a minimum working time of 11

    A. 45 seconds
    B. 60 seconds
    C. 75 seconds
    D. 90 seconds

12. Porosities caused by entrapped air on the inner surface of a dental casting ("back-pressure porosities") can usually be avoided through each of the following, EXCEPT 12

    A. vent rods in the investment
    B. good burnout
    C. sufficiently high water-to-powder ratio in the investment
    D. maximum investment thickness of 6.0 mm between the tip of the pattern and the end of the ring

13. The smallest cusp on all the maxillary molars is the 13

    A. distolingual
    B. distobuccal

C. mesiobuccal
D. mesiolingual

14. From the proximal view of a mandibular canine, the 14.____
    I. crown is longer faciolingually than incisocervically
    II. facial outline is slightly concave
    III. cusp tip is slightly lingual to the middle of the crown
    IV. lingual line has a flattened S shape with the cingulum extending to half the crown length

A. I and II
B. I, II and III
C. III and IV
D. I, II, II, and IV

15. After the wax pattern of a partial denture is made to full contour, the form is preserved by 15.____

A. taking exact measurements
B. making a casting
C. making a silicone impression
D. making a duplicate

16. Which of the following types of articulators is fully adjustable? 16.____

A. Hanau
B. Arcon
C. Stuart
D. Whip-Mix

17. The cusp of Carabelli is found on the ______ surface. 17.____

A. distofacial
B. mesiobuccal
C. mesiolingual
D. distolingual

18. The coronal length of a stock porcelain facing is typically adjusted by grinding the 18.____

A. gingival end
B. mesial and distal surfaces
C. bucco-occlusal edge
D. occlusal surface

19. Ceramic alloys are typically cast at a temperature not lower than 19.____

A. 700° C (1292° F)
B. 980° C (1796° F)
C. 1150° C (2102° F)
D. 1240° C (2264° F)

20. The first step in developing the axial contour of an artificial tooth is to 20._

A. remove half of the occlusal surface
B. locate the proximal contact areas
C. add wax to the height of contour
D. fill in the cervical area

21. The porosity of a porcelain restoration is sometimes reduced by introducing a diffusible gas into the furnace atmosphere during vitrification. Gases that can be used for this purpose include each of the following, EXCEPT 21._

A. helium
B. carbon dioxide
C. hydrogen
D. steam

22. What is the Universal Code designation for the mandibular left second premolar? 22._

A. 8
B. 12
C. 20
D. 35

23. For metal-ceramic crowns, a technician should consider ______ mm to be the absolute minimum depth of porcelain for esthetic areas. 23._

A. 0.50
B. 0.75
C. 1.0
D. 1.25

24. The main reason to avoid using acrylic resins as die materials is their 24._

A. expense
B. poor compressive strength
C. susceptibility to abrasion
D. excessive curing contraction

25. When the alumina content of porcelain core powder is more than 50%, 25._

I. strength is reduced
II. strength is increased
III. translucency is reduced
IV. translucency is increased

A. I only
B. I and III
C. II and III
D. II and IV

KEY (CORRECT ANSWERS)

1. A
2. C
3. B
4. B
5. D

6. A
7. B
8. C
9. C
10. C

11. C
12. A
13. A
14. C
15. C

16. C
17. C
18. C
19. C
20. B

21. B
22. C
23. B
24. D
25. D

TEST 4

DIRECTIONS: Each question or incomplete statement is followed by several suggested answers or completions. Select the one the BEST answers the question or completes the statement. *PRINT THE LETTER OF THE CORRECT ANSWER IN THE SPACE AT THE RIGHT.*

1. Typically, oxide and flux are removed from the surface of a soldered casting assembly by

   A. abrasive blasting
   B. pickling in hydrochloric acid
   C. ultrasonic detergent cleaning
   D. pickling in hydrogen peroxide

2. Each of the following factors is known to affect the bonding of porcelain and metal, EXCEPT

   A. electromagnetic bonding
   B. chemical bonding
   C. mechanical bonding
   D. molecular attraction

3. After glazing, a porcelain facing is returned to a working cast for construction of a stone matrix. This matrix is typically formed on the ______ surface(s) of the cast.

   A. facial
   B. lingual
   C. occlusal
   D. facial and lingual

4. Occasionally, standard trays won't cover the desired areas and must be modified with wax. For a patient with large jaws, a common area for this to occur is the

   A. third molar
   B. canine
   C. palatal
   D. incisai

5. Color frits are added to dental porcelain to impart various shades. The metallic oxide that would be added in order to add a yellowish brown tint is

   A. titanium
   B. copper
   C. iron
   D. nickel

6. The partial veneer crown is indicated on posterior teeth that have any of the following characteristics, EXCEPT

   A. greater than average crown length
   B. greater than average occlusal forces
   C. intact or minimally restored coronal structure
   D. normal crown form

7. A container of porcelain powder has been sitting on a shelf undisturbed for several weeks. The technician should 7.____

A. rotate the container end-over-end several times, and then wait a minute or so before opening it
B. rotate the container end-over-end several times, and then open and dispense immediately
C. scoop powder from the bottom of the container
D. shake the container up and down and side to side

8. A technician receives a wax transfer fork in which the maxillary teeth have been forced into the coating material beyond their heights of contour. The technician should 8.____

A. trim the wax to leave registrations only of cusp tips and incisal edges
B. send the fork back for re-registration
C. take a negative impression
D. refine the indentations with impression paste

9. Which of the following impression materials is generally the most difficult to use? 9.____

A. Condensation silicone
B. Polysulfide
C. Addition silicone
D. Reversible hydrocolloid

10. Typically, aluminous porcelain crowns are heated to glazing temperature at a rate of ______ ^{o}F per minute. 10.____

A. 25
B. 50
C. 100
D. 250

11. Spaces between teeth are denoted generally as 11.____

A. lamellae
B. leeway space
C. voids
D. diastemas

12. Postsoldering can be accomplished using either an oven or a gas-oxygen torch. Which of the following is an advantages associated with the use of a torch? 12.____

A. Prevention of overheating
B. Easier assurance of integrity of adjacent porcelain veneers
C. Easier monitoring of solder flow
D. Availability of vacuum to control oxidation

13. A technician is fabricating a porcelain-fused-to-metal crown for a posterior tooth in the maxillary arch. Usually, porcelain coverage should extend from 13.____

A. the facial surface over to one-third of the inner surface of the buccal cusp
B. the lingual surface over to one-third of the inner surface of the palatal cusp

C. the facial surface over to the entire inner surface of the buccal cusp
D. the lingual surface over to the entire inner surface of the palatal cusp

14. Typically, the sequence of cutback in forming a pattern for a metal-ceramic crown begins with the reduction of the ______ surface(s). 14.

A. incisal or occlusal
B. proximal
C. facial
D. gingival

15. Of the following tooth surfaces, the ______ a contact area. 15.

A. buccal
B. occlusal
C. mesial
D. lingual

16. In adding porcelain to a metal substructure, which of the following is applied FIRST? 16.

A. A layer of mixed dentin powder, modifier, and opaque powder
B. Translucent powder
C. Opaque powder
D. A thin, wet wash of dentin powder mix

17. A technician, using a dowel pin system, has just completed a cast and is preparing to separate the dies. The technician is sectioning the entire cast. In making saw cuts, the technician should AVOID making cuts that 17

I. penetrate the entire depth of the first pour
II. diverge slightly downward
III. converge slightly downward
IV. are parallel to the long axis of the tooth

A. I only
B. I and II
C. II and III
D. I,II, III and IV

18. Each of the following landmarks is found on the mandibular first molar, EXCEPT the 18

A. lingual groove
B. buccal pit
C. transverse ridge
D. triangular ridge

19. In the construction of a porcelain jacket crown, which of the following die materials involves the greatest risk during swaging? 19

A. Acrylic resin
B. Epoxy
C. Metal
D. Gypsum

20. The optimal thickness of the porcelain which forms the gingival surface of the pontic in a porcelain-fused-to-metal fixed partial denture is ______ mm. 20.____

A. 0.3
B. 0.5
C. 0.8
D. 1.0

21. Occlusocervically, the base of a triangular ridge is located 21.____

A. occlusally
B. toward the center of the tooth
C. cervically
D. facially

22. Of the following teeth, the ______ is most likely to have a proximal groove in its root. 22.____

A. mandibular central
B. maxillary central
C. mandibular lateral
D. maxillary lateral

23. Most base metal-ceramic alloys are composed primarily of 23.____

A. nickel and iron
B. chromium and cobalt
C. iron and chromium
D. nickel and chromium

24. Phosphate-bonded investment material is used for casting porcelain-fused-to-metal crowns because it 24.____

A. has better wetting properties than gypsum
B. releases wax more easily than gypsum
C. has a less variable rate of thermal expansion
D. can withstand the higher temperatures used for ceramic alloy casting

25. The casting of porcelain-bonding alloys differs from casting low-fusing gold alloys. With porcelain-bonding alloys, 25.____

I. no asbestos is used in the high-heat crucibles
II. no casting flux is used
III. the technician should have one crucible for each brand of alloy being cast
IV. greater casting pressures are generally required

A. I only
B. I and II
C. II, III and IV
D. I, II, III and IV

KEY (CORRECT ANSWERS)

1. B
2. A
3. A
4. A
5. A
6. B
7. A
8. A
9. D
10. B
11. D
12. C
13. A
14. A
15. C
16. C
17. C
18. C
19. D
20. B
21. C
22. D
23. D
24. D
25. D

EXAMINATION SECTION
TEST 1

DIRECTIONS: Each question or incomplete statement is followed by several suggested answers or completions. Select the one the BEST answers the question or completes the statement. *PRINT THE LETTER OF THE CORRECT ANSWER IN THE SPACE AT THE RIGHT.*

1. _______ acid is most commonly used to bond composite to porcelain. 1.____

   A. Hydrosulfuric
   B. Hydrofluoric
   C. Phosphoric
   D. Hydrochloric

2. The final step in recontouring a porcelain restoration of an anterior tooth would be to correct the 2.____

   A. facial surface
   B. incisal thickness
   C. restoration contour
   D. coronal length

3. Posterior tooth line angles include the 3.____

   I. distolinguoocclusal
   II. linguoincisal
   III. mesiolingual
   IV. distoocclusal

   A. I only
   B. I and II
   C. III and IV
   D. I, II, III and IV

4. A technician has poured an impression and left it in an alginate impression overnight. The likely result is that the cast will 4.____

   A. have a chalky surface
   B. need to be soaked in disinfectant for a period of at least 2 hours
   C. already have pulled away from the impression surface due to shrinkage
   D. have fused to the impression material

5. A technician is transferring a hinge-axis facebow relationship to an articulator. In mounting the maxillary cast, the first step will be to 5.____

   A. adjust the axis-indicating pins
   B. attach the facebow to the mounting stand
   C. raise the back of the articulator
   D. align the facebow and articulator axes

6. The main purpose of opaque powder in porcelain restorations is to 6.____

   A. lend an appropriate sub-tint to the enamel layer
   B. provide a substrate for dentin powder

C. seal cracks or voids in the dentin layer
D. mask the metallic color of the substructure

7. Some ______ alloys have demonstrated a sensitivity to phosphate-bound investments containing carbon, and therefore require a carbon-free investment. 7.

A. gold-platinum-palladium
B. gold-palladium
C. high-palladium-content
D. base metal

8. Which of the following elastic impression materials is typically LEAST accurate? 8.

A. Reversible hydrocolloid
B. Alginate
C. Condensation silicone
D. Addition silicone

9. When presoldering cast units, it is important to 9

A. solder the cast units after the porcelain is fired
B. use a solder than melts at the same point as porcelain's firing temperature
C. use a solder than melts at a point higher than porcelain's firing temperature
D. use a solder than melts at a point higher than porcelain's firing temperature

10. Torch soldering of dental castings has several disadvantages. Which of the following is NOT one of them? 10

A. Imprecise overall control of temperature
B. Uneven distribution of heat
C. Need for pressurized supply of gases
D. Imprecise control of oxidation and reduction reactions

11. When cutting the lining material for a casting ring, the technician should be sure that the liner is positioned to be about ______ mm short of the top of the ring, in order to make sure the investment can directly contact the ring. 11

A. 1
B. 3
C. 5
D. 7

12. A technician is fabricating a denture using the postporcelain veneer method. After the cutback procedure on the wax patterns, the technician waxes a lingual strut from the lingual surface of the pontic to the cast surface. Which of the following would NOT be a purpose of this strut? 12

A. Stabilizing the cast segment in the soldering investment during postsoldering
B. Serving as a handle during porcelain application
C. Stabilizing the wax patterns after separation
D. Serving as a sprue during casting from one pattern to another

13. Layers of opaque and core porcelain typically require about ______ minutes of drying before firing. 13.____

    A. 1 to 2
    B. 2 to 5
    C. 5 to 10
    D. 15 to 20

14. Restoring the posterior occlusal surfaces with porcelain is often avoided by technicians because it 14.____

    A. is too brittle to withstand occlusal forces
    B. uses costly material in an area that isn't likely to be seen
    C. is aesthetically unattractive
    D. may round over during firing and affect the accuracy of occlusal relationships

15. Which of the following porcelain addition procedures is most likely to be unique to porcelain jacket crown fabrication? 15.____

    A. Mesial grooving
    B. Incisal edge removal
    C. Proximal cutbacks
    D. Shoulder-relief adaptation

16. Which of the following is NOT a guideline for hand mixing dental stone? 16.____

    A. The interior of the bowl should be parabolic in cross-section
    B. The end of the spatula should be rounded.
    C. Mixing should stop as soon as the mixture is smooth and homogeneous in texture.
    D. A flexible rubber spatula should be used.

17. Which of the following anterior teeth have mesiodistal widths is greater than their distofacial widths? 17.____

    A. Mandibular canines
    B. Maxillary canines
    C. Mandibular incisors
    D. Maxillary incisors

18. Which of the following is NOT a guideline for the glazing of a porcelain facing? 18.____

    A. before applying the glazing mixture, dry glazing powder should be rubbed into the facing
    B. before firing, glazing should overlap any parts of the facing surface that will be backed with metal
    C. glazing powder should be mixed with liquid glycerine
    D. to check the completeness of the glazing application, the technician should dry the facing at the entrance of a heated oven

19. When used with polyether material, a properly selected impression tray should be deep enough to provide at least ______ mm of space beyond the incisal and occlusal surfaces of the teeth. 19.____

A. 1
B. 2
C. 3
D. 4

20. Each of the following is a substance that adds opacity to dental porcelain, EXCEPT 20

A. tin
B. zirconium
C. titanium
D. manganese

21. The spaces adjacent to the deciduous canines are known as 21

A. leeway space
B. the mesial step
C. primate space
D. the terminal plane

22. After it is removed from the investment, a dental casting has a surface that is uniformly rough. Of the following, which is LEAST likely to have created this condition? 22

A. improper orientation of the pattern in the investment
B. too-high casting pressure
C. excessive amount of wetting agent used during investment
D. too-high water-to-powder ratio in the investment

23. Advantages associated with electric melting of ceramic alloys include the prevention of 23

I. overheating
II. gaseous release
III. oxidation
IV. investment adhesion

A. I only
B. I and III
C. II and IV
D. I, II, III and IV

24. Typically, which of the following adjustments to a stock porcelain facing is made FIRST? 24

A. Placement of the bevel
B. Correction of the mesiodistal width
C. Correction of the interdental embrasure
D. Correction of the coronal length

25. A technician observes that the color of porcelain on a fixed partial denture varies from one tooth to the next, even though the same shade was used. Most likely, the difference is due to 25

A. improper firing temperature
B. nonuniform thickness of porcelain from tooth to tooth
C. inadequate bulk in the framework
D. too much reduction during contouring

KEY (CORRECT ANSWERS)

1. B
2. A
3. C
4. A
5. B

6. D
7. C
8. B
9. D
10. D

11. B
12. D
13. B
14. D
15. D

16. D
17. D
18. B
19. D
20. D

21. C
22. A
23. B
24. B
25. B

TEST 2

DIRECTIONS: Each question or incomplete statement is followed by several suggested answers or completions. Select the one that BEST answers the question or completes the statement. *PRINT THE LETTER OF THE CORRECT ANSWER IN THE SPACE AT THE RIGHT.*

1. A technician wants to melt a ceramic alloy quickly to avoid overheating. In order to achieve this, he preheats the crucible by placing it in the oven with the casting ring during burnout. Guidelines for heating the crucible in this way include using 1.____

    I. a silica crucible
    II. a clay crucible
    III. a ceramic fiber or asbestos crucible liner
    IV. flux

    A. I only
    B. I and III
    C. II, II, and IV
    D. II and IV

2. Which of the following terms is NOT synonymous with the others? 2.____

    A. Spheroid pontic
    B. Conical pontic
    C. Bullet pontic
    D. Hygienic pontic

3. The purpose of gum dammar, a component of dental wax, is to 3.____

    A. raise the melting range
    B. decrease the flow of wax
    C. add color to the wax
    D. resist flaking and allow for a smooth surface

4. Of the following, the lingual surface of the _____ most resembles that of mandibular lateral incisor. 4.____

    A. Maxillary central incisor
    B. Mandibular canine
    C. Maxillary canine
    D. Maxillary lateral incisor

5. Glass modifiers used in dental porcelains, which act as fluxes, include 5.____

    A. calcium
    B. sodium
    C. phosphorus
    D. potassium

6. A technician is investing a pattern into a ring for burnout. The height of the pattern should be adjusted so that it is _____ mm from the end of the ring. 6.____

A. 2 B. 3 C. 4 D. 6

7. Which of the following is NOT a guideline that should be followed in the finishing of a ceramic casting? 7.____

A. Small nodules and residual oxidation can be removed with rotary carbide burs.
B. Rouge sticks or Tripoli should not contact the surface to which porcelain will be added.
C. Resin-bound abrasives should be avoided.
D. The part of the casting that is to be veneered should be finished first.

8. Which of the following impression materials has the highest tear strength? 8.____

A. Polysulfide
B. Alginate
C. Addition silicone
D. Polyether

9. When either retainer of a fixed partial denture is made of a gold alloy, post-soldering should 9.____

A. not be used
B. use solder that melts at a point above the firing temperature of porcelain
C. be performed under vacuum
D. be performed with a gas-oxygen torch

10. To set the Whip-Mix articulator using a protrusive registration, the sideshift guides are initially set at about _____ degrees, so the condyles are free to move laterally. 10.____

A. 5 B. 15 C. 30 D. 45

11. Stones or discs used to prepare metal substructures for porcelain should be ______, in order to prevent contamination of the surface. 11.____

A. ceramic-bound
B. treated in mild acid solution
C. resinous
D. disinfected

12. Aluminous dentin and enamel porcelain powders have a fusing temperature of about _____°F. 12.____

A. 1740 B. 1922
C. 1652 to 1742 D. 2012 to 2356

13. Many high-palladium-content alloys omit silver because of concerns about 13.____

A. carbon sensitivity
B. porcelain discoloration
C. strength
D. castability

14. A technician has just completed an incisal wax crown, and is beginning to scribe the outline of the veneer. The first step in the deveneering process is to draw a horizontal line on the ______ that is ______mm cervical to the incisal edge. 14.____

A. facial; 1.0
B. lingual; 1.0
C. facial; 1.5
D. lingual; 1.5

15. When metal castings are heated with an oxygen-gas flame, solder should be placed over the joint area when the castings appear. 15.____

A. bright blue
B. orange
C. cherry red
D. dull white

16. Which of the following dental alloys generally has the HIGHEST silver content? 16.____

A. Type 1
B. Type II yellow gold
C. Type III palladium
D. Type IV silver palladium

17. The FDE designation for the maxillary left canine is 17.____

A. 3 B. 11 C. 23 D. 31

18. In dental ceramics, gold powders are used to 18.____

A. condition the porcelain surface for firing
B. encourage masking in the opaque layer
C. seal the surface of the metal to suppress the liberation of gases
D. improve the strength of the porcelain-metal bond

19. The MAIN advantage of polyether impression material over other elastomers is that it has 19.____

A. a longer working time
B. better rebound associated with undercuts
C. lower sensitivity to heat and moisture
D. good wetting properties

20. In the process known as ______, a technician holds a wet porcelain restoration firmly with a metal instrument and taps it lightly with another metal instrument. 20.____

A. condensation
B. glazing
C. slumping
D. vitrification

21. Which of the following is a posterior tooth point angle? 21.____

A. Distoocclusal
B. Mesiolinguoincisal
C. Distolingual
D. Distobuccoocclusal

22. The metal substrate of a porcelain-faced pontic should be thick enough to protect against potential fracture of the porcelain. For maxillary teeth, this means a minimum thickness of about ______ mm of metal; for mandibular teeth, about ______ mm. 22.____

A. 0.8; 1.5
B. 1.5; 3.0
C. 1.5; 0.8
D. 2.0; 1.0

23. The fewest cervical contact areas are found on the 23.____

A. third molars
B. premolars
C. central incisors
D. canines

24. Which of the following steps in soldering castings is typically performed LAST? 24.____

A. applying flux to the connector area
B. heating the soldering block
C. trimming the investment around the connector area
D. adding chloroform and rouge to the occlusal surfaces of the castings

25. Which of the following porcelain layers is/are typically fired under vacuum? 25.____

I. Opaque
II. Dentin
III. Enamel
IV. Glazing

A. I only
B. I, II and III
C. II and III
D. I, II, III and IV

KEY (CORRECT ANSWERS)

1. A
2. D
3. D
4. B
5. C
6. D
7. D
8. A
9. C
10. B
11. A
12. C
13. B
14. C
15. C
16. C
17. B
18. C
19. D
20. A
21. D
22. A
23. C
24. B
25. B

TEST 3

DIRECTIONS: Each question or incomplete statement is followed by several suggested answers or completions. Select the one the BEST answers the question or completes the statement. *PRINT THE LETTER OF THE CORRECT ANSWER IN THE SPACE AT THE RIGHT.*

1. Disinfectants appropriate for polyether impression materials include 1.____
   I. sodium hypochlorite
   II. complex phenolics
   III. glutaraldehydes
   IV. iodophors

   A. I only
   B. I, II and IV
   C. II, III and IV
   D. I, II, III and IV

2. Patients who prefer porcelain prosthetic teeth over plastic ones usually say it's because 2.____

   A. porcelain teeth can be more easily repolished
   B. they perceive a better ability to chew hard or fibrous foods
   C. they don't experience as much pain or discomfort
   D. porcelain teeth can occlude with natural teeth

3. The purpose of degassing metal substructures after casting is to 3.____

   A. produce an oxide film that will enhance the bond with porcelain
   B. rid the substructure of any voids
   C. prevent the release of toxic gases in the mouth after fitting
   D. increase the compressive strength of the substructure

4. The ______ groove pattern is the most commonly seen in mandibular second premolars. 4.____

   A. Y
   B. H
   C. W
   D. U

5. A technician is finishing the gingival end of a stock porcelain pontic. Each of the following is a guideline that may be used in this procedure, EXCEPT 5.____

   A. the facial surface should contact the edentulous ridge
   B. the lingual surface should contact the alveolar crest at an oblique angle
   C. the lingual surface should be finished to present a slight concavity
   D. the mesial and distal surfaces should be slightly open to the edentulous ridge

6. A technician is deveneering a wax incisor crown to make a casting for the metal coping. If the mandibular incisal edge contacts the incisal one-third of the maxillary incisor, it should be drawn 6.____

   A. proximally
   B. incisally

C. mesially
D. cervically

7. To increase the abrasive resistance of dental stone, "gypsum hardeners" are sometimes used instead of water during mixing. These substances include 7.

A. epoxy
B. alumina
C. calcium oxide
D. colloidal silica

8. Because of possible distortion in the joint areas during porcelain firing, presoldering is generally NOT recommended for 8

A. long-span fixed partial dentures
B. dentures that span from incisors to cuspids or cuspids to premolars
C. dentures that include pontics with reverse curvatures
D. incisal occlusions

9. In order for the matrix to be removed without distortion, there must be no undercuts on the surface of a porcelain jacket crown die within an area of ______ mm below the preparation margin. 9

A. 0.5
B. 1.5
C. 3
D. 5

10. A technician is making an anatomic reverse-pin facing from an existing denture tooth. The FIRST step in this procedure is to 10

A. grind the appropriate ridge contact
B. mark the location of pinholes
C. grind away the lingual half of the tooth
D. embed the facing in dental compound

11. Overglazing is a procedure most commonly used for 11

A. recontoured denture teeth and pontics
B. porcelain-fused-to-metal crowns
C. porcelain jacket crowns
D. acrylics

12. Of the following ceramic alloys, ones that contain high levels of ______ should never be pickled in acid solutions. 12

A. platinum
B. gold or palladium
C. silver
D. nonprecious nickel and chromium

13. Among the following anterior teeth, the one that varies most in its morphology is the 13.____

A. maxillary canine
B. maxillary lateral incisor
C. mandibular canine
D. mandibular central incisor

14. A technician has just wrapped platinum foil over a die. After it is pressed into place, the foil should be adapted to the die surface with a(n) 14.____

A. PKT #3 instrument
B. blunt scalpel
C. heat shrinker
D. orangewood burnishing tool

15. A technician plans to melt a ceramic alloy with a gas-oxygen torch. The technician should ignite the torch with the 15.____

A. gas and oxygen simultaneously at a low setting
B. gas supply only and then add the oxygen slowly
C. oxygen supply only and then add the gas supply slowly
D. gas supply only and then add the oxygen in a short, sudden burst

16. The ideal soldering joint space between pontic and retainer castings is about ______ mm. 16.____

A. 0.3 to 0.5
B. 0.5 to 0.8
C. 0.8 to 1.0
D. 1.0 to 1.3

17. Which of the following types of pontics is typically used to replace mandibular posterior teeth when a narrow alveolar ridge is present? 17.____

A. Hygienic
B. Ridge-lap
C. Saddle
D. Spheroid

18. Severely protruded maxillary incisors often create an excessive 18.____

A. crossbite
B. overbite
C. mesioclusion
D. overjet

19. Deviations in water-to-powder ratios in dental investment material affect 19.____

I. surface smoothness of the casting
II. hygroscopic expansion
III. setting expansion
IV. thermal expansion

A. I only
B. I, II and III

C. IV only
D. I, II, III and IV

20. Which of the following variables typically has the LEAST effect on the transverse strength of a dental porcelain restoration? 20._

A. Liquid-to-powder ratio
B. Firing temperature
C. Vacuum firing
D. Thickness of glaze

21. Of the following teeth, which is formed from five lobes? 21._

A. Mandibular first molar
B. Maxillary first premolar
C. Maxillary second molar
D. Mandibular second molar

22. "Slumping" during the buildup of porcelain layers is eliminated by 22._

A. applying an absorbent material to the mixture
B. frequent condensation
C. keeping layers thin and uniform
D. applying heat during application

23. A technician is fabricating a denture using the postporcelain veneer method. After positioning the cast retainers and pontic in the stone core, the technician may apply a layer of _______ to the porcelain to prevent investment material from touching the veneer. 23._

A. inlay or baseplate wax
B. sticky wax
C. separating solution
D. mineral oil

24. Which of the following is used as a strengthener in dental porcelains? 24._

A. Kaolin
B. Quartz
C. Potash
D. Soda

25. Advantages associated with the use of custom impression trays include 25._

I. standardized material viscosity
II. eliminating the need for surfactants
III. reduced amount of impression material
IV. minimal dimensional changes

A. I and II
B. II and III
C. III and IV
D. IV only

KEY (CORRECT ANSWERS)

1. B
2. B
3. A
4. A
5. B
6. D
7. D
8. A
9. D
10. C
11. A
12. D
13. B
14. D
15. B
16. A
17. D
18. D
19. D
20. C
21. A
22. A
23. A
24. B
25. C

TEST 4

DIRECTIONS: Each question or incomplete statement is followed by several suggested answers or completions. Select the one the BEST answers the question or completes the statement. *PRINT THE LETTER OF THE CORRECT ANSWER IN THE SPACE AT THE RIGHT.*

1. A technician has just finished scribing the outline of a veneer. The next step is to reduce the incisal edge of the crown 1

   A. at a slight angle toward the labial surface
   B. perpendicularly, 1.0 mm from the incisal edge
   C. at angles to the mesial and distal surfaces
   D. at a slight angle toward the lingual surface

2. Which of the following is NOT a step involved in the fabrication of a custom acrylic impression tray? 2

   A. Placing a sheet of warmed baseplate wax on the cast
   B. Applying petroleum jelly to gloved hands
   C. Forming resin mixture into a thick, wide rope that fits the entire ridge
   D. Cutting away excess tray material with a cast trimmer

3. The crowns of the mandibular molars are typically 3

   A. inclined mesiolingually
   B. inclined distofacially
   C. inclined facially but otherwise upright
   D. upright in all directions

4. A consideration unique to the fabrication of porcelain jacket crowns is 4

   A. presoldering
   B. porcelain shading
   C. incisal strength
   D. die strength

5. A casting ring filled with investment material is placed on the shop bench for about an hour, after which the technician removes a shiny outside layer from the investment. The effect of this procedure will most likely 5

   A. expedite the release of gases during burnout
   B. reduce the need for vibration
   C. accelerate the setting process of the investment
   D. create a poor seat for the wax pattern

6. Porcelain can be mixed with distilled water or a special liquid medium. The primary disadvantage associated with the use of distilled water to mix porcelain is 6

   A. clumping or incomplete mixing
   B. weak bonding during buildup
   C. rapid drying
   D. bubbles and voids

7. A modified ridge-lap pontic 7.____

   I. is intended to prevent food from impaction and retention
   II. provides a convexity lingual to the pontic tip
   III. has a T-shaped area of tissue contact
   IV. creates a limited concavity in the faciolingual direction

   A. I and II
   B. I, III and IV
   C. II and III
   D. I, II, III and IV

8. Of the following teeth, which has the most prominent cingulum? 8.____

   A. Maxillary canine
   B. Maxillary lateral incisor
   C. Mandibular canine
   D. Maxillary central incisor

9. The total cross-sectional area of a connector for a porcelain-fused-to-metal fixed partial denture should not be less than ______ square millimeters. 9.____

   A. 2
   B. 3
   C. 4
   D. 6

10. Which of the following is a type of anatomic pontic? 10.____

   A. All-metal
   B. Occlusal bar
   C. Spheroid
   D. Reverse-pin

11. To what class of materials do poly vinyl impression materials belong? 11.____

   A. Elastomers
   B. Inelastics
   C. Hydrocolloids
   D. Mucostatics

12. The danger of melting castings during soldering procedures stems from the fact that 12.____

   A. porcelain will vary in thickness over the metal surfaces
   B. the melting point of most solders is within 70°-90°F of the cast metal's melting point
   C. small bits of investment material may adhere to the castings before soldering
   D. the melting point of fluxes is unpredictable

13. Vacuum investment is not generally performed with phosphate-bonded investment materials because they 13.____

   A. are thin and form voids and bubbles under vacuum
   B. are used in high-fusion applications

C. tend to adhere to patterns under vacuum
D. have a high viscosity that can trap air in nooks and corners

14. Teeth described as "retruded" are inclined 14.___

A. facially
B. distally
C. mesially
D. lingually

15. The airbrush is the preferred method of applying opaque powder in the construction of a porcelain jacket crown, because it 15.___

A. is more precise
B. does not require heat during application
C. can be done with or without the coping
D. provides a more uniform thickness

16. A technician places a metal substructure on a tray, heats it in a furnace under vacuum for 10 minutes, and then rapidly cools it to room temperature. The technician is 16.___

A. pickling
B. tempering
C. degassing
D. degreasing

17. A technician has just finished making corrections to a stock porcelain facing. The next step would be to 17.___

A. smooth the facing with a polishing point and/or rubber wheel
B. rub glazing powder into the surface pores
C. scrub the facing with a brush and liquid detergent
D. clean the facing ultrasonically in a beaker of diluted detergent

18. Dental alloys are sometimes measured in pennyweights (dwt). 10 dwt is approximately equal to _______ grams. 18.___

A. 8
B. 10
C. 12
D. 16

19. Which of the following has a contour that would be altered by an open contact between maxillary central incisors? 19.___

A. Lingual embrasure
B. Cementoenamel junction
C. Cingulum
D. Interdental papilla

20. Each of the following is potential use of chloroform in a dental laboratory, EXCEPT 20.____

A. with rouge or disclosing wax, to aid in seating a porcelain facing onto a metal backing
B. with rouge, as an antiflux in soldering pontics and retainers
C. as a pickling agent
D. to clean porcelain veneers

21. A technician wants to create a die that is slightly larger than the prepared tooth. This can be accomplished by adding the gauging water 21.____

A. colloidal silica
B. borax
C. cyanoacrylate
D. potassium sulfate

22. An alginate impression has set prematurely. Possible explanations include each of the following, EXCEPT 22.____

A. Tray incompletely seated
B. Too much water
C. Prolonged mixing time
D. Room too warm

23. The development of a liquid phase during the melting of porcelain is known technically as 23.____

A. vitrification
B. sintering
C. condensation
D. fritting

24. After the postsoldering investment of a casting has set, all wax residues should be removed by 24.____

A. using a scalpel
B. flushing with boiling water
C. burnout
D. applying a solvent

25. Which of the following metal-ceramic alloys have the lowest strength? 25.____

A. Gold-platinum-palladium
B. Gold-palladium
C. High-palladium-content
D. Base metal

KEY (CORRECT ANSWERS)

1. D
2. D
3. A
4. D
5. A

6. C
7. D
8. A
9. C
10. D

11. A
12. B
13. D
14. D
15. D

16. C
17. A
18. D
19. D
20. C

21. A
22. B
23. A
24. B
25. A

EXAMINATION SECTION
TEST 1

DIRECTIONS: Each question or incomplete statement is followed by several suggested answers or completions. Select the one the BEST answers the question or completes the statement. *PRINT THE LETTER OF THE CORRECT ANSWER IN THE SPACE AT THE RIGHT.*

1. Which of the following wire forms is used to provide mechanical retention for an acrylic base? 1.____

   A. Deflection bend
   B. Helical finger spring
   C. Smooth curve bend
   D. Zigzag bend

2. Which of the following types of clasps offers the best retention? 2.____

   A. Circumferential
   B. Ball
   C. Adams
   D. Arrowhead

3. Diagnostic casts are typically NOT used for 3.____

   A. making orthodontic appliances
   B. treatment tracking
   C. educating patients
   D. legal documentation

4. After soldering a wire to a clasp, a technician observes that the solidified solder is porous. The most likely reason is that 4.____

   A. the solder was overheated
   B. the technician did not use flux
   C. there were impurities on the wire surface
   D. the technician used too much flux

5. One of the purposes of a palatal arch is to keep the molars from tipping ______ in response to forces from an occipital pull facebow headgear. 5.____

   A. mesially
   B. distally
   C. buccally
   D. facially

6. The preferred method of adding a spring action to a wire is to form a(n) 6.____

   A. right-angle bend
   B. helical bend
   C. smooth curve bend
   D. semicircular bend

7. Uses of the Hawley appliance include 7.
   I. maintaining space
   II. correcting crossbites
   III. closure of interdental spaces
   IV. rehabilitation of cleft palates

   A. I and II
   B. II only
   C. I, II and III
   D. I, II, III and IV

8. A wire designated "26 gauge" is ______ mm wide. 8.

   A. 0.15
   B. 0.35
   C. 0.65
   D. 0.90

9. The main difference between cobalt-chromium wires and typical stainless steel wires is that cobalt-chromium wires 9.

   A. are initially more bendable
   B. are useful in different phases of treatment
   C. do not require heat-treating for stiffening
   D. deliver about half the force levels for the same deflection

10. An orthodontic working cast is being poured into alginate impression material. Which of the following is true? 10.

   A. The bands should be pinned into place in the impression before pouring.
   B. The bands should be waxed into place in the impression before pouring.
   C. The technician should use plaster, not stone.
   D. Acrylic resin should be adapted to the appliance before pouring.

11. For the most part, springs are used with removable appliances to move teeth 11.
   I. buccolingually
   II. mesiodistally
   III. occlusogingivally

   A. I only
   B. I or II
   C. II or III
   D. I, II or III

12. When trimming a diagnostic cast, a technician should be careful not to trim any closer than about ______ cm from the vestibular areas. 12.

   A. 0.5
   B. 1.5
   C. 3.0
   D. 5.0

13. Which of the following types of clasps is most useful on the most distal teeth in the upper arch? 13.____

A. Circumferential or C
B. Arrow
C. Resta
D. Ball

14. Which of the following appliances would be used for deep bite correction for a patient with a deep overbite or excessive maxillary incisor display at rest? 14.____

A. Intrusion arch
B. Labial bow
C. Palatal arch
D. Herbst appliance

15. A labial bow spring is formed around the ______ anterior teeth. 15.____

A. 4
B. 6
C. 8
D. 10

16. A technician is examining a cast for asymmetry. The best way to do this is to 16.____

A. mount both casts in centric occlusion
B. observe the cast at a 90-degree angle, with grids for improving visualization
C. observe the casts from directly in the front and the back
D. mount one cast and tilt it forward about 30 degrees

17. Before finishing and polishing a diagnostic cast, a technician should fill small surface voids with plaster or stone. Just prior to doing this, the cast should be 17.____

A. soaked in clear slurry water
B. open out the void margins with a plaster knife
C. roughed up with fine sandpaper in the areas of correction
D. dried thoroughly

18. The term "functional appliance" means that the focus of the appliance is on the position of the 18.____

A. anterior teeth
B. mandible
C. palate
D. posterior teeth

19. A child needs a transpalatal arch, but will soon lose both second primary molars. Which of the following appliances is most appropriate as a substitute? 19.____

A. Modified Nance
B. Lingual arch
C. W-arch
D. Herbst

20. The labial bow of a Hawley retainer is typically made of ______ gauge stainless steel wires. 20

A. 16 to 18
B. 22 to 24
C. 28 to 30
D. 32 to 36

21. The side cut of the maxillary cast should be at an angle of about ______ degrees to the heel cut. 21

A. 25
B. 63
C. 87
D. 120

22. What is the term for the force system in a fixed appliance that provides control in three planes of space? 22

A. Moments
B. Arms
C. Couples
D. Mediation

23. Which of the following requires an edentulous area for placement? 23

A. Deflection bend
B. Labial bow spring
C. Lingual bow spring
D. Dumbbell spring

24. A technician is manufacturing a Bionator functional appliance. For most patients, the acrylic body of the appliance should allow for an interocclusal clearance of about ______ mm. 24

A. 1 to 2
B. 3 to 4
C. 5 to 6
D. 6 to 7

25. Advantages of removable appliances over bonded retainers include 25

I. reduced likelihood of breakage
II. variability of design
III. better oral hygiene
IV. flexibility in the amount of wear time

A. I and II
B. II, III and IV
C. III only
D. I, II, III and IV

KEY (CORRECT ANSWERS)

1. D
2. C
3. A
4. A
5. C

6. B
7. C
8. C
9. A
10. A

11. B
12. B
13. A
14. A
15. B

16. B
17. A
18. B
19. A
20. C

21. B
22. C
23. D
24. B
25. B

TEST 2

DIRECTIONS: Each question or incomplete statement is followed by several suggested answers or completions. Select the one the BEST answers the question or completes the statement. *PRINT THE LETTER OF THE CORRECT ANSWER IN THE SPACE AT THE RIGHT.*

1. Generally, the circumferential clasp 1.

   A. cannot be adapted to primary teeth
   B. has better retention than a ball clasp
   C. is difficult to form
   D. should be used only as an auxiliary clasp

2. A child has adequate space in the primary arch perimeter for the permanent teeth, but will lose her primary posterior teeth prematurely. This child is a candidate for the ______ appliance. 2.

   A. Hawley
   B. Transpalatal
   C. Herbst
   D. W-arch

3. Type ______ gypsum materials are most appropriate for orthodontic casts. 3.

   A. I
   B. II
   C. III
   D. IV

4. If the acrylic on a Hawley appliance is distorted, it is usually because 4.

   A. the impression was poured improperly
   B. wires were activated prematurely
   C. the resin was overheated during finishing and polishing
   D. a pressure cooker wasn't used

5. The "omega loop" of a labial bow spring should extend about ______ mm past the gingival margin. 5

   A. 1
   B. 2
   C. 3
   D. 4

6. Which of the following terms, applicable to the load deflection of orthodontic wires, is NOT synonymous with the others? 6

   A. Elastic limit
   B. Yield strength
   C. Proportional limit
   D. Ultimate tensile strength

7. Uses of a labial bow spring include 7._____
   - I. correcting minor rotations
   - II. positioning anterior teeth labiolingually (with a lingual finger spring)
   - III. closing spaces
   - IV. serving as a retention clasp in the anterior region

   A. I and III
   B. I, II and III
   C. II and IV
   D. I, II, III and IV

8. A technician wants to use an Adams clasp, but interocclusal space is available on only the mesial and distal sides of the tooth to be clasped. The next best choice for the technician would be a(n) ______ clasp. 8._____

   A. ball
   B. Resta
   C. circumferential
   D. arrow

9. Corner cuts on diagnostic casts are made on the maxillary and mandibular casts simultaneously, at an angle of ______ degrees to the heels. 9._____

   A. 25
   B. 63
   C. 120
   D. 142

10. The ______ consists of a wire embedded in an acrylic button on the anterior palate and soldered to bands on the maxillary first molars. 10._____

    A. Modified Hawley appliance
    B. Rapid palatal expander
    C. Herbst appliance
    D. Nance holding arch

11. The typical labial bow of a Hawley retainer passes through the occlusion between the 11._____

    A. lateral incisors and canines
    B. canines and first premolars
    C. first premolars and second premolars
    D. second premolars and first molars

12. When soldering a stainless steel wire to an orthodontic clasp, the fluxed solder joint should be heated for about ______ before adding the solder. 12._____

    A. 3 seconds
    B. 15 seconds
    C. 45 seconds
    D. 3 minutes

13. Many orthodontic technicians believe that it is often unnecessary to mount orthodontic casts because for most patients, 13.

A. orthodontic therapy will be completed before final maturation of the condyle/fossa relationship
B. they will not occlude in a useful way at any rate
C. a significant interarch discrepancy exists that will be easily observed
D. intercuspation is a secondary goal of treatment

14. Which of the following terms is used most often to refer to the relative mesiodistal movement of the anterior and posterior teeth? 14.

A. Extrusion
B. Anchorage control
C. Torque
D. Activation

15. Which of the following should be adapted to the patient's teeth BEFORE making an impression for the working cast? 15

A. Bands
B. Clasps
C. Wires
D. Acrylic resin base

16. Finger springs used with a removable appliance are typically formed from ______ -gauge stainless steel wires. 16

A. 12 to 14
B. 18 to 20
C. 22 to 26
D. 28 to 32

17. The main advantage associated with the Herbst appliance is 17

A. excellent retention of mandibular incisors
B. full-time wear
C. light "footprint" in patient's mouth
D. durability

18. No. 139 orthodontic pliers would be used to form each of the following, EXCEPT a 18

A. semicircular bend
B. closed end loop
C. deflection bend
D. zigzag bend

19. Differences between orthodontic casts and other dental casts include the 19

I. amount of the alveolar process displayed
II. degree to which the bases are symmetrical
III. way in which they are mounted on articulators
IV. level of detail on the occlusal surfaces

A. I and II
B. II only
C. II and III
D. I, II, III and IV

20. The heel cut of the maxillary cast should be perpendicular to the palatal midline and stopped about ______ mm distal to the deepest point of the pterygomaxillary notch area on either side. 20.____

A. 2
B. 4
C. 6
D. 8

21. Compared with stainless steel wires, nickel-titanium wires 21.____

A. are more rigid
B. bond better to acrylic resin
C. deliver lighter forces for large deflections
D. are composed of multiple strands

22. Probably the most widely used interceptive orthodontic device is the ______ appliance. 22.____

A. Transpalatal
B. Hawley
C. Herbst
D. Lingual arch

23. Which of the following is NOT a type of fixed appliance? 23.____

A. Maxillary expander
B. Lower lingual arch
C. Edgewise appliance
D. Hawley with jackscrew

24. Semicircular bends are used in orthodontic wires when 24.____

A. a spring action is needed
B. mechanical clasp retention is needed
C. the direction of the wire must change abruptly
D. teeth and soft tissues need to be avoided

25. The uses of transpalatal arches include 25.____
I. establishing and maintaining arch widths
II. preventing molar rotations
III. correcting mesiodistal asymmetries
IV. correcting third-order axial inclinations

A. I only
B. I and IV
C. I, III and IV
D. I, II, III and IV

KEY (CORRECT ANSWERS)

1. D
2. B
3. C
4. C
5. B

6. D
7. D
8. B
9. C
10. D

11. B
12. B
13. A
14. B
15. A

16. B
17. B
18. D
19. A
20. C

21. C
22. B
23. D
24. A
25. D

TEST 3

DIRECTIONS: Each question or incomplete statement is followed by several suggested answers or completions. Select the one the BEST answers the question or completes the statement. *PRINT THE LETTER OF THE CORRECT ANSWER IN THE SPACE AT THE RIGHT.*

1. Which of the following devices consists of a wire passing over the palatal vault and soldered to the first molars? 1.____

   A. Hawley appliance
   B. Edgewise appliance
   C. Palatal arch
   D. Herbst appliance

2. Because of its elasticity and tendency to retain its original shape, ______ orthodontic wire is usually difficult to adapt as an arch wire. 2.____

   A. nickel-titanium
   B. gold
   C. stainless steel
   D. chrome nickel

3. The acrylic resin base for an orthodontic appliance, such as a Hawley retainer, should be built up on a working cast to a thickness of about ______ mm. 3.____

   A. 1
   B. 2
   C. 3
   D. 4

4. On a Hawley retainer, occlusal rests 4.____

   A. are essential for mandibular appliances
   B. should be avoided in most situations
   C. are essential for maxillary appliances
   D. often substitute for circumferential clasps

5. A wire designated "18 gauge" is ______ mm wide. 5.____

   A. 0.30
   B. 0.45
   C. 0.65
   D. 0.80

6. When a wire for a modified Nance appliance is fitted into the palatal vault, there should be about ______ mm of space between it and the lingual surfaces of the maxillary teeth. 6.____

   A. 1 to 2
   B. 3 to 5
   C. 6 to 8
   D. 10 to 12

7. Which of the following is NOT a component of a typical Hawley appliance? 7.

   A. Springs
   B. Occlusal rests
   C. Clasps
   D. Labial bow wire

8. To return strength to an annealed wire, a technician should heat-treat it until it takes on a(n) ______ appearance. 8.

   A. cherry red
   B. bright orange
   C. amber or straw-colored
   D. dull white

9. When trimming a cast, the ______ cut is usually made first. 9

   A. heel
   B. base
   C. side
   D. anterior

10. The two most common "stress raisers" in orthodontic wires are 10

   A. gradual curves and loops
   B. sharp bends and coils
   C. coils and nicks
   D. nicks and sharp bends

11. As a general rule, the maximum distance for lip bumpers to placed away from the anterior teeth is about ______ mm. 11

   A. 1
   B. 2
   C. 3
   D. 4

12. Which of the following would be formed with a No. 200 orthodontic pliers? 12

   A. Semicircular loop
   B. Closed end loop
   C. Right-angle bend
   D. Smooth curve bend

13. The flexibility of stainless steel wires is modified by varying each of the following, EXCEPT their 13

   A. cross-sectional dimensions
   B. shape
   C. length
   D. alloy type

14. Before cementing a W-arch appliance, the appliance should be activated by 14.____

A. elongating the W shape anteroposteriorly 4 to 6 mm
B. spreading the W shape laterally 3 to 5 mm
C. spreading the W shape laterally 6 to 10 mm
D. heat-treating the wires

15. Which of the following is indicated when distal movement of a posterior tooth is needed to regain lost arch length? 15.____

A. T loop
B. Labial bow spring
C. Ball clasp
D. Slingshot spring

16. The point at which any greater force leads to permanent distortion of a wire is known as the 16.____

A. ultimate tensile strength
B. failure point
C. elastic limit
D. permanent bend point

17. Which of the following is a looped wire used to upright and extrude a tipped lower second molar? 17.____

A. Helical spring
B. T-loop
C. Dumbbell spring
D. Finger spring

18. Soldering flux used for stainless steel typically contains 18.____

I. Boric acid
II. Boric glass
III. Silica
IV. Fluoride

A. I and III
B. II, III and IV
C. II and IV
D. I, II, III and IV

19. Advantages of the arrowhead clasp include 19.____

I. no need to alter the working cast
II. excellent retention
III. no need for manufactured clasp material
IV. no need to add solder

A. I and II
B. I, II and III
C. II, III and IV
D. I, II, III and IV

20. The side cuts on a mandibular cast should be at an angle of ______ degrees to the heels. 20.

A. 25
B. 55
C. 120
D. 142

21. T-loops are useful for 21.

I. controlling buccolingual inclination of uprighted teeth
II. rotating molars
III. uprighting molars
IV. distalizing molars

A. I only
B. II only
C. I, III and IV
D. I, II, III and IV

22. Which of the following wire forms is used primarily to adapt wire to soft tissue and teeth? 22.

A. Zigzag bend
B. Deflection bend
C. Smooth curve bend
D. Right-angle bend

23. Adams clasps are typically bent from ______ -gauge stainless steel wires. 23.

A. 12 to 14
B. 18 to 20
C. 22 to 24
D. 26 to 28

24. When adapting a wire to make a lingual arch, the technician should first place the wire so that it 24.

A. extends 4 or 5 mm past the banded teeth
B. ends on the mesiolingual surfaces of the banded teeth
C. curves around the distal ends of the banded teeth
D. meets the bands in a butt joint

25. The acrylic body of a Hawley retainer should be polished smooth on the surfaces that touch the 25.

I. tongue
II. palate
III. alveolar ridges
IV. lingual surfaces of teeth

A. I only
B. I and IV
C. II and III
D. I, II, III and IV

KEY (CORRECT ANSWERS)

1. C
2. A
3. C
4. A
5. B
6. B
7. A
8. C
9. B
10. D
11. C
12. C
13. D
14. B
15. D
16. C
17. A
18. D
19. C
20. B
21. C
22. C
23. B
24. A
25. A

TEST 4

DIRECTIONS: Each question or incomplete statement is followed by several suggested answers or completions. Select the one the BEST answers the question or completes the statement. *PRINT THE LETTER OF THE CORRECT ANSWER IN THE SPACE AT THE RIGHT.*

1. Disadvantages associated with annealed orthodontic wires include 1.

   I. ease of distortion
   II. inelasticity
   III. relatively thin diameter
   IV. brittleness

   A. I and II
   B. II only
   C. III and IV
   D. IV only

2. Which of the following appliances is used to prevent mesial shift of the mandibular posterior teeth? 2

   A. Hawley appliance
   B. Modified Nance appliance
   C. Lingual arch
   D. W-arch

3. When applying the resin base to a working cast, the technician should 3

   A. build up the entire width at the same time
   B. extend the resin slightly past the outline form of the appliance
   C. vary the thickness of the resin along the lingual or palatal ridge
   D. use sticky wax on the lingual or palatal area to hold the wires in place

4. Most commonly, functional appliances are used to hold the mandible 4

   A. in a retrusive position to correct a Class II occlusion
   B. in a retrusive position to correct a functional anterior crossbite
   C. off to one side to correct an asymmetrical occlusion
   D. in a protrusive position to correct a Class II occlusion

5. The anchor teeth for a removable appliance are ideally clasped with a(n) ______ clasp. 5

   A. Adams
   B. C
   C. arrow
   D. ball clasp

6. Occlusal rests for a Hawley retainer are typically made of ______ gauge stainless steel wires. 6

   A. 18
   B. 24
   C. 28
   D. 32

7. Which of the following is NOT a procedure involved in bonding orthodontic brackets? 7.____

   A. Bonding with resin adhesive
   B. Etching the enamel with phosphoric acid solution for 30 seconds
   C. Rinsing enamel and leaving it moist
   D. Cleaning the tooth surface with pumice

8. What is the term for the maximum force a wire can withstand before it begins to weaken? 8.____

   A. Elastic limit
   B. Ultimate tensile strength
   C. Base shear
   D. Failure point

9. The force of a finger spring in a removable appliance should be applied at the level of the 9.____

   A. gingiva
   B. cervical third
   C. height of contour
   D. occlusal or incisal third

10. A technician is fabricating a lingual arch on the working cast. Care should be taken to keep the solder joint in the 10.____

   A. mesial aspect
   B. incisal third
   C. height of contour
   D. cervical third

11. Anterior cuts on a maxillary cast should be at angles of ______ degrees to the heel cuts. 11.____

   A. 25
   B. 63
   C. 120
   D. 142

12. The acrylic body of a Hawley retainer should be trimmed so that leaves a 12.____

   A. space of 0.5 to 1.5 mm short of the gingival margin
   B. space of 1.5 to 2.5 mm short of the gingival margin
   C. 1.5- to 2-mm band of acrylic touching the lingual surfaces of the teeth
   D. 2.5- to 3-mm band of acrylic touching the lingual surfaces of the teeth

13. Solder used to connect orthodontic wires and clasps differs from solder used with most dental precious metals. One of the most significant differences is that orthodontic solder 13.____

   A. does not require flux
   B. contains silver
   C. has a wider melting range
   D. has a lower melting point

14. In a lower lingual holding arch, the wire with adjustment loops is soldered to bands on the 14.____

   A. second premolars
   B. first molars

C. second molars
D. third molars

15. When forming a zigzag bend, the technician usually forms a series of bends at a(n) _______ -degree angle. 15.

A. 30
B. 45
C. 90
D. 135

16. When trimming a diagnostic cast, a technician should be careful to keep at least _______ cm from the pterygomaxillary notch areas of the maxillary cast and the retromolar pad areas of the mandibular cast. 16.

A. 2
B. 4
C. 6
D. 8

17. Forming the _______ clasp does NOT require the technician to create a depression in the embrasure area of the working cast. 17.

A. Adams
B. ball
C. arrowhead
D. circumferential

18. Which of the following types of appliances is used to correct posterior functional cross-bites in the primary and early mixed dentition? 18.

A. W-arch
B. Rapid palatal expander
C. Hawley
D. Modified Nance

19. Which of the following terms is used to describe the movement of a tooth toward the occlusal plane? 19

A. Eruption
B. Retrusion
C. Uprooting
D. Extrusion

20. Which of the following wire forms is used primarily to provide mechanical retention for clasps? 20

A. Closed end loop
B. Helical bend
C. Right-angle bend
D. Semicircular bend

21. Which of the following steps in forming an indirect lingual wire on a cast would be performed FIRST? 21.____

A. Positioning the wire with utility wax
B. Pumicing and cleaning the lingual surfaces of the lower anterior teeth
C. Bending the wire to conform to the lingual arch
D. Etching the lingual surface of the canines

22. Which of the following is NOT an advantage associated with the Hawley appliance? 22.____

A. Good oral hygiene
B. Excellent long-term retention
C. Allowance for settling of teeth after the removal of appliances
D. Facilitation of occlusion during wear

23. The omega loop of a labial bow spring begins at the middle of the 23.____

A. lateral incisor
B. first molar
C. first premolar
D. canine

24. Which of the following is a fixed appliance that helps expand the maxilla bilaterally to correct mild to moderate crossbites? 24.____

A. Utility arch
B. Quad helix
C. Lingual arch
D. W-arch

25. Selection of the proper wire size for an orthodontic appliance is based primarily on the 25.____

A. magnitude of forces and moments needed
B. difference in play between two similar wires
C. the load-deflection rate required
D. maximum elastic deflection required

KEY (CORRECT ANSWERS)

1. A
2. C
3. B
4. D
5. A
6. D
7. C
8. B
9. A
10. B
11. A
12. C
13. D
14. B
15. D
16. A
17. D
18. A
19. D
20. A
21. C
22. D
23. D
24. B
25. C

ORTHODONTICS / PEDODONTICS
EXAMINATION SECTION
TEST 1

DIRECTIONS: Each question or incomplete statement is followed by several suggested answers or completions. Select the one that BEST answers the question or completes the statement. *PRINT THE LETTER OF THE CORRECT ANSWER IN THE SPACE AT THE RIGHT.*

1. Properly contoured restorations for primary teeth serve to maintain 1.____

   A. interarch relationship
   B. proximal contacts and length of the dental arch
   C. vertical dimension by preventing overeruption of teeth
   D. all of the above
   E. none of the above

2. When the gingival wall of a Class II cavity preparation in a primary molar extends too far gingivally, a satisfactory gingival wall is difficult to obtain because the 2.____

   A. facial pulp horn is endangered
   B. proximal contact is broad and flat
   C. cervical enamel rods incline occlusally
   D. facial and the lingual surfaces are tapered
   E. primary molar has a marked cervical constriction

3. Defensive reactions of the tooth to dental caries include 3.____

   A. remineralization of enamel
   B. formation of reparative and sclerotic dentin
   C. formation of reparative dentin and salivary ions
   D. formation of sclerotic dentin and salivary enzymes
   E. formation of sclerotic dentin and salivary ions

4. Small, irregular, bright red spots on a child's buccal mucosa, with bluish-white specks in the centers, may be seen at the onset of 4.____

   A. mumps B. herpes C. leukemia
   D. rubeola E. rubella

5. Primary teeth discolored by trauma with no clinical signs of infection should 5.____

   A. be bleached
   B. be pulp tested
   C. receive root canal therapy
   D. be examined by periodic radiograph
   E. remain untreated

6. Cephalometrics is used in orthodontics to 6.____
   I. treat malocclusions
   II. study growth changes
   III. aid in diagnosis and case analysis

   The CORRECT answer is:

A. I, II
B. I, III
C. II, III
D. All of the above
E. III *only*

7. Placing the beaks of the forceps into the bifurcation of a primary mandibular second molar is CONTRAINDICATED when extracting th'e tooth of a 6-year-old patient because of the 7.___

A. thinness and the divergence of roots
B. proximity of the succedaneous tooth bud
C. possibility of crushing the facial plates of bone
D. marked convergence of the crown toward the occlusal surface
E. relatively large pulp chamber and the possibility of fracturing the crown

8. Ectodermal cells are responsible for 8.___

A. alveolar bone
B. periodontal tissue
C. cementum formation
D. determining crown and root shape
E. none of the above

9. Following removal of a relatively large area of decay in a recently erupted permanent molar, an exposure of the pulpal tissue is noted. The dentist decides to perform a pulpotomy using calcium hydroxide to treat the tissue remaining in the root canals. 9.___
The dentist would expect a dentin bridge to form at

A. a level somewhat below the amputation
B. a level halfway between the apex and the amputation
C. the exact level of the amputation
D. the apical site
E. any of the above

10. When handling an uncooperative child in the dental office, the BEST method of obtaining cooperation is to 10.___

A. use favors to persuade the child to cooperate
B. allow the parent to punish the child while in the dental chair
C. instruct the parent to return with the child when cooperation can be expected
D. display authority and command respect of the child by continuing with treatment
E. use physical force to keep the child in the chair so as not to harm himself

11. When dealing with decayed primary teeth, the BEST space maintainer is a 11.___

A. lingual arch
B. band and loop
C. properly restored tooth
D. functional, removable type
E. any of the above

12. A 7-year-old child has localized gingival recession between two teeth only. 12.___
The dentist should suspect

A. an oral habit
B. a chronic disease
C. a hereditary factor
D. poor eating habits
E. periodontosis simplex

13. An 11-year-old patient who is wearing a full-banded orthodontic appliance has inflamed gingiva. 13.____
The family dentist should

A. encourage better oral hygiene
B. perform deep scaling and curettage
C. perform gingivoplasty after the bands are removed
D. ask the orthodontist to remove the bands so healing can occur
E. none of the above

14. Crowding that occurs with mandibular incisors after age 18 is MOST often the result of 14.____

A. orthodontic relapse
B. periodontal disease
C. impacted third molars
D. a physiologic maturational change
E. impacted second molars

15. The BEST procedure to gain the cooperation of a child patient with a different cultural background is to 15.____

A. attempt to speak in his language
B. provide treatment under general anesthesia
C. communicate through an auxiliary who understands
D. demonstrate the procedure prior to performing it
E. ask his parent to explain the procedure to him

16. Pulp extirpation in primary teeth is mechanically difficult because of 16.____

A. sensitivity of primary pulps
B. lack of cooperation of children
C. tortuous anatomy and branching of canals
D. all of the above
E. none of the above

17. The 4-year-old child who is aggressive in his behavior in the dental office is USUALLY manifesting a basic 17.____

A. fear reaction
B. spoiled nature
C. reaction to rejection
D. reaction to underaffection
E. resentment against dentistry

18. In patients with severe Class II skeletal malocclusion, the cephalometric ANB angle MOST often approximates 18.____

A. -3° B. 0° C. 2° D. 8° E. -8°

19. Amalgam is most often the restorative material of choice for primary teeth. 19.____
The MOST important modification in its use for children is in the

A. cavity preparation
B. use of a rubber dam

C. use of a zinc-free alloy
D. condensation of the alloy
E. placement of matrix bands

20. An aphthous ulcer should be treated by 20._

A. palliation and patience
B. 50 mg. tetracycline q.i.d.
C. 125 mg, penicillin V q.i.d.
D. topical ethyl chloride spray
E. topical application of Mycostatin q.i.d.

21. An anatomic crossbite, as contrasted with a functional crossbite USUALLY demonstrates 21._

A. marked wear facets
B. smooth closure to centric occlusion
C. deviated closure to centric occlusion
D. symmetrical individual dental arches
E. none of the above

22. Clinical examination of a 15-year-old girl reveals permanent central incisors, permanent canines, and primary canines anterior to premolars.
This suggests 22._

A. a thumb-sucking habit
B. ankylosed primary canines
C. impacted permanent lateral incisors
D. congenitally missing permanent lateral incisors
E. slow erupting permanent lateral incisors

23. Among Americans, Angle Class II malocclusions occur 23._

A. rarely
B. in less than 15 percent of the population
C. in about 25 percent of the population
D. in almost 50 percent of the population
E. in more than 75 percent of the population

24. During routine examination, it is noted that a permanent tooth is trying to erupt while the primary tooth is still firmly in place.
The BEST course of treatment is to 24._

A. allow the primary tooth to exfoliate
B. luxate the primary tooth to facilitate its exfoliation
C. remove the primary tooth and allow the permanent successor to erupt
D. remove the primary tooth and place a corrective appliance immediately
E. any of the above

25. After age 6, the GREATEST increase in size of the mandible occurs 25.____

A. at the symphysis
B. between the canines
C. along the lower border
D. distal to the first molars
E. distal to the second molars

KEY (CORRECT ANSWERS)

1.	B	11.	C
2.	E	12.	A
3.	B	13.	A
4.	D	14.	D
5.	D	15.	D
6.	C	16.	C
7.	B	17.	A
8.	D	18.	D
9.	A	19.	A
10.	D	20.	A

21. B
22. D
23. C
24. C
25. D

TEST 2

DIRECTIONS: Each question or incomplete statement is followed by several suggested answers or completions. Select the one that BEST answers the question or completes the statement. *PRINT THE LETTER OF THE CORRECT ANSWER IN THE SPACE AT THE RIGHT.*

1. The undesirable side-effect MOST commonly associated with the use of a finger spring to tip the crown of a tooth is 1._

   A. pain
   B. gingival irritation
   C. tendency for the tooth to intrude
   D. severe mobility of the tooth
   E. tendency for the root apex to move in the direction opposite from the crown

2. A serious complication that can develop as a result of juvenile diabetes mellitus is 2._

   A. ataxia
   B. aphasia
   C. deafness
   D. blindness
   E. motor paralysis

3. A distal shoe space maintainer is indicated when a primary 3._

   A. canine is in crossbite
   B. first molar is prematurely lost
   C. second molar is lost after eruption of a permanent first molar
   D. second molar is lost prior to eruption of a permanent first molar
   E. none of the above

4. A 9-year-old epileptic has a petit mal seizure in the office. No other member of the office staff is available to render assistance. 4._
   The PROPER course of management is to

   A. administer oxygen
   B. inject a barbiturate
   C. wait until the episode passes
   D. inject epinephrine subcutaneously
   E. call the local emergency code for assistance

5. A radiograph of a 4-year-old child reveals no evidence of calcification of mandibular second premolars. 5._
   This means that

   A. these teeth may develop later
   B. the child will probably never develop second premolars
   C. it is too early in life to make final predictions concerning development of any permanent teeth
   D. primary second molars should be extracted to allow permanent first molars to drift forward
   E. any of the above

6. When treating rampant dental caries, the FIRST step is to 6.____

   A. restore all teeth with stainless steel crowns
   B. excavate softened tooth structure and temporize with zinc oxide-eugenol
   C. perform a diet analysis and apply topical fluoride solution to all teeth
   D. perform a prophylaxis, instruct in oral hygiene, and watch for improved habits
   E. apply topical fluoride, instruct in oral hygiene, and recall in three months

7. Gonion, menton, and pogonion are cephalometric landmarks located on the 7.____

   A. midline
   B. mandible
   C. bony chin
   D. skeletal profile
   E. none of the above

8. An EFFECTIVE method to determine the vitality of primary incisors after trauma is to use 8.____

   A. transillumination
   B. ultraviolet radiometry
   C. an electric pulp tester
   D. ice or hot gutta-percha
   E. none of the above

9. A MAJOR disadvantage of treatment using cervical headgear is 9.____

   A. impaction of maxillary canines
   B. extrusion of maxillary incisors
   C. extrusion of maxillary molars
   D. potential deformity of the neck
   E. psychologic trauma due to appearance

10. To minimize gagging and overcome fear in a child when taking alginate impressions, it is recommended to 10.____

    A. rinse the child's mouth with water
    B. secure the maxillary impression first
    C. secure the mandibular impression first
    D. discuss the procedure thoroughly beforehand
    E. none of the above procedures is particularly helpful

11. A periapical radiograph reveals a mesiodens in a 7-year-old boy. His maxillary right central incisor has erupted only partially. The maxillary left central incisor has not yet appeared. 11.____
    The PROPER procedure is to

    A. remove the mesiodens and observe progress carefully
    B. allow the mesiodens to erupt before attempting extraction .
    C. remove the mesiodens, band the unerupted central incisor, and institute orthodontic therapy
    D. allow the mesiodens and the right central incisor to erupt into the oral cavity to determine their relative positions
    E. any of the above

12. Chronic pulpal infection in primary molars is usually FIRST noted radiographically as 12.____

    A. internal resorption
    B. periapical bony change
    C. changes in the bony furcation

D. widening of the apical periodontal ligament space
E. none of the above

13. An early prepuberal growth spurt indicates 13._

A. a longer treatment time
B. a fast maturing child
C. a slow maturing child
D. nothing of interest
E. an endocrine dysfunction, such as hyperthyroidism

14. A purulent lesion in the facial vestibule of an 8-year-old patient is MOST likely a(n) 14._

A. pyogenic granuloma
B. odontogenic fistula
C. infected aphthous ulcer
D. isolated herpetic lesion
E. none of the above

15. A corrected anterior crossbite is BEST retained by 15._

A. overcorrection
B. normal incisor relation
C. placing a Hawley retainer
D. placing an acrylic palatal appliance with no labial arch wire
E. none of the above

16. Recurring tooth rotations occur MOST frequently after orthodontic correction because of 16._

A. density of the cortical bone
B. persistence of tongue and finger habits
C. persistence of free gingival and transseptal fibers
D. persistence of oblique fibers of the periodontal ligament
E. lack of follow-up retainer treatment

17. A light bluish, dome-shaped lesion on the inside lip of a 2-year-old child is MOST likely a 17._

A. mucocele
B. melanoma
C. hematoma
D. hemangioma
E. sucking callous

18. A maxillary central incisor erupting in a lingually directed path should be 18._

A. corrected before it reaches the occlusal plane
B. allowed to erupt until all incisors can be banded
C. allowed to erupt into crossbite and then corrected
D. ignored because pressures of the tongue will correct it as it erupts
E. ignored because pressures of the lip will cause the problem to recur

19. In an individual whose mandible is growing forward less than it should, the mandibular incisors will PROBABLY be inclined 19.

A. forward
B. backward
C. normally
D. backward and flared out
E. there is little relationship between mandibular growth and incisor inclination

20. The permanent maxillary first molar of an 8-year-old patient is extracted because of caries. 20.____
The BEST approach to manage this situation is to

A. place a space maintainer
B. surgically reposition the second molar
C. wait for the second molar to erupt and drift mesially into the space
D. extract the contralateral maxillary first molar to maintain integrity of the midlines
E. extract the contralateral maxillary first molar and place a space maintainer on each side

21. The downward and forward direction of facial growth results from 21.____

A. upward and backward growth of the maxillary sutures and the mandibular condyle
B. vertical eruption and mesial drift of the dentitions
C. interstitial growth in the maxilla and the mandible
D. epithelial induction at the growth centers
E. downward and backward growth of the maxillary sutures and the mandibular condyle

22. Radiographs of the jaws of a newborn child ORDINARILY indicate calcification of ______ teeth. 22.____

A. 12 B. 16 C. 20 D. 24 E. 28

23. Mesioangular ectopic eruption of a permanent maxillary first molar causing resorption of distal surfaces of the roots of the primary second molar should be treated by 23.____

A. extracting the primary second molar
B. disking the distal surface of the primary second molar
C. tipping the permanent first molar distally using a separating device
D. removing the soft tissue overlying the occlusal surface of the permanent molar
E. extracting the permanent maxillary first molar

24. The MOST frequent cause of fracture of root tips in extracting a primary molar is 24.____

A. ankylosis of the tooth
B. improper use of cowhorn forceps
C. presence of a supernumerary premolar
D. root resorption between the apex and the bifurcation
E. asymmetrical root resorption in which only one root is completely resorbed

25. An apparent unilateral crossbite involving the permanent maxillary first molar may be 25.____

A. associated with a mandibular shift
B. a bilateral constriction of the maxilla
C. corrected with palatal expansion
D. all of the above
E. none of the above

KEY (CORRECT ANSWERS)

1. E
2. D
3. D
4. C
5. A

6. B
7. B
8. E
9. C
10. C

11. A
12. C
13. B
14. B
15. B

16. C
17. A
18. A
19. A
20. C

21. A
22. D
23. C
24. D
25. D

TEST 3

DIRECTIONS: Each question or incomplete statement is followed by several suggested answers or completions. Select the one that BEST answers the question or completes the statement. *PRINT THE LETTER OF THE CORRECT ANSWER IN THE SPACE AT THE RIGHT.*

1. Radiographic examination of a 9-year-old patient reveals the pre-eruptive position of a mandibular second premolar tipped 20° from vertical. 1.____
The MOST appropriate action is to

   A. consider a surgical procedure to upright the tooth bud
   B. remove the primary second molar and place a space maintainer
   C. warn the parent that ectopic eruption will probably occur
   D. expect the tooth bud to correct itself as the tooth erupts
   E. extract the second premolar before it erupts

2. The MOST effective immediate action for a child who has accidentally swallowed 10 cc. of a 10 percent fluoride solution is to 2.____

   A. have the child drink copious quantities of water to dilute the solution
   B. have the child drink 10 percent sodium bicarbonate solution
   C. have the child drink milk or some other calcium-containing liquid
   D. send the child immediately to the emergency room of a hospital
   E. have the child drink water and send him home with the parents, instructed to watch for signs of reaction

3. At birth, jaws are large enough to accommodate 3.____

   A. primary incisors *only*
   B. all primary teeth, if they were to erupt simultaneously
   C. no teeth
   D. primary incisors and canines
   E. none of the above

4. An 11-year-old child is confined to a wheelchair. He has continuous involuntary movement of his head and extremities and difficulty in vocal communication. 4.____
The MOST probable cause of his condition is

   A. grand mal epilepsy
   B. muscular dystrophy
   C. ataxic cerebral palsy
   D. athetoid cerebral palsy
   E. none of the above

5. A dentist performing services for children should expect some youngsters to be frightened of dental procedures. The BEST way to help the patient overcome his fear is to 5.____

   A. ignore the fear
   B. identify the fear
   C. shift the patient's attention
   D. ridicule the child for being frightened
   E. tell him you will not hurt him

6. A 3-year-old patient is scheduled for extraction of a primary maxillary second molar. Adequate local anesthesia may be secured by administering 6.

A. a tuberosity block alone
B. buccal infiltration alone
C. buccal and palatal infiltration
D. a tuberosity block plus an anterior palatine block
E. a tuberosity block plus subperiosteal infiltrations for lingual and mesiofacial roots

7. Enlarged tonsils in a 6-year-old child are, at age 12, MOST likely to be 7.

A. larger
B. smaller
C. the same size
D. purulent
E. hyperemic

8. Impacted maxillary canines MUST be managed because 8.

A. they are apt to become ankylosed
B. they may damage roots of other teeth
C. good function is impossible without them
D. they will not erupt after root formation is complete
E. all of the above

9. The MOST common cause of Class I malocclusion is 9.

A. lack of sufficient tooth material
B. crossbite in the posterior segments
C. discrepancy between tooth material and supporting bone
D. improper eruption of permanent first molars
E. improper eruption of primary mandibular first molars

10. The condyle of the mandible grows by 10.

A. membrane bone growth
B. interstitial bone growth.
C. appositional bone growth
D. proliferation of cartilage
E. none of the above

11. Asymmetrical anterior open bite with normal posterior occlusion is characteristic of 11.

A. thumb-sucking
B. mouth breathing
C. abnormal swallowing habits
D. tongue- thrust ing
E. none of the above

12. A 9-year-old patient has marked crowding of anterior teeth. A space analysis indicates that maxillary and mandibular arches will be deficient 6 mm. of space for succedaneous teeth. 12
The dentist should

A. initiate serial extraction
B. refer the patient to an orthodontist
C. place active lingual arch appliances to align the teeth correctly

D. observe the patient carefully since the crowded teeth may improve with growth
E. none of the above

13. Relative to primary mandibular incisors, permanent mandibular incisors erupt 13.____

A. lingually
B. facially
C. distally
D. mesially
E. apically

14. Direct pulp capping is indicated for a primary molar with an exposure when there is 14.____

A. pain from the tooth when eating
B. a history of unprovoked or spontaneous toothache
C. radiographic evidence of internal resorption
D. little or no hemorrhage from the exposure site
E. pain from tooth only when in contact with something cold

15. In completing a medical history questionnaire, a mother indicates that her child is currently receiving Ritalin and Chlor-Trimeton daily. 15.____
To BEST manage this child, the dentist should

I. increase the doses of both drugs the day of treatment
II. increase the dose of Ritalin only the day before and the day of treatment
III. contact the child's physician
IV. further question the mother to determine the child's ability to undergo treatment
V. make no changes in the child's drug regimen

The CORRECT answer is:

A. I, III
B. II, III
C. II, III, IV
D. II, IV
E. III, V

16. A child with congenital heart disease requires special treatment planning for dental care because of potential problems with 16.____

I. bleeding
II. local infection
III. systemic infection
IV. enamel hypoplasia

The CORRECT answer is:

A. I *only*
B. I, II, III
C. I, III
D. III *only*
E. All of the above

17. Accepted methods for closing a diastema between maxillary central incisors include using 17.____

I. a lingual arch with finger springs
II. a rubber elastic around the two teeth
III. a steel ligature around the two teeth
IV. a Hawley appliance with finger springs
V. cemented orthodontic bands with intertooth traction

The CORRECT answer is:

A. I, II, III
B. I, III, IV
C. I, IV, V
D. II, III, V
E. II, IV, V

18. Continuous, heavy orthodontic forces employed in moving . teeth may cause 18._
    I. resorption of cementum
    II. resorption of dentin
    III. resorption of enamel
    IV. devitalized teeth
    V. undermining resorption of alveolar bone

The CORRECT answer is:

A. I, II, III B. I, II, IV, V C. I, IV, V
D. II, IV, V E. III, IV, V

19. A 12-year-old child has a normal complement of erupted permanent teeth with the exception of the mandibular left second premolar. The primary mandibular left second molar is still present. 19._
The prolonged retention may have resulted from
    I. trauma
    II. a nonvital pulp
    III. ankylosis
    IV. a missing left second premolar

The CORRECT answer is:

A. I, III B. I, IV C. II, III
D. II, IV E. III, IV

20. The crown of the permanent maxillary left central incisor of an 8-year-old child is discolored. The tooth was injured two weeks ago. It gives a negative response to ice and electric pulp tests. 20._
Which of the following can be said with REASONABLE assurance?
    I. There is hemorrhage into the pulp chamber.
    II. The tooth is nonvital.
    III. Nerve conduction from the pulp is impaired

The CORRECT answer is:

A. I, II B. I, III C. II, III
D. All of the above E. None of the above

21. A patient's chin and mandible deviate to the right upon opening. 21._
Which of the following is a POSSIBLE cause?
    I. Hyperplasia of the right condyle
    II. Hyperplasia of the left condyle
    III. Ankylosis of the right condyle
    IV. Ankylosis of the left condyle

The CORRECT answer is:

A. I, III B. I, IV C. II, III
D. II, IV E. III *only*

22. Which of the following is the PROPER sequence of procedures for molar uprighting? 22._
    I. Band
    II. Bridge
    III. Perform periodontal surgery
    IV. Separate
    V. Upright

The CORRECT answer is:

A. I, IV, III, V, II
B. III, I, V, IV, II
C. III, IV, I, V, II
D. IV, I, V, II, III
E. IV, I, V, III, II

23. Which of the following is the order of tooth extraction in a serial extraction procedure? 23.____

I. Primary canines
II. Selected premolars
III. Primary first molars

The CORRECT answer is:

A. I, II, III
B. I, III, II
C. II, I, III
D. II, III, I
E. III, I, II

24. The cranial vault increases rapidly in size the first few years postnatally and completes approximately 90 percent of its growth by 6 years of age. 24.____
This is typical of which of the following types of tissues?

A. Neural
B. Dental
C. Genital
D. Lymphoid
E. General (somatic)

25. How is tooth development affected by severe congenital heart disease? 25.____

A. It is delayed.
B. It is advanced.
C. Cyst formation is likely, but the effect is unpredictable.
D. Development of posterior teeth is advanced; development of anterior teeth is delayed.
E. It is unaffected.

KEY (CORRECT ANSWERS)

1. D
2. C
3. B
4. D
5. B

6. C
7. B
8. B
9. C
10. D

11. A
12. B
13. A
14. D
15. E

16. D
17. C
18. B
19. E
20. B

21. C
22. E
23. B
24. A
25. A

EXAMINATION SECTION
TEST 1

DIRECTIONS: Each question or incomplete statement is followed by several suggested answers or completions. Select the one that BEST answers the question or completes the statement. *PRINT THE LETTER OF THE CORRECT ANSWER IN THE SPACE AT THE RIGHT.*

1. An 8-year-old patient with all primary molars still present exhibits a cusp-to-cusp relationship of permanent maxillary and mandibular first molars. 1.____
The dentist should

   A. continue regular recalls
   B. plan serial extractions for more normal adjustment of the occlusion
   C. refer the patient to an orthodontist for consultation
   D. place a cervical headgear to reposition maxillary molars
   E. disk the distal surfaces of primary mandibular second molars to allow normal adjustment of permanent molars

2. A radiopaque area is observed in the dentin underlying a three-month-old Class II amalgam restoration. 2.____
Which of the following bases was used in this restoration?

   A. Calcium hydroxide
   B. Zinc oxyphosphate cement
   C. Zinc oxide and eugenol
   D. Zinc oxide and eugenol and formocresol
   E. Zinc phosphate paste

3. Stainless steel orthodontic arch wire can be hardened by 3.____

   A. tempering
   B. work hardening
   C. age hardening
   D. precipitation hardening
   E. heating

4. If the chronological age of the patient whose dental film is labeled A (see next page) is 10 years, his dental developmental age is 4.____

   A. delayed
   B. normal
   C. advanced
   D. precocious
   E. there is inadequate information to determine

5. The MOST probable diagnosis for the condition illustrated in the photograph labeled B (see next page) is 5.____

   A. scurvy
   B. leukemic gingivitis
   C. herpetic gingivitis
   D. gingival dehiscence
   E. juvenile periodontitis

Question 4 refers
to photograph A
at the right

A

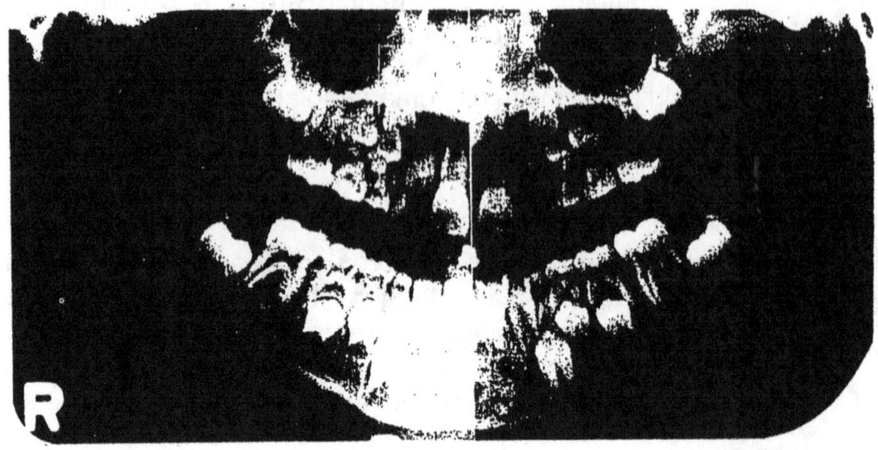

Question 5 refers
to photograph B
at the right

B

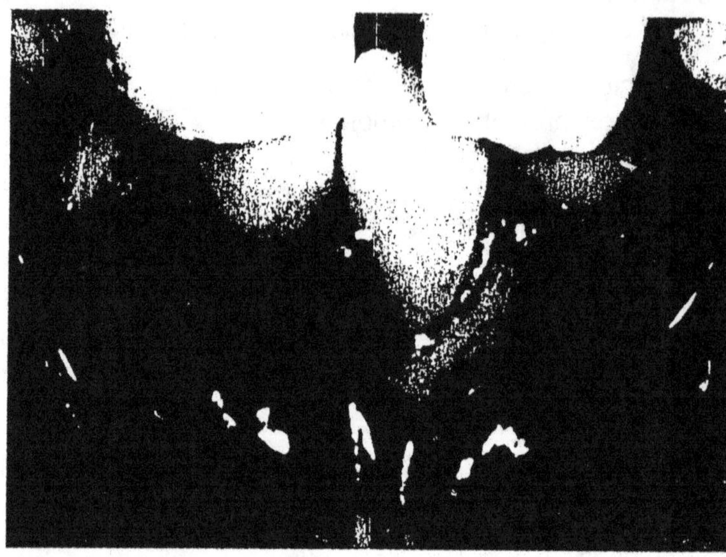

6. A 10-year-old patient exhibits slight crowding of mandibular anterior teeth with primary molars in various stages of exfoliation. 6.
The MOST appropriate approach to management is to

   A. observe the patient at six-month intervals
   B. observe the patient at yearly intervals
   C. obtain study casts and perform an arch length analysis
   D. delay treatment until all permanent teeth have completely erupted
   E. any of the above

7. In which of the following situations is space maintenance MOST difficult to manage? 7.
A ______-year-old patient with loss of a ______.

   A. 9 1/2; permanent maxillary first molar
   B. 5; primary maxillary central incisor
   C. 6; primary mandibular first molar

D. 7; primary maxillary second molar
E. 5; primary mandibular second molar

8. An early prepuberal growth spurt indicates 8.____

A. a longer treatment time
B. a fast maturing child
C. a slow maturing child
D. nothing of interest
E. an endocrine dysfunction, such as hyperthyroidism

9. When the orthodontic force applied is light, resorption will PROBABLY be 9.____

A. apical
B. direct
C. indirect
D. undermining
E. none of the above

10. A MAJOR disadvantage of treatment using a cervical headgear is 10.____

A. impaction of maxillary canines
B. extrusion of maxillary incisors
C. extrusion of maxillary molars
D. potential deformity of the neck
E. psychological trauma due to appearance

11. One of the GREATEST advantages of using extraoral anchorage is that 11.____

A. more force can be applied
B. it has a direct reciprocal action of the opposing arch
C. it permits posterior movement of teeth in one arch without adversely disturbing the opposite arch
D. it has parallel action of the opposing arch
E. none of the above

12. During the history-taking and interview with the parent of an 8-year-old patient, the information is elicited that the child is head-strong, willful, and given to temper tantrums. In his approach to the training of his child for the acceptance of treatment, the dentist will be required to 12.____

A. use a firm approach
B. depend upon mixed premedication
C. use physical measures to control the child
D. depend upon general anesthesia to treat this child
E. either B or D above

13. Following the growth rate curve typical for lymphoid tissue, tonsillar and adenoid tissue masses can be expected to show 13.____

A. continuous growth throughout life
B. a rapid increase in size at the time of puberty
C. a decrease in size beginning in the circumpubertal period
D. a progressively decreasing rate of growth from birth to adulthood
E. no significant increase in size between 4 and 10 years of age

14. Which of the following conditions is USUALLY present in a Class II, Division 2 malocclusion? 14.____

A. Open bite
B. Steep mandibular plane
C. Mesiocclusion of permanent first molars
D. Lingual inclination of maxillary central incisors
E. Lateral inclination of maxillary central incisors

15. An 8-year-old girl is admitted to the hospital for treatment of *swollen gums* of three weeks' duration. Oral examination reveals markedly edematous and erythematous gingivae. Her parents state that the child has been well although, in the past month, some malaise, anorexia, and occasional fever were noted. 15.____
The MOST appropriate course of action is to

A. refer the child to a periodontist
B. request a hematologic consultation
C. scale and curet the affected areas and prescribe mild rinses
D. prescribe a 10-day course of oral penicillin (1 million units per day)
E. enroll the child in an active prevention program that emphasizes adequate home care

16. A dentist performing services for children should expect some youngsters to be frightened of dental procedures. The BEST way to help the patient overcome his fear is to 16.____

A. ignore the fear
B. identify the fear
C. shift the patient's attention
D. ridicule the child for being frightened
E. have the parent talk to the child

17. Which of the following is the preferred procedure to anesthetize primary mandibular molars for restorative procedures? 17.____

A. Mental nerve block
B. Inferior alveolar nerve block
C. Infiltration around the teeth and the mental foramen
D. Buccal and lingual infiltration around the teeth
E. None of the above

18. A 9-year-old child has crowding of mandibular anterior teeth, an end-to-end molar relationship, and a Class II facial profile. The mixed dentition analysis shows a -4.4 mm. tooth size-arch length discrepancy in the mandible. 18.____
Which of the following is BEST management at this time?

A. Refer the child to an orthodontist.
B. Begin a serial extraction program to create room for posterior teeth.
C. Remove a mandibular lateral incisor to allow crowded anterior teeth to align themselves.
D. Do nothing because the probability is good that the child's apparent malocclusion is a transitional stage and future growth spurts will correct the problem.
E. Observe on a six-month recall basis.

19. On the first dental visit, the basic fear of a child under the age of 2 is related to 19.____

A. fear of an injection
B. anxiety over being separated from a parent
C. anxiety regarding the instruments used to perform dental treatment
D. not understanding the reason for dental treatment
E. fear of pain

20. An anatomic crossbite, as contrasted with a functional crossbite, USUALLY demonstrates 20.____

A. marked wear facets
B. smooth closure to centric occlusion
C. deviated closure to centric occlusion
D. symmetrical individual dental arches
E. none of the above

21. If the eruption sequence of permanent teeth is normal, one can expect maxillary 21.____

A. second premolars to precede maxillary first premolars
B. second premolars to precede maxillary canines
C. canines to precede mandibular canines
D. both A and C
E. both B and C

22. Treatment of a root fracture in the apical third of a permanent central incisor includes 22.____

A. extraction
B. calcium hydroxide pulpotomy
C. immobilization for 2-4 weeks
D. immobilization for 2-4 months
E. any of the above

23. A 9-year-old patient exhibits a lingually locked permanent maxillary left central incisor. Supporting bone is in harmony with tooth size, and there are no basic discrepancies in other relationships.
The MOST probable etiologic factor is v 23.____

A. premature extraction of the primary maxillary right central incisor
B. prolonged retention of the primary maxillary left central incisor
C. premature extraction of the primary maxillary left central incisor with space loss in the area
D. pronounced facioversion on eruption of the permanent mandibular left central incisor
E. none of the above

24. A child with Down Syndrome is characterized as being 24.____

A. affectionate
B. fearful of quick movements
C. capable of learning dental procedures
D. all of the above
E. none of the above

25. A 10-year-old patient has an end-on molar relationship in the mixed dentition. This will PROBABLY become a Class I molar relationship by 25._

A. the maxillary molar drifting posteriorly 0.9 mm.
B. the mandibular molar drifting forward 3.4 mm.
C. both molars drifting forward with the mandibular molar drifting about twice as far as the maxillary molar
D. orthodontic intervention *only*
E. it will never become a Class I molar relationship

26. Which of the following is the BEST indicator of success of a pulpotomy in an immature permanent tooth? 26._

A. Patient comfort
B. Stable vitality readings
C. Continuation of root formation
D. Formation of a dentinal bridge covering the pulp stumps in the root canal
E. All of the above

27. Excessive orthodontic force used to move a tooth may 27._

A. cause hyalinization
B. cause undermining resorption
C. crush the periodontal ligament
D. all of the above
E. only A and C above

28. The MOST stable area from which to evaluate craniofacial growth is the 28._

A. nasal floor
B. cranial vault
C. occlusal plane
D. nasomaxillary complex
E. anterior cranial base

29. How will extraction of a primary maxillary central incisor in a 5-year-old child with incisal spacing affect the size of the intercanine space? 29._

A. The intercanine space will increase in size.
B. The intercanine space will decrease in size.
C. No change will occur in the size of the intercanine space.
D. The change in space will depend on the spacing in the rest of the mouth.
E. None of the above

30. Severely crowded mandibular incisors USUALLY result from 30.

A. mesial migration of teeth
B. premature loss of primary teeth
C. presence of supernumerary teeth
D. tooth size-arch length discrepancy
E. any of the above

KEY (CORRECT ANSWERS)

1. A
2. A
3. B
4. A
5. D

6. C
7. E
8. B
9. B
10. C

11. C
12. A
13. C
14. D
15. B

16. B
17. B
18. A
19. B
20. B

21. B
22. D
23. B
24. D
25. C

26. C
27. D
28. E
29. C
30. D

TEST 2

DIRECTIONS: Each question or incomplete statement is followed by several suggested answers or completions. Select the one that BEST answers the question or completes the statement. *PRINT THE LETTER OF THE CORRECT ANSWER IN THE SPACE AT THE RIGHT.*

1. A healthy 8-year-old child has a fractured permanent central incisor. The pulp is widely exposed and vital. From radiographs, root ends appear incompletely calcified. The recommended procedure is to 1.___

   A. cap the pulp
   B. extract the tooth
   C. perform a pulpotomy
   D. remove the entire pulp
   E. place a sedative dressing and administer antibiotics

2. Surgical procedures on the maxilla may alter its 2.___

   A. anterior portion *only*
   B. posterior height *only*
   C. length and anteroposterior position *only*
   D. length, width, and height
   E. length and posterior height *only*

3. The permanent anterior tooth that is MOST often atypical in size is the 3.___

   A. mandibular canine
   B. mandibular central incisor
   C. maxillary canine
   D. maxillary central incisor
   E. maxillary lateral incisor

4. Which of the following procedures is used to prevent relapse after correction of a rotated permanent maxillary canine? 4.___

   A. Recontour of the crown
   B. Supracrestal fiberotomy
   C. Establishment of cuspid-protected occlusion
   D. Removal of all functional contacts with the canine in lateral and protrusive excursions
   E. None of the above

5. A 3-year-old child has a primary central incisor that has been completely intruded into alveolar structures without perforation of the labial plate. Radiographic examination reveals no root fracture or contact with the permanent successor. 5.___
   Treatment of choice is to

   A. prescribe antibiotic therapy and tetanus injection
   B. bring the tooth into position and ligate it
   C. perform a modified endodontic procedure immediately
   D. observe periodically for re-eruption
   E. extract the central incisor and place a space maintainer

6. Before eruption, the position of permanent mandibular incisor buds relative to primary incisors is _______ an 6.____

A. superior; facial
B. superior; lingual
C. inferior; facial
D. inferior; lingual
E. none of the above

7. Using a topical fluoride rinse before acid etch direct bonding of orthodontic brackets is contraindicated because fluoride 7.____

A. decreases the solubility of enamel
B. increases the pH of the etching agent
C. causes copious amounts of saliva
D. directly reacts chemically with the bonding agent
E. all of the above

8. If a 7-year-old patient loses a primary mandibular canine about the same time the adjacent lateral incisor is erupting or shortly thereafter, the dentist should be alert to the possibility of 8.____

A. a tongue habit
B. a developing crossbite
C. early eruption of the permanent canine
D. lingual collapse of mandibular anterior teeth
E. any of the above

9. Premature exfoliation of a primary canine may indicate a(n) 9.____

A. arch length excess
B. arch length deficiency
C. skeletal malocclusion
D. any of the above
E. none of the above

10. Fractured maxillary anterior teeth occur MOST often in children with 10.____

A. maxillary retrusion
B. Class I malocclusion
C. Class II, Division 1 malocclusion
D. Class II, Division 2 malocclusion
E. Class III malocclusion

11. Prognosis following fracture of the root of a permanent maxillary incisor is MOST favorable if the fracture is in the ______ of the root. 11.____

A. apical third
B. middle third
C. coronal third
D. either apical or coronal third
E. none of the above

12. When comparing cementum to bone in their responses to orthodontic forces, cementum resorbs 12.____

A. more readily
B. less readily
C. not at all

D. under lighter loads
E. by indirect (undermining) resorption

13. Which of the following is the BEST space maintainer? A 13.___

A. Nance holding arch
B. fixed lingual arch
C. band and loop appliance
D. removable acrylic appliance
E. pulpectomized primary molar

14. The gray color often seen in a traumatized primary incisor is the result of 14.___

A. pulpal hemostasis
B. internal resorption of dentin
C. diffusion of biliverdin into dentinal tubules
D. development of a heavy layer of secondary dentin
E. none of the above

15. At what stage of development of a tooth does dentinogenesis imperfecta occur? 15.___

A. Initiation
B. Proliferation
C. Histodifferentiation
D. Morphodifferentiation
E. Apposition

16. Calcification of teeth begins during which stage of pregnancy? 16.___

A. First trimester
B. Second trimester
C. Third trimester
D. Begins differently with each pregnancy
E. Either first or second trimester

17. A 9-year-old epileptic patient has a petit mal seizure in the office. No other member of the office staff is available to render assistance. 17.
The PROPER course of management is to

A. administer oxygen
B. inject a barbiturate
C. wait until the episode passes
D. inject epinephrine subcutaneously
E. call the local emergency code for assistance

18. Anodontia, diagnosed in a 5-year-old child, PRIMARILY affects the growth of the 18.___

A. midface
B. maxilla
C. mandible
D. alveolar bone
E. midface and the mandible

19. What is the recommended filling material for root canals of primary teeth? 19.___

A. Gutta-percha
B. Barium sulfate
C. Calcium hydroxide
D. Zinc oxide and eugenol
E. Zinc phosphate

20. The area in a Class II restoration in a primary molar MOST likely to fracture is the 20.____

A. isthmus
B. gingival margin
C. lingual margin of the occlusal aspect
D. facial margin of the interproximal aspect
E. any of the above

21. A 4-year-old child has a normal complement of primary teeth, but they are gray and exhibit extensive occlusal and incisal wear. Radiographic examination indicates some extensive deposits of secondary dentin in these teeth. 21.____
This condition is

A. neonatal hypoplasia
B. amelogenesis imperfecta
C. cleidocranial dysostosis
D. dentinogenesis imperfecta
E. none of the above

22. The average age at which calcification of crowns of permanent central incisors is completed is 22.____

A. birth
B. 2-3 years of age
C. 4-5 years of age
D. 6-7 years of age
E. 9-10 years of age

23. Which of the following statements BEST describes the relationship between fluorides and dental caries? 23.____

A. Children living in areas of endemic mottling tend to show a higher DMF index than those living in areas where mottling is rare.
B. Children living in areas of endemic mottling tend to show a lower DMF index than those living in areas where mottling is rare.
C. Children drinking optimal quantities of fluoridated water have about the same number of interproximal carious lesions but significantly fewer pit and fissure caries than do children who drink the same quantities of nonfluoridated water.
D. Optimal effects of fluorides can be achieved only at levels where mottled enamel also occurs.
E. None of the above

24. A 3 1/2-year-old child has an acute fever, diarrhea, oral vesicular lesions, and gingival tenderness. 24.____
The MOST likely diagnosis is

A. thrush
B. drug allergy
C. aphthous ulcerations
D. acute herpetic stomatitis
E. necrotizing ulcerative gingivitis

25. A 10-year-old girl with clinically normal occlusion reports for examination immediately after losing a primary mandibular second molar. 25.____
The dentist should

A. keep the patient under observation
B. place a lingual arch space maintainer
C. place a functional space maintainer
D. place a removable partial denture
E. base his choice of treatment upon radiographic findings

26. The MOST common response to frustration is 26._

A. denial
B. fantasy
C. aggression
D. submission
E. compensation

27. The MAJOR criterion to differentiate between a true Class III and a pseudo-Class III malocclusion is 27._

A. degree of anterior crossbite
B. presence of a bilateral crossbite
C. existence of a forward shift of the mandible during closure
D. occlusal relationship between maxillary and mandibular first molars
E. all of the above

28. When elastics are used to move teeth, they should be 28._

A. changed at least weekly
B. attached directly to the appliance components
C. placed directly around the teeth if possible
D. stretched to the maximum for controlled movement
E. both B and D

29. Caries activity is directly proportional to each of the following EXCEPT 29.

A. oral retention of fermentable carbohydrates eaten
B. frequency of eating fermentable carbohydrates
C. total daily intake of fermentable carbohydrates
D. physical form of food items eaten containing fermentable carbohydrates
E. all of the above

30. Which of the following is LEAST likely to result from persistent long-term thumb-sucking? 30._

A. A deep overbite
B. Protrusion of maxillary incisors
C. Constriction of maxillary arch
D. Rotation of maxillary lateral incisors
E. Lingual inclination of mandibular incisors

KEY (CORRECT ANSWERS)

1. C
2. D
3. E
4. B
5. D

6. D
7. A
8. D
9. B
10. C

11. A
12. B
13. E
14. C
15. C

16. B
17. C
18. D
19. D
20. A

21. D
22. C
23. B
24. D
25. E

26. C
27. C
28. B
29. C
30. A

TEST 3

DIRECTIONS: Each question or incomplete statement is followed by several suggested answers or completions. Select the one that BEST answers the question or completes the statement. *PRINT THE LETTER OF THE CORRECT ANSWER IN THE SPACE AT THE RIGHT.*

1. A bimaxillary protrusion occurs when 1.

   A. a large horizontal overlap with bilateral crossbite exists
   B. the maxillary dentition is forward with respect to basal bone
   C. both dental arches are forward with respect to basal bone
   D. both dental arches are posterior with respect to basal bone
   E. none of the above

2. Radiographic examination of a child reveals several missing primary and permanent teeth. No teeth have been extracted. Medical history indicates practically no perspiration during hot, summer months. 2.
   These facts suggest a preliminary diagnosis of

   A. achondroplasia
   B. osteogenesis imperfecta
   C. cleidocranial dysostosis
   D. anhidrotic ectodermal dysplasia
   E. diabetes mellitis

3. Which of the following dental sequelae is LIKELY in a child with a history of generalized growth failure (*failure to thrive*) in the first six months of life? 3.

   A. Retrusive maxilla
   B. Enamel hypoplasia
   C. Retrusive mandible
   D. Small permanent teeth
   E. Dentinogenesis imperfecta

4. Spread of odontogenic infection into the lymphatic chain of the neck is detected by 4.

   A. angiography
   B. laminography
   C. hematologic examination
   D. biopsy of cervical nodes
   E. palpation of the cervical region

5. Prolonged retention of a primary tooth may cause 5

   A. resorption of roots of adjacent teeth
   B. warping of the alveolar bone in the area
   C. ankylosis of succeeding permanent tooth buds
   D. a change in the path of eruption of the succeeding tooth
   E. any of the above

6. The MAJOR source of anchorage in a maxillary Hawley appliance is the 6

A. molar clasp
B. labial bow
C. acrylic portion
D. interproximal clasp
E. bracket of the band

7. Orthodontic correction of which of the following is MOST easily retained? 7.____

A. Diastema
B. Rotation
C. Expansion
D. Posterior crossbite
E. Anterior crossbite

8. Genetic influences on physical growth of a child are 8.____

A. apparent from examination of the parents
B. apparent from examination of the siblings
C. easily isolated by examination of the child
D. not necessarily apparent from examination of the parents or the siblings
E. only apparent from examination of both parents and siblings

9. Radiographic examination of a permanent first molar with an early acute pulpal abscess in a 9-year-old child would reveal 9.____

A. involvement of the bifurcation
B. little change from normal structure
C. a large area of periapical bone rarefaction
D. a disturbance in the integrity of the periodontal ligament
E. none of the above

10. A distal shoe space maintainer is indicated when a primary 10.____

A. incisor is avulsed
B. first molar is prematurely lost
C. second molar is lost after eruption of a permanent first molar
D. second molar is lost before eruption of a permanent first molar
E. none of the above

11. The MOST frequent cause of fracture of a root tip during extraction of a primary molar is 11.____

A. ankylosis of the tooth
B. improper use of cowhorn forceps
C. presence of a supernumerary premolar
D. root resorption between the apex and the bifurcation
E. asymmetric root resorption in which only one root is completely resorbed

12. A permanent maxillary first molar of an 8-year-old patient is extracted because of caries. Appropriate treatment is to 12.____

A. place a space maintainer
B. reposition surgically the second molar
C. wait for the second molar to erupt and drift mesially into the space
D. extract the contralateral maxillary first molar to maintain integrity of the midlines
E. any of the above

13. An 11-year-old girl complains of discomfort in her primary maxillary right second molar when masticating. The tissue is slightly inflamed in the immediate area. There is no swelling, but the tooth is quite mobile. A large mesio-occlusal restoration is present. There is no pain upon application of hot or cold. 13.___
The MOST probable diagnosis is

A. hyperemic pulpitis
B. traumatic occlusion
C. acute serous pulpitis
D. an exfoliating tooth
E. advanced internal resporption

14. In serial extraction procedures, concerns about eruption sequence are USUALLY related to the eruption pattern of 14.___

A. primary first molars
B. permanent maxillary canines
C. permanent mandibular first molars and incisors
D. permanent mandibular canines and first premolars
E. all molars

15. An 8-year-old girl with Class I occlusion lost both maxillary central incisors in an accident. 15.___
The BEST treatment is to

A. observe
B. move lateral incisors into central incisor positions
C. construct and place a space maintainer with bands cemented on lateral incisors
D. construct and place a permanent prosthesis using lateral incisors as abutments
E. place a temporary prosthesis supplying artificial crowns for the lost central incisors

16. In a child, a combination of malnutrition, steatorrhea, chronic respiratory infections, thyroid deficiency, a great salt loss through the skin, and functional disturbances in secretory mechanisms of various glands is indicative of 16.___

A. cystic fibrosis
B. starch intolerance
C. Pierre Robin syndrome
D. immune deficiency syndrome
E. hereditary fructose intolerance

17. Transillumination of soft tissues is useful in detecting which of the following problems in a child? 17.___

A. Koplik's spots
B. Sialolithiasis
C. Aortic stenosis
D. Sickle cell disease
E. Abnormal frenum attachment

18. Treatment of severe intraoral infections in children differs from that in adults because 18.___

A. allergy to penicillin is more common in children than in adults
B. the incidence of bleeding diathesis is greater in children than in adults

C. leukocytopenia develops more frequently in children than in adults
D. dehydration occurs more rapidly and more severely in children than in adults
E. children are more anxious than adults

19. In festooning and trimming a stainless steel crown, greater length is necessary in the region of the mesio-facial bulge in a primary 19.____

A. first molar
B. second molar
C. maxillary canine
D. maxillary lateral incisor
E. central incisor

20. Cephalometrics is an aid in orthodontic treatment planning because it provides information about the 20.____

I. relationship of maxillary and mandibular basal bone to the cranial base
II. relationship of maxillary anterior teeth to the maxillary basal bone
III. relationship of mandibular anterior teeth to the mandibular basal bone
IV. relationship of maxillary and mandibular teeth to one another
V. progress of orthodontic treatment

The CORRECT answer is:

A. I, II, III
B. I, II, III, IV
C. I, IV, V
D. II, III, V
E. All of the above

21. Nitrous oxide-oxygen analgesia is of value in behavior management of children because it 21.____

I. prolongs the effects of local anesthesia
II. shortens treatment time by eliminating the need for tell-show-do
III. calms children who are uncooperative and defiant at the beginning of treatment
IV. can be counted on to provide the same effect on each patient and, therefore, make the dentists' job easier

The CORRECT answer is:

A. I, III
B. II, III
C. II, IV
D. III, IV
E. None of the above

22. Which of the following are LIKELY to occur during orthodontic therapy? 22.____

I. Gingival irritation
II. Cementum resorption
III. Increased mobility of teeth
IV. Demineralization of enamel adjacent to appliances in patients with poor oral hygiene

The CORRECT answer is:

A. I, III, IV
B. I, IV
C. II, III
D. II, III, IV
E. All of the above

23. An 8-year-old girl has a 2 mm. diastema between permanent maxillary central incisors. Permanent maxillary lateral incisors are in position. 23.____
The diastema is PROBABLY the result of

I. thumb-sucking
II. an abnormal frenum attachment
III. a normal developmental process

The CORRECT answer is:

A. I *only* B. I, II C. I, III
D. II *only* E. III *only*

24. The normal downward and forward direction of facial growth results from 24._
   I. upward and backward growth of maxillary sutures and the mandibular condyle
   II. vertical eruption and mesial drift of the dentitions
   III. interstitial growth in the maxilla and the mandible
   IV. epithelial induction at growth centers

   The CORRECT answer is:

   A. I, II B. I, III C. I, IV
   D. II, III E. II, IV

25. Dens in dente is FREQUENTLY associated with 25._
   I. supernumerary teeth
   II. errors in apposition
   III. maxillary lateral incisors
   IV. pulp exposures

   The CORRECT answer is:

   A. I, II B. I, III C. I, IV
   D. II, IV E. III, IV

26. In planning treatment for an 8-year-old child, a history of thumb-sucking until age 4 should lead the dentist to suspect 26._
   I. behavior problems due to maternal dependence
   II. behavior problems due to unusual independence
   III. malocclusion problems due to severe open bite
   IV. malocclusion problems due to retarded growth of the mandible

   The CORRECT answer is:

   A. I, III B. I, IV C. II, III
   D. II, IV E. None of the above

27. Which of the following should be described in an orthodontic examination? 27._
   I. Tongue
   II. Gingivae, faucial pillars, and throat
   III. Malposed individual teeth and occlusal relationships of teeth
   IV. Number of teeth, size of teeth, and sequence and position of erupting teeth

   The CORRECT answer is:

   A. I, II, III B. I, II, IV C. I, III, IV
   D. II, III, IV E. All of the above

28. After approximately 7 years of age, the mandible increases in size by 28._
   I. generalized deposition of bone on free surfaces of the mandible
   II. condylar growth
   III. interstitial growth
   IV. growth on the posterior border of the ramus
   V. deposition of bone on the alveolar process

   The CORRECT answer is:

   A. I, II, V B. I, III, IV C. II, III, IV
   D. II, IV, V E. III, IV, V

29. The MAIN advantages of using a rubber dam are that it 29.____
    I. muffles cries of a child
    II. aids in management of child behavior
    III. reduces the danger of aspiration of debris
    IV. reduces the necessity to burnish amalgam margins
    V. permits greater control of the operating field

The CORRECT answer is:

A. I, II, III B. I, IV C. II, III, V
D. II, IV, V E. III, IV, V

30. Which of the following are appropriate for managing children in the dental office? 30.____
    I. Reward appropriate behavior
    II. Be prepared and expect the child to be a problem
    III. Set limits on undesirable behavior
    IV. Point out to the child that it is silly to be afraid of going to the dentist
    V. Obtain adequate anesthesia where indicated

The CORRECT answer is:

A. I, II, IV B. I, III, IV C. I, III, V
D. II, IV, V E. II, III, V

KEY (CORRECT ANSWERS)

1.	C	16.	A
2.	D	17.	B
3.	B	18.	D
4.	E	19.	A
5.	D	20.	E
6.	C	21.	E
7.	E	22.	E
8.	D	23.	E
9.	B	24.	A
10.	D	25.	E
11.	D	26.	E
12.	C	27.	E
13.	D	28.	D
14.	D	29.	C
15.	E	30.	C

BASIC FUNDAMENTALS OF DENTAL HISTOLOGY

CONTENTS

BASIC FUNDAMENTALS OF
DENTAL HISTOLOGY

Section I. INTRODUCTION

1. General

Histology is a branch of anatomy which deals with the microscopic study of the structure, composition, and functions of tissues. Dental histology concerns this type of study of dental tissues. A knowledge of the nature, composition, arrangement, and function of the tissues of the teeth and their supporting structures is essential to an understanding of the effects of disease, and of various dental treatment procedures, on these tissues.

2. Tissues of the Tooth

A tooth is made of four separate tissues. One of these, the dental pulp, is a soft tissue which occu-

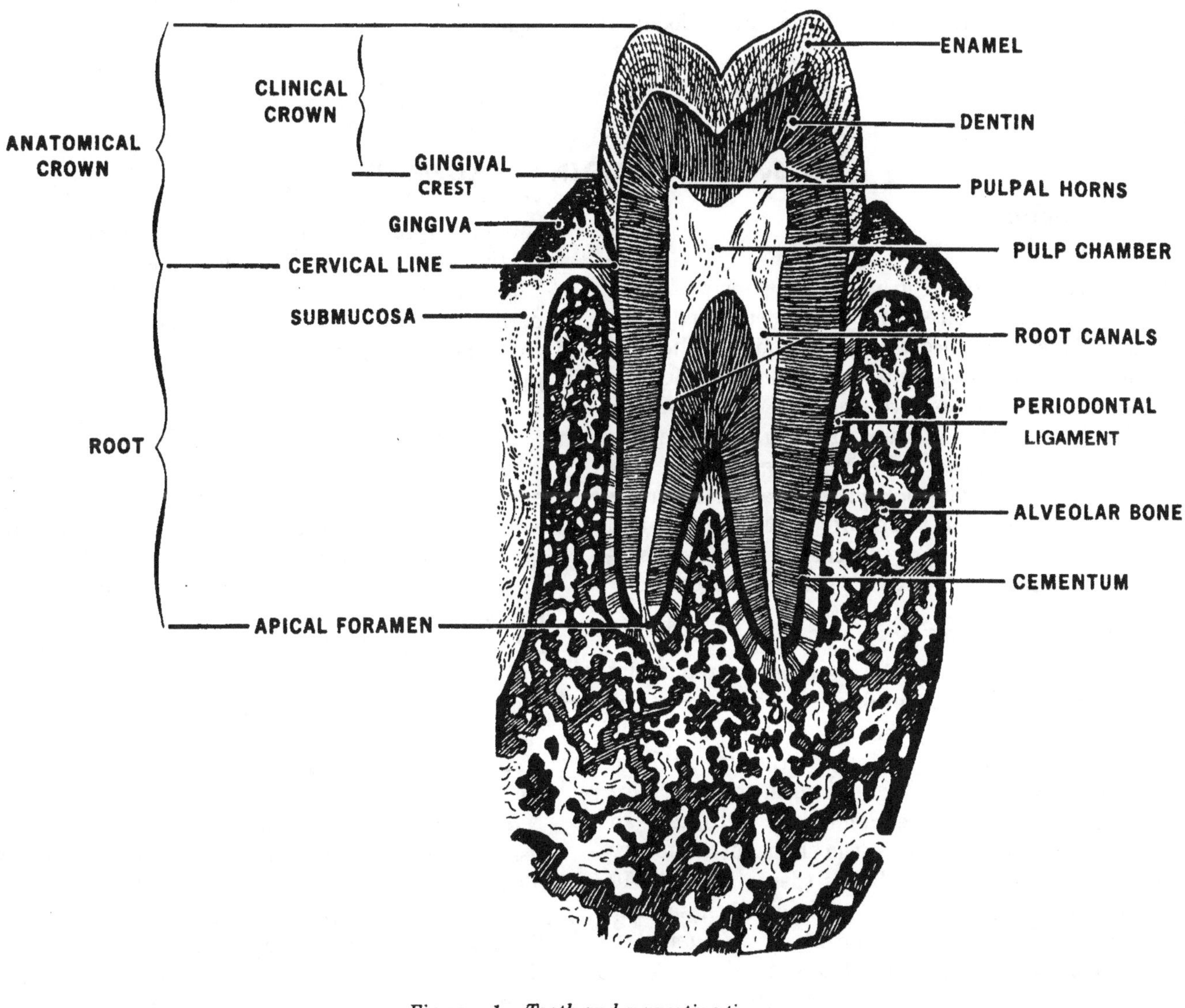

Figure 1. Tooth and supporting tissues.

pies a space within the body of the tooth. This space takes the form of a chamber within the crown of the tooth (pulp chamber) and of canal-like extensions running through each root of the tooth (root canals). The other three tissues—dentin, enamel, and cementum—are hard tissues containing a high percentage of mineral salts. Dentin comprises the bulk of the tooth, entirely enclosing the pulp except at the apex of the root where blood vessels and nerves enter the tooth through an opening called the apical foramen. Enamel, the hardest of the body tissues, covers the crown of the tooth. Cementum, which is similar to bone in its chemical composition and structure, covers the root of the tooth.

3. Tissues Which Support the Teeth

Certain tissues which are adjacent to the teeth provide their support and are related to their functions. These tissues are the alveolar bone, the periodontal ligament, and the gingiva (gum tissue). The roots c teeth are embedded in bony sockets (alveoli) in th alveolar processes of the jaws (fig. 1). Microscop cally, there is normally a space between the cemer tal covering of a tooth root and the walls of its a veolus. This space is occupied by the periodont ligament, a white fibrous connective tissue. Th fibers of this ligament actually serve to suspend th tooth in its socket (para 27). Thus, the tooth i allowed a slight movement in every direction, whic absorbs the shock of mastication. The gingivae that part of the soft oral mucous membran (epithelial tissue lining the oral cavity) that cove the alveolar process of the jaws and surrounds th necks of the teeth. The marginal gingiva encircle the necks of the teeth and, being closely adapted t the tooth in its healthy state, prevents particles c food from lodging and impinging on the periodont ligament (fig. 1).

Section II. TOOTH DEVELOPMENT

4. General

(fig. 2)

The processes involved in the development of teeth are closely interrelated, interdependent, and complex. Enamel is formed from embryonic epithelium. Dentin, dental pulp, and cementum are formed from embryonic connective tissue, but the processes by which these three tissues are formed correspond closely to, and appear to be influenced by, the various stages in the development of enamel. Even the formation of root dentin apparently is initiated, and the outline determined, by extensions of the enamel-forming epithelium (Hertwig's epithelial sheath).

5. Dental Lamina

a. Tooth development is preceded at about the sixth week of intra-uterine life by the extension or growth of bands of epithelium of the embryonic mouth into the underlying connective tissue. Two such bands of epithelium, one to form the maxillary teeth and one to form the mandibular teeth, take an archlike form to conform to the shape of the future jaws. From each of these bands (dental lamina) 10 budlike growth centers develop. Each of these buds of epithelium is the tissue from which the enamel of a primary (temporary or deciduous) tooth will arise.

b. Further extensions of the dental lamina will give rise to epithelial tooth buds which are destined to be enamal-forming organs of the permanent molar teeth. Enamel of the six anterior permanent teeth and the permanent bicuspids is formed by epithelial outgrowths from the enamel-forming organ of the temporary teeth which they later replac The epithelium which is to give rise to enamel c permanent teeth remains relatively dormant unt the time for permanent tooth development to tak place.

6. Enamel Formation

The buds of epithelium which are to give rise t enamel undergo a period of cell differentiation an arrangement preparatory to the formation of enam el. In its final form, just before formation of th first identifiable tooth structure, the enamel-formin epithelium has differentiated and become arrange into a specialized bell-shaped structure known a the enamel organ. The epithelium lining the ename organ has assumed the outline of the inner layer c the future enamel, and the innermost cells at the ti of the cusp or incisal edge have differentiated int columnar, enamel-forming cells called ameloblasts.

a. Ameloblasts begin to lay down partly calcifie tissue in the form of rods. This is the first ename formed on the newly developing teeth. Each amelc blast continues to lay down its individual rod fror the inside outward at approximate right angles t the inner surface of the developing enamel. A each ameloblast begins to form enamel, adjacen cells differentiate into ameloblasts and enter int the formative process. Enamel, then, is deposited i the shape of rods, starting on the inside and prc gressing toward the surface. It starts in the incisa

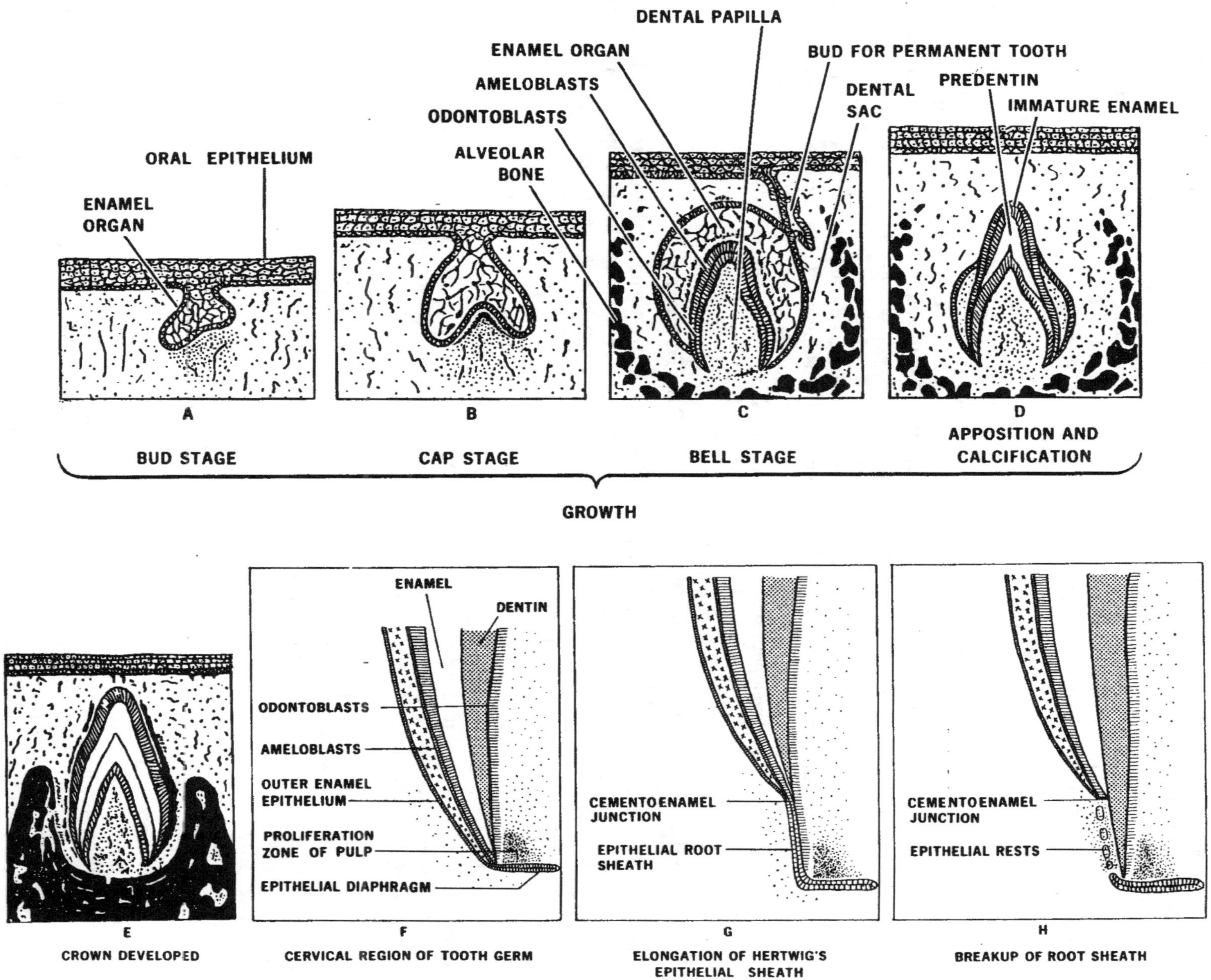

Figure 2. Early stages in tooth development (diagrammatic).

or occlusal area and progresses toward the root to end at the future junction of the enamel with the cementum of the root (cementoenamel junction).

b. Final calcification of enamel takes place after the ameloblasts have completed formation of the partly calcified enamel. The first portions of enamel to be completely calcified are those portions forming the incisal edges or the tips of cusps.

7. Dentin Formation

a. Crown. Formation of enamel organ to assume the shape of the future dentinoenamel junction is accompained by cell multiplication (proliferation) and cell specialization (differentiation) of the adjacent connective tissue. That connective tissue which pushes into, and becomes enclosed within, the "hollow" of the enamel organ becomes known as the dental papilla. The dental papilla gives rise to the dentin and to the pulp of the developing tooth.

(1) Immediately following the differentiation of epithelial cells into ameloblasts, connective tissue cells of the dental papilla adjacent to the ameloblasts elongate to form a layer of dentin-forming cells called odontoblasts. Formation of ameloblasts continues to be followed by formation of odontoblasts within the crown of the tooth.

(2) As each odontoblast is formed, it begins to lay down an incompletely calcified form of dentin known as predentin. Each odontoblast moves from without inward leaving a fibrous extension covered with immature dentin behind it. Predentin is converted to mature dentin through a continuing process of calcification which follows the formation of predentin.

(3) As the approximate size and shape of the normal pulp chamber is approached, the rate of dentin formation is diminished. Dentin formation continues to some extent throughout the life of the tooth, however, as a means of protecting the pulp and as a natural aging process.

(4) Dentin formation, then, takes place from without inward, and as this occurs, each odontoblast leaves behind a protoplasmic extension which is called Tomes' fiber. The Tomes' fibers occupy spaces within the dentin which are known as dentinal tubules. Tomes' fibers are believed to be associated with the transmission of pain sensation and with physiologic changes which sometimes occur in the dentin.

b. Root. Although ameloblasts differentiate before odontoblasts in the crown of the tooth, the first identifiable tooth tissue formed is dentin. The formation of enamel seems to depend on the presence of some previously formed dentin. Similarly, the differentiation of odontoblasts and the outline of the initial layer of newly formed dentin seems to be influenced by the presence of epithelium. In the crown this influence is provided by the enamel organ. Following formation of enamel, epithelium from the enamel organ extends rootward into the underlying connective tissue in the form of a sheath (Hertwig's epithelial sheath) having the outline of the future root dentin. Development and growth of this sheath is followed by differentiation of odontoblasts and laying down of dentin in a continuation of, and in the same manner as in the development of the dentin in the crown. Remnants of Hertwig's epithelial sheath may cause cysts of epithelial origin later in life.

8. Pulp Formation

That connective tissue of the dental papilla which becomes inclosed within the developing dentin continues to occupy the space within the dentin and becomes the dental pulp.

9. Cementum, Periodontal Ligament, and Bone Formation

During the development of enamel and dentin, surrounding connective tissue begins to take on a fibrous form and is known as the dental sac. As the root sheath extends and stimulates the production of odontoblasts and as dentin formation of the root begins, the connective tissue of this dental sac begins to proliferate and extends between the cells of the epithelial sheath of Hertwig, causing it to break into a network of epithelial strands. The connective tissue cells of the sac then undergo differentiation and specialization to form the cementum, periodontal ligament, and alveolar bone. The multipotential fibroblast cells of the dental sac first differentiate into cementoblasts which deposit a bone-like tissue (cementum) upon the dentin of the root of the tooth. Fibroblasts also synthesize and secrete collagen to form the periodontal ligament. Other fibroblasts differentiate into osteoblasts to form the alveolar bone which will support the tooth.

Section III. TOOTH ERUPTION

10. General

Many theories have been presented on the causes of tooth eruption. Among the factors which have been considered are growth of the root, growth of dentin, pressure from muscular action, formation and resorption of bone, proliferation of dental tissues, and pressure from blood vessels of the pulp and periapical tissue. Conflicting theories indicate the actual cause of tooth eruption is not known. However, the various steps in the process of tooth eruption can be described. Tooth eruption occurs in two phases, active and passive.

a. Active eruption is the first phase. During this phase the tooth moves from a position imbedded in the tissues of the jaws to a position in which the crown portion of the tooth has penetrated the mucous membrane of the mouth and come into its functional relationship with the teeth of the opposing jaw. The age at which active eruption of each tooth occurs is fairly consistent from person to person.

b. Passive eruption is a normal process in which the epithelial attachment recedes upon the surface of the tooth to expose more and more of the tooth surface. The rate and degree of passive eruption vary widely from person to person and tooth to tooth.

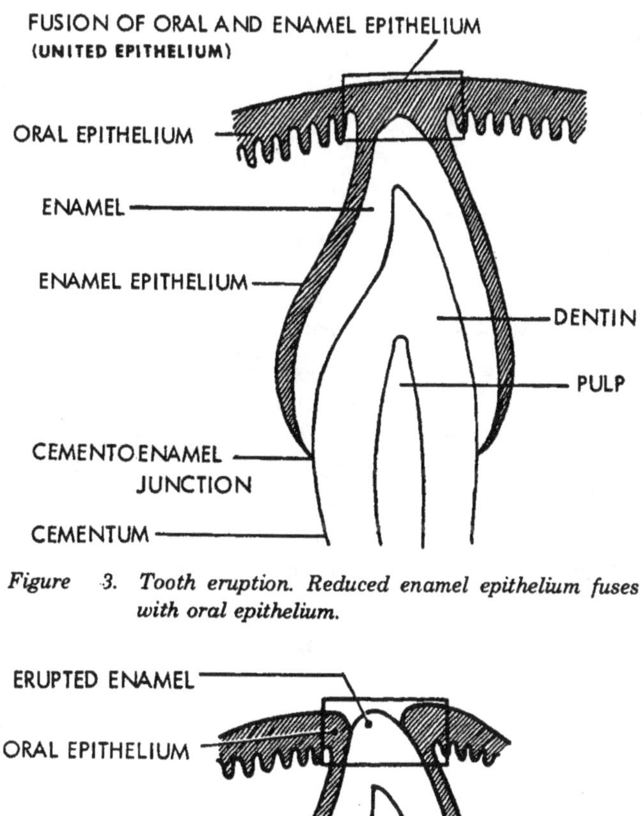

Figure 3. Tooth eruption. Reduced enamel epithelium fuses with oral epithelium.

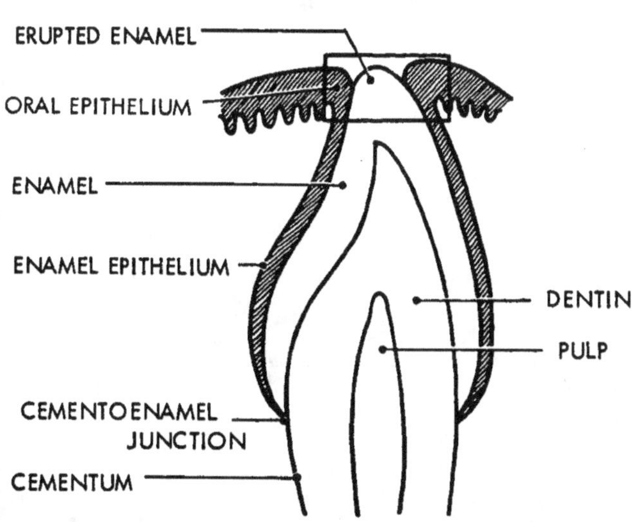

Figure 4. Tooth eruption. Tooth emerges through perforation in the fused epithelium.

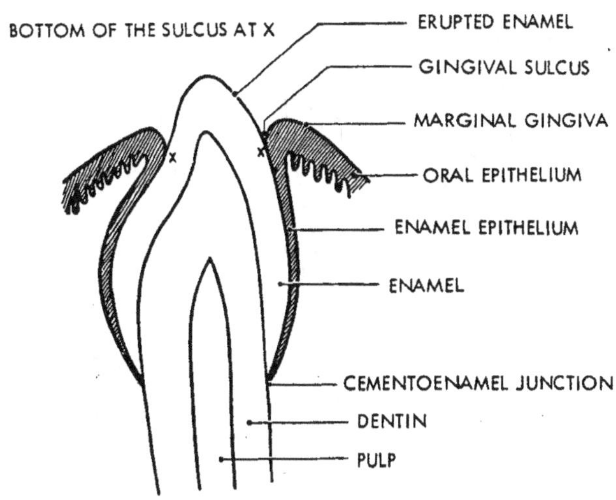

Figure 5. Tooth eruption. Gingival sulcus at an early stage.

11. Active Eruption

(figs. 3, 4, and 5)

As the formation of enamel is completed, the cells of the enamel organ including the ameloblasts compress to form a thin layer upon the surface of the enamel. Their final function is the deposition of a thin cuticular layer known as the primary enamel cuticle (Nasmyth's membrane). The ameloblasts then degenerate. The remaining epithelial tissue of the enamel organ becomes the "reduced enamel epithelium" which is attached to the entire enamel surface of the crown of the tooth. As the tooth continues to push or erupt toward the oral cavity, the reduced enamel epithelium contacts epithelium of the oral cavity and the reduced enamel epithelium and the oral epithelium unite and grow together. As the tooth erupts and finally breaks through this united epithelium, the remaining attachment to the tooth is called the epithelial attachment (figs. 3 and 4). Later during passive eruption, the epithelial attachment shifts apically on the cementum.

12. Passive Eruption

Passive eruption is one of the body's normal physiological aging processes. It should not be confused with recession of the gingiva, or in a shift of the position of the epithelial attachment upon the surface of the tooth which is caused by disease, or some other pathological process.

a. Stages (fig. 6). For clarity of discussion, the process of passive eruption is described as occurring in four stages. As it passes to each successive stage,

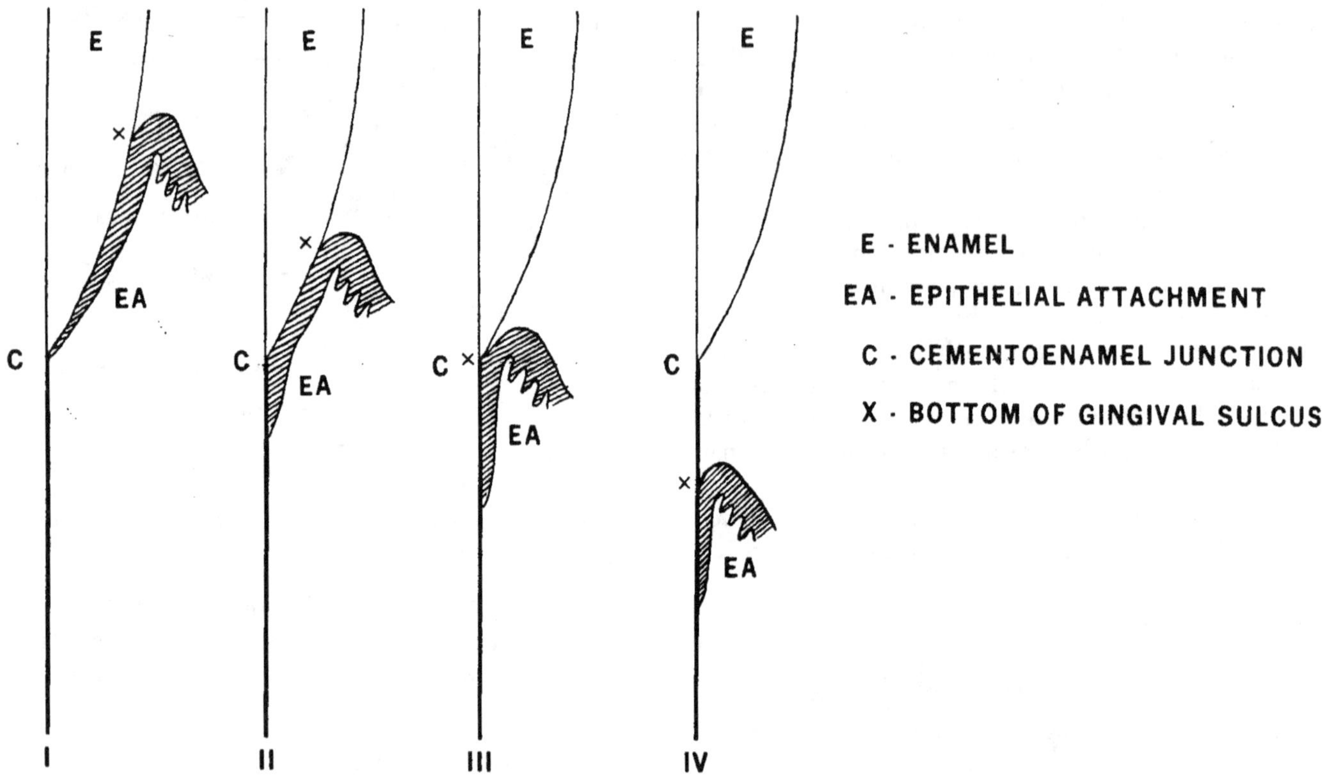

Figure 6. Four stages of passive tooth eruption.

the depth of the epithelial attachment gradually becomes less.

(1) In the first stage the epithelial attachment is located largely on the enamel, with the deepest part of the attachment lying at or near the cementoenamel junction.

(2) The second stage is reached when the epithelial attachment is partly on enamel and partly on cementum.

(3) As the process continues, the third stage is reached when the epithelial attachment is entirely on cementum and the base of the gingival sulcus approximates the level of the cementoenamel junction.

(4) The fourth stage of passive eruption is reached when the epithelial attachment has receded upon the cementum to the extent that the root portion of the tooth is exposed.

b. Rate. The rate of passive tooth eruption varies greatly. In some individuals the fourth stage may be reached between the 20th and 30th years, while in others the teeth may still be in the second stage at the 50th year. A too rapid recession of the gingiva is indicative of a pathological recession and not a normal passive eruption. The color and tone of the gingiva, plus the depth of the gingival sulcus, are signs which aid in differentiating a pathological recession from passive eruption.

13. Periods of Eruption

Table 1 gives the usual periods of active eruption of deciduous and permanent teeth. This table is not absolute; in some cases teeth may erupt either sooner or later than stated. If the variation is not too great, it is usually insignificant. As indicated below, mandibular teeth usually erupt somewhat earlier than do their maxillary counterparts.

Table 1. Approximate Ages of Tooth Eruption

Eruption of Deciduous Teeth	
Mandibular central incisors	6 months
Maxillary central incisors	7½ months
Mandibular lateral incisors	7 months
Maxillary lateral incisors	9 months
First molars	12 to 14 months
Cuspids	16 to 18 months
Second molars	20 to 24 months

Eruption of Permanent Teeth	
First molars	6 to 7 years
Central incisors	6 to 8 years
Lateral incisors	7 to 9 years
Cuspids	9 to 12 years
First bicuspids	10 to 12 years
Second bicuspids	10 to 12 years
Second molars	11 to 13 years
Third molars	17 to 21 years

Section IV. MATURE ENAMEL

14. General

Enamel is the hardest tissue of the body. It is composed of approximately 96 percent inorganic matter (mineral salts) and 4 percent substance and water. It forms a resistant covering of the tooth crown and does not wear away readily under the stress of mastication. The enamel can withstand crushing stresses to about 100,000 pounds per square inch. Enamel is completely formed at the time of eruption. Once it is formed it cannot be replaced.

15. Structure

(fig. 7)

Enamel is made up of enamel rods or prisms, rod sheaths, and a cementing inter-rod or interprismatic substance. Only through the microscope can these elements of enamel be detected. It is estimated there are 12 million enamel rods in the average upper first molar. These rods run outward from the dentino-enamel junction to the periphery of the crown in a curled, corkscrew-like fashion. Around the periphery of each rod is a thin layer which seems to have more organic substance and to be less calcified. This layer is known as the rod sheath. The enamel rods are held together by a cementing or interprismatic substance, which seems less calcified than the rod itself but more calcified than the rod sheath. It is harder at its periphery than at the dentino-enamel junction and harder at the tips of the cusps than at the gingival line. Because of its structure, it is cleavable and splits along the general direction of the enamel rods.

16. Enamel Cuticle

a. Formation of the enamel cuticle is described in paragraph 11.

b. Mastication soon wears away the cuticle on the incisal edges and occlusal surfaces. On the other exposed surfaces, it may be worn away by mechanical means, such as the brushing of the teeth. In protected areas, such as the surface between the teeth, it may persist for many years. Stains form on this cuticle, especially in the mouths of children. This is the green stain most commonly seen on the facial surfaces of the anterior teeth. It is produced by color-forming bacteria which collect on the cuticle when mouth hygiene is poor. The stain can usually be removed with pumice, and once removed it seldom returns.

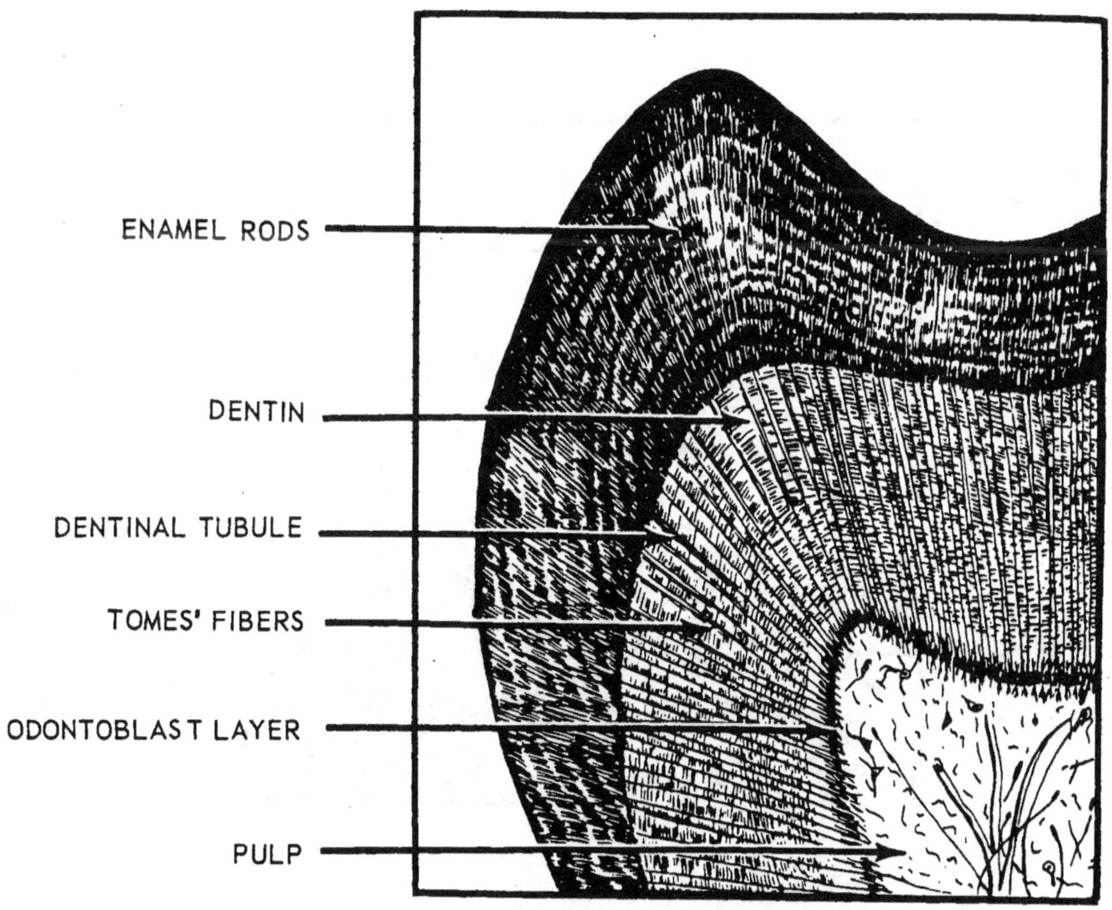

Figure 7. Semidiagrammatic sketch of enamel and dentin.

Section V. MATURE DENTIN

17. General

Next to enamel, dentin is the hardest tissue of the body. It is composed of approximately 65 percent inorganic matter and 35 percent organic substance and water. It constitutes the bulk of both the crown and the root of the tooth, and it completely surrounds the dental pulp except at its apical opening. Dentin is yellowish in color. The crown part of dentin is covered by enamel and its root part is covered by cementum. Dentin can withstand crushing stresses to about 30,000 pounds per square inch.

18. Structure
(fig. 7)

Mature dentin consists of calcified organic matrix containing many microscopic tubules running from the periphery of the dentin to the layer of odontoblasts which line the pulpal wall. Each tubule contains a fiberlike process (Tomes' fibers) which does not undergo calcification. Most observers deny the existence of nerve fibers in the substance of dentin, but attribute to Tomes' fibers the transmission of painful impulses.

19. Secondary Dentin

When the formation of primary dentin is completed, the odontoblasts do not disappear but remain as a layer of cells of the dental pulp lying adjacent to the dentin of the pulpal wall. They may in later years deposit additional dentin, known as secondary dentin, in response to external irritation. This is a commonly observed process in the progress of dental caries (decay) in which the odontoblasts deposit secondary dentin in the path of the invading caries to protect the dental pulp.

Section VI. THE DENTAL PULP

20. General

A portion of the dental papilla of the developing tooth remains within the pulp chamber and the root canals of the matured tooth as the dental pulp. It is largely connective tissue but contains a network of

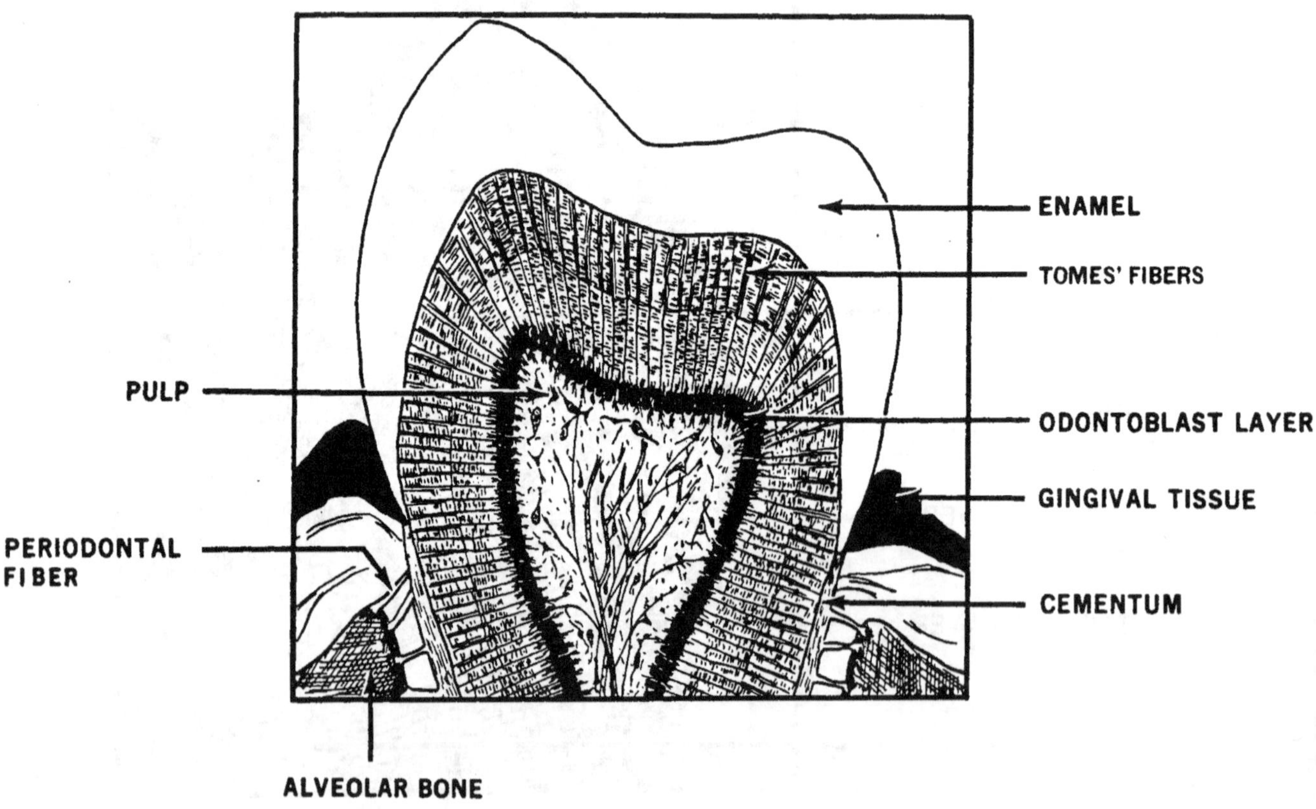

Figure 8. Odontoblast layer (diagrammatic).

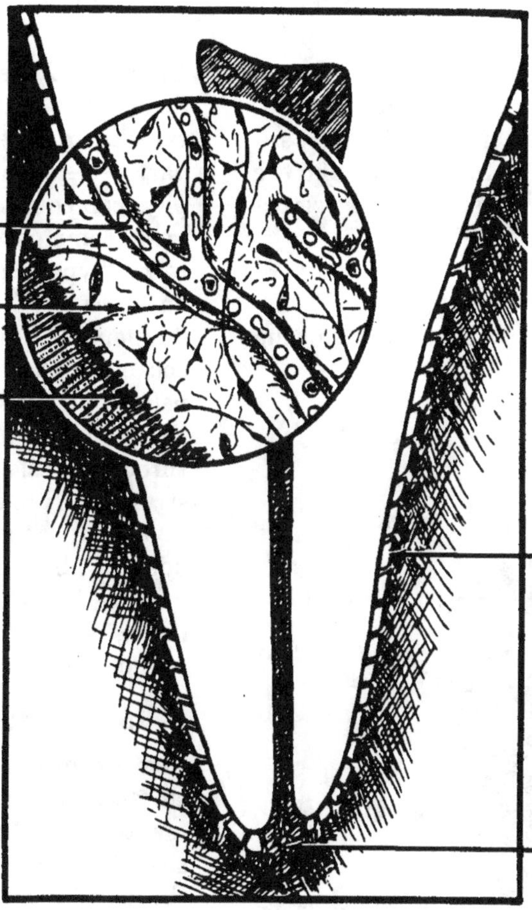

Figure 9. Pulp (diagrammatic).

blood vessels, nerves, and lymphatics to carry out the vital processes of the tooth.

21. Structures and Function
(figs. 8 and 9)

The odontoblasts of the original papilla remain as an outer layer adjacent to the dentin which forms the walls of the pulp chamber and root canals. When the structure of the tooth has been completed, the basic formative function of the odontoblasts ceases, but these cells still can produce secondary dentin and continue to do so throughout life in response to various stimuli (para 19). The body of the pulp contains a network of connective tissue fibers rich with many small blood vessels and nerves. Some of the nerves supply sensation to the tooth, and others regulate the blood supply to the tooth through their endings in the muscular layer of the walls of the blood vessels. The pulpal nerves are unusual in that pain is their only response to any stimulus.

22. Blood Supply

The position of the dental pulp is unique in that it is a highly vascular soft tissue enclosed within unyielding bony walls. Consequently, inflammation which produces an increase in blood supply (hyperemia) causing an exudate into the soft tissue (edema) will usually injure the pulp. As a result of the swelling, the blood vessels entering the narrow apical foramen are constricted. Blood supply is, in turn, restricted or cut off and pulp tissue dies because of lack of nourishment. Often the result of advanced decay, this is one of the processes involved in the development of a dental abscess at the root end of the tooth.

Section VII. CEMENTUM

23. General

Cementum covers the surfaces of the roots of teeth. Its principal function is as an attachment for periodontal ligament fibers (fig. 4-10) which hold the tooth in proper relationship to surrounding structures.

24. Secondary Cementum

Cementum, like dentin, can continue growing throughout the life of the tooth. The original cementum is called primary cementum. Later additions are referred to as secondary cementum. Secondary cementum is usually laid down as the result of physical, chemical, or bacterial injury, but is caused most commonly by physical injury or stress. The term "hypercementosis" refers to a condition where an unusually large amount of secondary cementum develops. The erupted tooth is suspended in its bony socket by the periodontal ligament (para 4-28). Fibers of the periodontal ligament are embedded in the cementum. Teeth undergo minute movement throughout life and often change position because of stresses of mastication. Consequently, secondary layers of cementum are needed to reattach periodontal fibers or to add support to counterbalance unnatural occlusal stresses. Cementum is also laid down, especially in the apical area, as teeth and surrounding structures wear down.

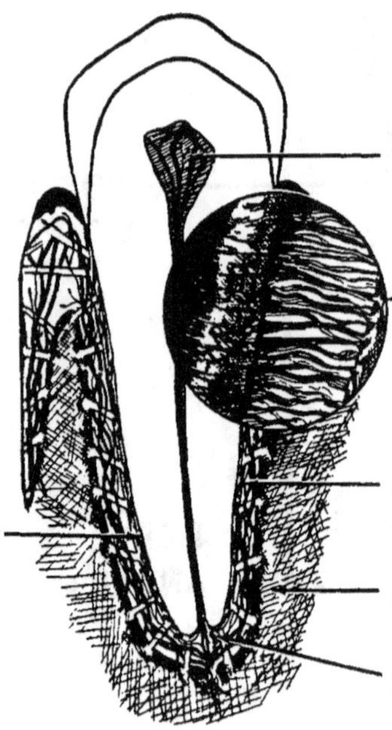

Figure 10. Periodontal ligament (diagrammatic).

25. Structure

Cementum is a bonelike structure which covers the surfaces of the roots of the teeth. The primary cementum is only a thin layer, but, because of successive deposits of secondary cementum, it may be thickened considerably. The thickening may not be uniform but may be noticeable in certain areas, depending upon the cause. It is light yellow. By its color it can be distinguished from enamel and dentin, being of a darker hue than the enamel and lighter than the dentin.

Section VIII. GINGIVA

26. General

Normal gingiva is pale coral pink, has a firm, knife-edged interdental papilla, and is demarcated from the lining oral mucous membrane by a clearly defined line which marks the muco-gingival junction. The color of the gingiva is the result of rich vascular blood supply, the degree of keratinization of the epithelium, and the presence or absence of pigment-containing cells. Keratinization is a normal microscopic protective adaptation to function. Increased keratinization may be produced by stimulation of the gingival surface. Another important characteristic of the gingiva is the stippled or "orange peel" appearance of attached gingiva. This stippling results from the depression of the connective tissue gingival fibers attaching the gingiva to the underlying alveolar bone.

27. Structures
(fig. 11)

a. The marginal or free gingiva surrounds the tooth like a collar. This thin border of gingiva at the gingival crest is not attached to the tooth and forms the outer soft tissue wall of the gingival sulcus.

b. The gingival sulcus is a shallow crevice or space (less than 3 mm) which develops between the gingiva and the surface of the tooth around its circumference. It is bound by the surface of the tooth on one side and by the marginal gingiva on the other. The bottom of the sulcus is at the epithelial attachment to the tooth.

c. The epithelial attachment is that portion of the united epithelium (union of reduced and oral epithelium) which is attached or adapted to the tooth sur-

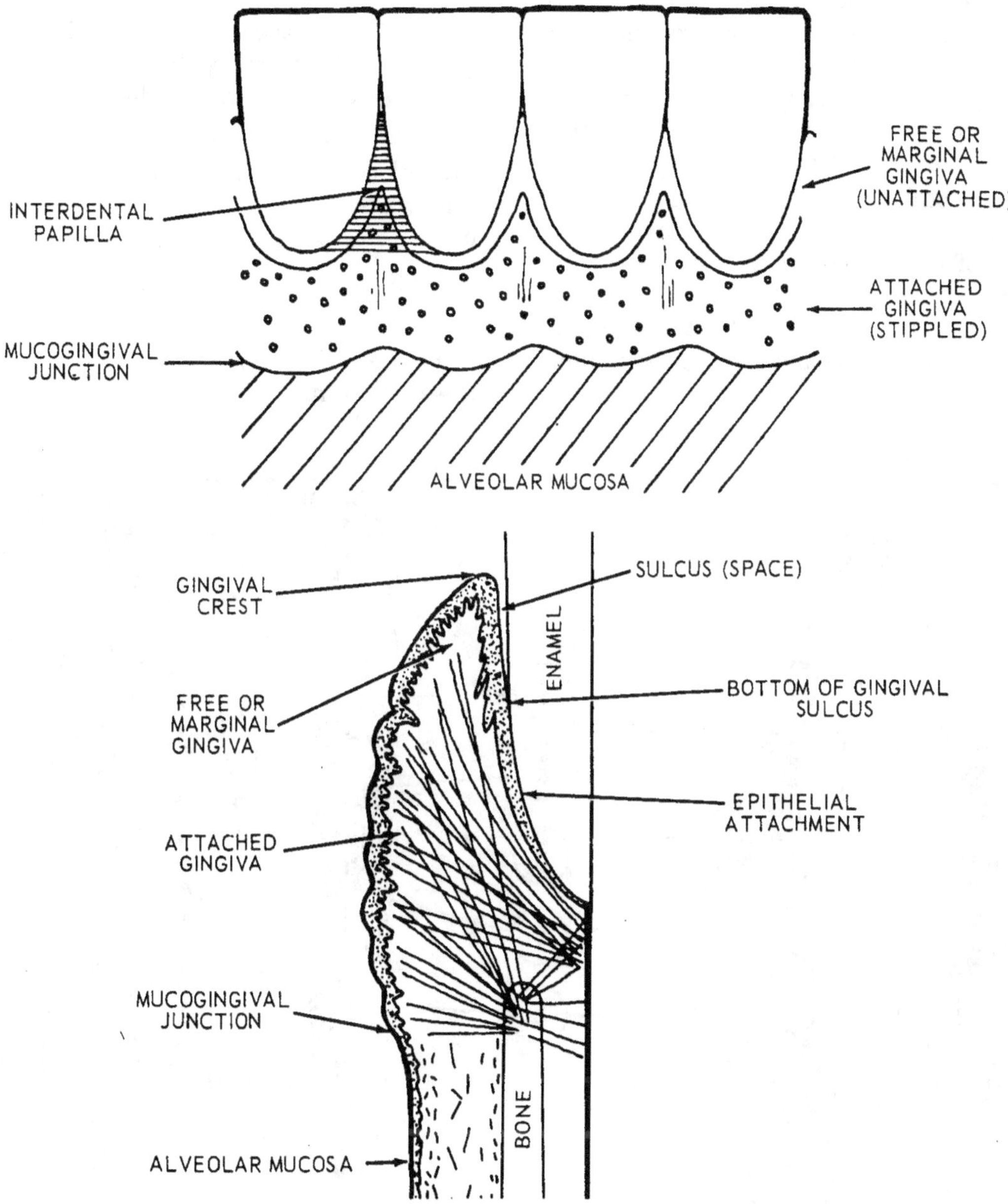

Figure 11. Structures of the gingiva.

face from the base of the sulcus and for some variable distance apically.

d. Attached gingiva is that portion of the gingiva which is attached by gingival, transseptal, and alveolar fibers. It extends from the apical boundary of the marginal gingiva to the muco-gingival junction.

Section IX. PERIODONTAL LIGAMENT

28. General

The periodontal ligament (fig. 10) is a fibrous connective tissue which serves to support the teeth and to maintain the proper positional and functional relationship between the teeth and adjacent tissues.

29. Structures

The completely developed periodontal ligament is made up of dense, hard, closely wound fibrous tissue (fig. 12). The fibers are arranged in bundles, whose ends are attached to cementum, alveolar bone, and gingival tissue. They support the tooth in its socket and hold the marginal or free gingiva firmly against the tooth. These fiber bundles run in different directions and are classified into seven groups as follows:

a. The free gingival fibers, which pass from the cementum in an occlusal direction to be inserted into the gingivae to support it.

b. The transseptal fibers, which pass from the cementum of one tooth across the alveolar crest to the cementum of the adjacent tooth to support the interproximal gingivae.

c. The alveolar crest fibers, which pass from the cementum to the crest of the alveolar process around the tooth.

d. The horizontal fibers, which arise from the occlusal third of the cementum and pass at right angles to the long axis of the tooth to be inserted into the alveolar bone forming the tooth socket.

e. The oblique fibers, which arise from the cementum of the apical two-thirds of the root and pass somewhat occlusally to be inserted into the alveolar bone.

f. The apical fibers, which radiate from the apex of the root to the adjacent alveolar bone.

g. The interradicular fibers which pass between the roots of multirooted teeth.

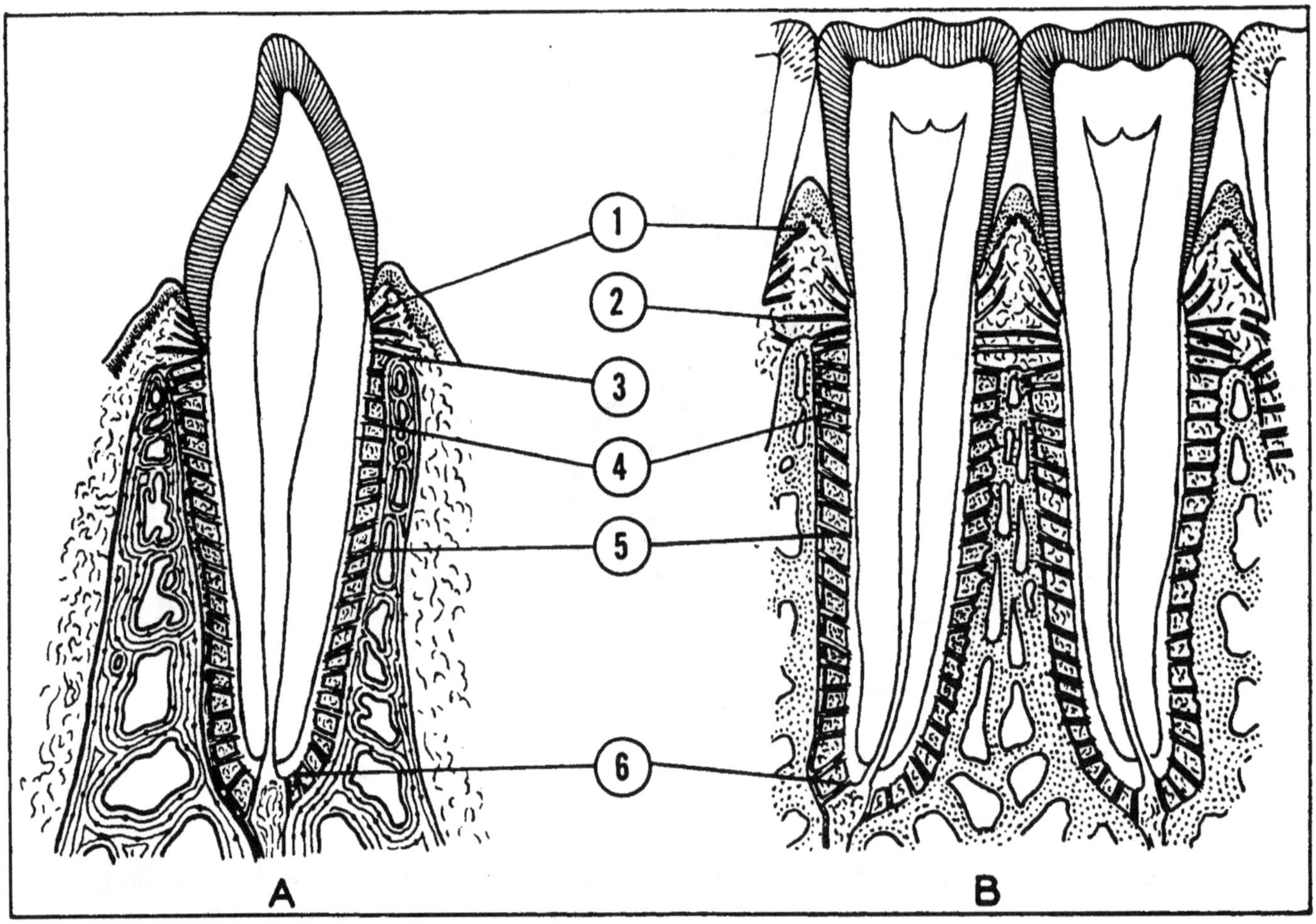

A. FACIAL AND LINGUAL FIBERS

B. MESIAL AND DISTAL FIBERS

1. GINGIVAL FIBERS
2. TRANSSEPTAL FIBERS
3. ALVEOLAR CREST FIBERS
4. HORIZONTAL FIBERS
5. OBLIQUE FIBERS
6. APICAL FIBERS

Figure 12. Principal fibers of the periodontal ligament.

30. Cellular Elements

The cellular elements of the periodontal ligament are fibroblasts, osteoblasts, cementoblasts, and osteoclasts.

a. Fibroblasts, which are connective tissue-forming cells, are found throughout the ligament, lying between the fibers which they have previously formed. These cells decrease in number with the age of the individual.

b. Osteoblasts, which are bone-forming cells, are found covering the surface of the alveolar bone of the tooth socket and lying between the embedded fibers of the periodontal ligament. In the elderly person they are either absent or greatly reduced in number and function.

c. Cementoblasts, previously described as cementum-forming cells, cover the surface of the root and lie between the fibers which are embedded in the cementum.

d. Osteoclasts, which are tissue-destroying cells, may or may not be present. They appear and disappear in response to various forms of stimuli. They may destroy the fibrous tissue, alveolar bone, or cementum.

31. Blood Supply

The blood supply of the ligament is derived from two sources. Part of the supply comes from the blood vessels which enter the dental pulp through the apical foramen. Before they enter the foramen, branches are given off which pass occlusally through the fibers of the ligament. A second source of blood is the vessels which supply the surrounding alveolar bone and give off branches which pierce the alveolar wall and enter the ligament to anastomose with vessels arising from the apical region.

32. Nerve Supply

The nerve supply, like the blood supply, is derived from two sources: first, from the nerves just before entering the apical foramen and, second, from nerves which supply the surrounding alveolar bone.

33. Functions

The functions of the periodontal ligament may be classed as formative, supportive, sensory, and nutritive.

a. Formative functions are those related to the formation of cementum, bone, and periodontal ligament fibers by cementoblasts, osteoblasts, and fibroblasts.

b. The supportive function is that of maintaining the tooth in its socket in a normal relationship to the surrounding soft and hard tissue. An important part of the supportive function is the manner in which it is performed. Because of the arrangement and curvature of the periodontal fibers, the tooth is suspended in the alveolar socket and protected from normal mechanical shock by the cushion-like action produced by the previously described arrangement.

c. The sensory function is that of supplying the tooth a sense of touch. Without the nerve supply of the ligament the sense of touch would be absent.

d. The nutritive function is exerted through the blood vessels of the ligament.

Section X. ALVEOLAR PROCESS

34. General

The alveolar process is that part of the mandible and maxillae which supports the teeth. It forms the tooth alveoli and surrounds the teeth. It fulfills the functional demand of supporting the teeth, but it disappears partly when the teeth are lost and the functional demand ceases.

35. Structure

The structure of the alveolar process is basically the same as that of other bone tissue. Because of variations in its structural arrangement, however, the alveolar process may be divided into three parts for description. These parts are called the cortical plate, the alveolar bone, and the spongiosa.

a. The cortical plate is the hard, dense outer surface of the alveolar process. It varies in thickness and is generally thinner on the facial surface than on the lingual surface.

b. The alveolar bone lines the socket of the teeth. It is a dense, calcified, thin layer of bone similar to the cortical plate with which it unites at the crest of the alveolar process. In a radiograph, alveolar bone appears as a thin, white line lining each socket and is called the lamina dura. Anatomically, it is referred to as the cribriform plate because of its many sieve-like openings which pierce it and provide passage for blood vessels and nerves that communicate with the periodontal ligament.

c. The spongiosa is a softer, more sponge-like bone in structure and occupies the space between the cortical plate and the alveolar bone. The spongiosa is also called the cancellous part of the process because of its lattice-like structure. It makes up the bulk of the alveolar process.

BASIC FUNDAMENTALS OF DENTAL MATERIALS

CONTENTS

BASIC FUNDAMENTALS OF DENTAL MATERIALS

Section I. INTRODUCTION

1. General

This chapter covers dental materials which are commonly handled or prepared by the dental specialist as part of his duties in assisting the dentist. The composition, properties, manipulation, and uses of these materials are discussed in this chapter. Dental materials which are peculiar, or which have greater application, to the dental laboratory and the work of the dental removable or fixed prosthetic specialists are discussed elsewhere.

2. Importance of Knowledge of Materials

The dental specialist may perform many procedures at the chair without having a comprehensive understanding of the materials being used. Yet he attains a far higher standard of accomplishment if he understands the nature and scientific composition of the materials, the reason for definite methods of manipulation, the results of improper handling or manipulation, and the reasons why faulty dental procedures result from such improper handling or manipulation. Our knowledge of materials used in dentistry is largely the result of continuing extensive scientific investigations. Specifications formulated for certain categories of dental materials and published by the American Dental Association serve to insure their suitability. Additional standards for quality are developed as further knowledge is gained. Optimum properties of dental materials can only be achieved through careful attention to details in their preparation and manipulation. Manufacturer's directions accompanying materials should be followed carefully. The techniques of manipulation discussed in this chapter are general and normally will give satisfactory results. However, if the manufacturer gives specific instructions regarding temperatures, mixing times, and ratios, they should be followed closely.

Section II. DENTAL SILVER ALLOY AND DENTAL AMALGAM

3. General

Silver and silver alloys mixed with mercury have been used more than a century for filling cavities in teeth. Little was known of the properties of the material or of how handling would affect them, so that early results of its uses were largely unsatisfactory and the materials fell into disfavor with the profession. About 1895 Dr. G. V. Black, often called the father of modem dentistry, began investigating the properties of amalgams. His studies showed the effects of chemical composition and physical structure on the properties of amalgam restorations. In 1919 the National Bureau of Standards began studies leading to the formulation of specifications for the selection and grading of dental amalgams, the first phase of a continuing extensive research program designed to improve dentistry through increased knowledge of the properties of dental materials. Due largely to the work done by Dr. Black, the National Bureau of Standards, and others, amalgam is used more than any other material for the restoration of posterior teeth.

4. Definition of Alloy and Amalgam

An alloy is a mixture of two or more metals. When mercury is one of the metals, the mixture is known as an amalgam. A dental amalgam is a combination of mercury with a specially prepared silver alloy for use as a dental restorative material. Amalgam is used also in making dies. In dentistry, a die is an exact, positive reproduction of an individual tooth and is used mainly for the fabrication of crowns, inlays, or fixed partial dentures.

5. Chemical Composition

Each metal incorporated into a dental silver alloy possesses specific properties when combined with mercury. Some properties are desirable and some are undesirable. An acceptable alloy is balanced so that the combined effects of the properties of its ingredients will provide the most satisfactory restorative material. Like other restorative materials, dental amalgam must meet the standards and requirements set by the National Bureau of Standards. The silver alloy composition, as well as the size of the fillings or shavings, varies slightly among manufacturers. Usually the silver alloy consists of silver and tin and perhaps other materials such as copper and zinc in limited amounts. Each manufacturer of silver alloy insures that his product meets the requirements of the National Bureau of Standards and American Dental Association. The composition of the alloy must include a minimum of 65 percent silver and 25 percent tin and must not contain more than 6 percent copper and 2 percent zinc. Some alloys are entirely zinc-free while others contain such additional materials as platinum or gold. The alloy is mixed with pure mercury, which is commonly known as "quicksilver" or "white liquid silver."

6. Physical Properties of Amalgam

The most important properties of amalgam are crushing strength, flow, and thermal conductivity.

a. *Crushing Strength.* The crushing strength of amalgam approaches 45,000 pounds per square inch (psi), which is completely acceptable when compared with other restorative materials and enamel and dentin. Enamel has a crushing strength of about 100,000 psi, dentin about 30,000 psi. These figures show amalgam to be an acceptable restorative material, even for restorations on stress-bearing areas of the teeth.

b. *Flow.* The amount of flow in amalgam is of a relatively low rate. Flow is the property of a material to flow or deform in shape when it is under stress or load for an extended time.

c. *Thermal Conductivity.* Thermal conductivity is the ability to transmit changes in temperature. Dental amalgam has a relatively high thermal conductivity. This becomes a distinct disadvantage when amalgam is placed close to the pulp. Amalgam allows heat or cold to pass through readily and irritate the pulp. To combat this disadvantage, an intermediate base with low thermal conductivity is placed under the amalgam.

7. Advantages and Disadvantages of Amalgam

a. Amalgam has many advantages over other materials for use as a restorative material. It is used more than any other material to restore carious teeth. It is easy to insert into the cavity preparation and adapts readily to cavity walls. In obtaining its initial set, or hardness, amalgam allows time for condensing and carving. It has an acceptable crushing strength and long life as a restoration. Before its final set, amalgam is easy to shape by carving.

b. Amalgam has several major disadvantages. First, its color does not match the color of teeth. It will tarnish with time no matter how well the amalgam restoration is prepared and inserted. To avoid or to reduce tarnish, the restoration is smoothed and highly polished a day or two after its insertion. The restoration may be reshined later at any time with little effort.

Because of its color, amalgam is used on the visible surfaces of anterior teeth only in exceptional circumstances. Another disadvantage is its inadequate edge strength. The edges of amalgam will fracture if unsupported by a bulk of amalgam. A third disadvantage of amalgam is its high thermal conductivity.

8. Elements and Their Effects on Amalgam

Each element composing amalgam imparts certain properties to the finished product. Silver imparts strength, durability, and color; gives the alloy desirable setting expansion; decreases flow; and accelerates the setting time. Tin makes the amalgam easier to work, controls excessive setting expansion, and increases both flow and setting time. Copper increases hardness, contributes to setting expansion, reduces flow, and decreases setting time. Zinc increases workability and cleanliness of the amalgam during trituration and condensation. Mercury, although an indispensable ingredient, imparts undesirable properties to the amalgam if added in incorrect proportions.

9. Setting Changes

The mixing of finely cut particles of silver alloy with mercury initiates the formation of a new alloy. Mixing (trituration) produces a soft mass in which all particles have been wetted with mercury. The mercury goes into solution with some of the particles of alloy and the hardening (setting) of amalgam is similar to the hardening process of the cements. Reactions which take place during hardening result in a cored structure consisting of a core of undisclosed alloy surrounded by a matrix of crystallized phases of the solution. As long as free mercury is present in excessive amounts, the amalgam will not set completely. For that reason, hardness of amalgam restorations is increased by eliminating as much excess mercury as possible during manipulation and placement of the material.

10. Properties Determined by the Manufacturer

a. Many factors controlled by the manufacturer influence the properties of dental silver alloys. Among them are purity of ingredients, proportioning of ingredients, controlled melting conditions, particle size, and proper heat treatment.

b. The effects of the ingredients upon the properties of a silver alloy were described in paragraph 8. Conditions under which these ingredients are melted to form the alloy must be controlled to prevent contamination through the introduction of oxides and other impurities. Particle size is important because as it decreases, the crushing strength of restorations made from the alloy is increased and setting expansion is reduced. Heat treatment to anneal (soften) the alloy after the formation of particles is essential to produce uniform crystalline structure of the material. When the metals composing a dental silver alloy are melted together and allowed to cool, the crystal composition of the alloy is subjected to tremendous strains. The molten mass solidifies or cools first on the outside. The crystals inside the mass, which solidify last, are of different composition. Thus the size of the crystals differs throughout the mass. To correct this, the alloy filings or shavings are annealed by heating slowly to 100°C (212°F). This method allows the crystalline structure to reorganize and produces an alloy of greater uniformity. This alloy requires less mercury for amalgamation and has less expansion and flow and greater crushing strength than the annealed material.

11. Properties Determined by the Operator

The following factors must be controlled by the dentist and his assistant to achieve satisfactory results.

a. Proper Ratio of Mercury to Alloy. The directions furnished by the manufacturer should be followed. These directions cover the proportions of alloy and mercury, trituration pressure, and trituration time. Too little mercury in a mix will produce a grainy, weak amalgam which is readily tarnished and corroded. Too much mercury in an amalgam restoration causes excessive expansion and weakens the material.

b. Proper Trituration. Both over trituration and under trituration are undesirable. Over trituration results in shorter setting time and increases shrinkage. Under trituration results in increased expansion, a lengthened setting time, and a weakened amalgam.

c. Proper Condensation. Condensation is the procedure of packing an amalgam mix by the dentist into a tooth cavity preparation. Time and pressure are important in achieving best results. Trituration of the amalgam should be so timed that the mix is ready at the exact time when the dentist desires to start the condensation. The longer the time between trituration and condensation is, the weaker the amalgam is, due to fracturing of forming crystals. Condensation should be completed in 3 1/2 minutes. Generally, the more pressure that is used, the stronger the restoration will be. Pressure of 8 to 10 pounds with a hand condenser is recommended.

d. Addition of Mercury. Addition of extra mercury should be avoided. If one drop of mercury is added to a partially set mix of average size, the compressive strength of the resulting amalgam will be about one-tenth of the normal strength. Once amalgam has begun to crystallize or harden, the addition of mercury lowers crushing strength tremendously.

e. Contamination by Moisture. Moisture should be avoided. Contact with any form of moisture contaminates freshly triturated amalgam. Moisture may cause excessive expansion, pain beginning several days after insertion of the restoration, lowered crushing strength, and blister formation on the amalgam surface. Moisture can be introduced into amalgam by mulling (working) the triturated amalgam in the palm of the hand, by trituration below the dew point (temperature at which moisture collects on a surface), by the presence of moisture in the cavity being filled, or by accidental contact with saliva. To avoid such contamination all instruments and equipment touching the amalgam should be dry. Mulling of amalgam should be done in a piece of rubber dam, a squeeze cloth, or a piece of clean linen but not in the palm of the hand. The temperature of equipment and materials should be kept high enough that no moisture collects. Saliva should be kept out of the cavity during insertion of the material. Amalgam that has accidentally contacted moisture in any form should be discarded.

12. Importance of Properly Mixed Amalgam

The dental specialist has the direct responsibility for the correct manipulation and preparation of amalgam for use as a restorative material. Incorrect manipulation may produce a faulty restoration which can cause or contribute to the loss of a tooth.

Therefore, the dental specialist must use extreme care in preparing a good mix of amalgam that will provide the best qualities obtainable from the alloy. Procedures in the manipulation of amalgam normally performed by dental specialists include proportioning the amounts of mercury to alloy; trituration to produce the amalgam; mulling; expressing free mercury; and assisting the dentist during insertion and condensation of the prepared amalgam.

13. Proportioning Alloy and Mercury

To proportion and mix dental alloy and mercury, the size of the mix and the alloy-mercury ratio must be known. The size of the mix is determined by the dentist. Dental alloy in pellets is the form used most in the restorative service of the dental clinic. The pellets are composed of silver alloy filings compressed under great pressure without a binding agent. They are supplied in weights ranging from 4.8 to 6 grains per pellet. A special dispenser is used to drop the pellets individually Pellets crush easily under light pressure of the pestle in a mortar or automatically by an amalgamator. Since the pellets are reformed in a set amount of silver alloy, only the amount of mercury used with each pellet needs to be measured. The mercury dispenser is equipped with four interchangeable plungers lettered A through D. The A plunger dispenses the most mercury; the D plunger the least. Changing the plunger allows for the individual preference of the dentist regarding the wetness or dryness of the amalgam when it is mixed. The manufacturer's instructions accompanying the pellets should be followed in selecting the size of plunger to use to provide the desired ratio of alloy to mercury.

14. Trituration

Trituration (mixing of amalgam is accomplished by the use of an electrically activated mechanical amalgamator or by hand trituration using a glass mortar and pestle.

a. Mechanical Trituration. This method employs a mechanical amalgamator which mixes the amalgam in a capsule by rapid shaking or vibration. It produces more consistently uniform mixes than does the hand trituration because it eliminates most human variables. It is much faster than the hand method, reducing trituration time to a matter of seconds. The operator must avoid setting the machine into action before the proper time is adjusted and must be careful not to over-triturate. It is important to follow the manufacturer's directions for both amalgamator and alloy.

(1) Special capsules are furnished with the mechanical amalgamator for holding the alloy mercury mixture during trituration. Each capsule is fitted with a cap and a small, rod-like pestle. A small funnel is furnished to help in pouring the previously proportioned alloy-mercury mixture into the capsule. When the mixture has been poured into the capsule, the pestle is inserted, its cap fitted in place, and the capsule is placed into the holder on the vibrating arm of the amalgamator. When using the pellet method, first insert the pestle in the capsule, dispense the required mercury, and then dispense the pellets. Usually one pellet is used for a small mix and two pellets for a large mix.

(2) Trituration is accomplished by setting the time according to the manufacturer's instructions for the alloy and for the type of amalgamator used. The time varies according to the size of the mix being manipulated. The average mixing time is 8 to 12 seconds per pellet. When the selected time has elapsed, the automatic timer will stop the machine.

b. Mortar and Pestle Trituration. In this method, trituration of the alloy-mercury mixture is done by hand with a ground glass or metal mortar and pestle the glass mortar has a ground inner surface to match the ground ends of the pestle. Mortar and pestle must mate to insure complete mixing. Each new mortar and pestle should be mated before use. An old mortar and pestle being used by an operator for the first time after prolonged use by another person must be remated to meet the particular angle at which the operator holds the pestle to the mortar. To mate a mortar and pestle, place a small amount of abrasive paste in the mortar and rotate the pestle in it just as in mixing the alloy and mercury. Repeat the procedure as needed until the two surfaces match perfectly. Then wash and dry the mortar and pestle completely before using them for manipulating alloy and mercury.

(1) Hand pressure, speed of mix, and mixing time all affect the properties of amalgam and should be as directed by the manufacturer. The pestle should be hold in a pen grasp rather than in a palm grasp. Speed of trituration is usually expressed in revolutions per minute. The recommended trituration pressure is 2 to 4 pounds per square inch, which is about the same as

the normal weight of the hand with no additional pressure. The pestle is revolved in the mortar at about 180 revolutions per minute.

(2) Properly proportioned and triturated amalgam results in a soft mass in which all alloy particles have been coated with mercury. To be a good mix the completed mix should show these characteristics-

(a) It does not stick to mortar or pestle. Sticking indicates the mortar and pestle were not mated accurately or too much pressure was applied to the pestle.

(b) The amalgam tends to climb the walls of the mortar but readily drops back into the base of the mortar.

(c) It has no particles of undissolved alloy. The presence of particles indicates insufficient mercury or incomplete mix.

(d) It has a silvery, flaky appearance.

15. Mulling the Mix

a. If mulling of the mix is desired after using the mechanical amalgamator, remove the pestle from the capsule and replace the mix in the capsule. Place the capsule back on the machine and vibrate it for 1 to 2 seconds. Or the mix may be mulled by placing it on a cotton squeeze cloth or a piece of rubber dam or into a finger stall to protect the amalgam from contamination by the fingers. Then the amalgam is rubbed or rolled for a few seconds to produce the consistency desired by the dental officer.

b. If mulling is desired after using the mortar and pestle method, empty the mix directly from the mortar onto a cotton squeeze cloth. Fold the squeeze cloth about the amalgam and rub or roll it as in an above. The rubber dam or finger stall also may be used.

16. Elimination of Free Mercury

a. After trituration and mulling, the amalgam mix will contain free mercury which must be expressed by squeezing. To do this, the mix is placed on a squeeze cloth, which is folded over the mix. Then the squeeze cloth is twisted with finger pressure, forcing free mercury out of the amalgam. The dentist will tell the dental assistant how much mercury to express. Depending upon the requirements of insertion, he may have the assistant express a slight amount of mercury or none and then, about halfway through the insertion, have all the free mercury expressed in a single action before continuing insertion of the amalgam into the cavity preparation. After the free mercury has been expressed, the mix is ready for insertion into the cavity preparation. The squeeze cloth is opened and the amalgam carrier loaded by forcing the open cylinder of the amalgam carrier into the balled amalgam.

b. Some dentist divides the mulled amalgams into segments before or after squeezing. If the mix is divided before squeezing, each segment then is squeezed just before it is used.

17. Special Precautions in Preparing Amalgam

a. Any portion of amalgam which is too dry or has begun to crystallize must be discarded. Its use would result in a weak, nonhomogeneous mass. For large restorations it may be necessary to prepare two or more mixes, preparing each mix as needed.

b. Amalgam should be mixed carefully. Free mercury in the restoration will cause excessive expansion and flow and decrease crushing strength. Over trituration by any method will result in decreased expansion or contraction and shorter setting time. Conversely, under trituration will result in excessive expansion and lengthened setting time. Mercury must never be added after mixing has started.

c. Contamination of the amalgam by moisture must be avoided.

Section III. DENTAL CEMENTS

18. General

Dental cements are generally low strength materials prepared by mixing a powder with a liquid. These cements vary in chemical composition, properties, and uses. They are more natural in appearance, are easy to manipulate, and have lower heat conductivity than metallic restorative materials. Dental cements, however, have the disadvantages of a relatively low crushing strength, varying degrees of solubility in mouth fluids, and setting shrinkage. Although used extensively in restorative dentistry, dental cements are among the least permanent restorative materials. Three types of cement are commonly used in dentistry: zinc phosphate cement, silicate cement, and zinc oxide and eugenol cement.

19. Zinc Phosphate Cement

a. General. Zinc phosphate cement is a nonpermanent material which may be used to restore teeth in any part of the mouth but is used most often for cementing crowns, fixed partial dentures (bridges), inlays, and certain dental appliances into place. It is also used widely for temporary restorations and intermediate bases. It is made in different shades to match tooth color beneath a translucent restoration. Zinc phosphate cement is supplied as powder and liquid which are mixed to obtain the desired product.

b. Chemical Composition.

(1) The composition of zinc phosphate cement powder varies from manufacturer to manufacturer but usually contains between 75 and 100 percent zinc oxide. The powder may also contain modifiers such as silica dioxide, magnesium oxide, copper silicate, bismuth trioxide, and pigments to alter its color.

(2) The liquid used with this powder is phosphoric acid and water in the ratio of about two parts acid to one part water. The solution contains aluminum hydroxide and often zinc oxide. Water content is critical. Water gain hastens setting time. Water loss lengthens setting time. The water content of the liquid is adjusted by the manufacturer to provide satisfactory setting. Care must be taken to preserve this established balance in water content. Liquids exposed in open bottles or on mixing slabs absorb moisture from the air if humidity is high and lose moisture if humidity is low. The liquid bottle should be kept tightly stoppered except when liquid is being withdrawn. Liquid which has been left unstoppered for a long period, is discolored, or is the last 25 percent in the bottle should be discarded.

(3). The manufacture of zinc phosphate cement is carefully controlled. Although cements made by different manufacturers are similar, satisfactory results cannot be attained by mixing the powder of one brand of cement with the liquid of another brand.

c. Properties.

(1) The advantages of zinc phosphate cement are its inconspicuous appearance, speed and ease of manipulation, and enough flow to form a very thin layer for the cementing of closely adapted crowns, fixed partial dentures, and inlays. One reason for using zinc phosphate beneath a metallic restoration is that its low thermal conductivity makes it an excellent insulator. This protects the pulp from sudden temperature changes transmitted by the permanent restoration.

(2) One disadvantage of zinc phosphate cement is its low crushing strength, which varies between 12,000 and 19,000 pounds per square inch. Another disadvantage is that it is slightly soluble in mouth fluids. In time, a zinc phosphate cement restoration would be washed from the cavity preparation. Its setting shrinkage also limits the use of the cement as a restorative material. Due to its opacity, zinc phosphate cement is not a lifelike restorative material on visible surfaces.

(3) The strength of phosphate cements can be increased to a certain point by increasing the ratio of powder to liquid in the mix. For this reason, the dental specialist should use as thick a mix as is practical for the work being performed. Although most of the acidity of phosphate is dissipated after several hours of setting, freshly mixed cement is extremely acid and the thinner the mix is the greater is its early acidity. This acidity sometimes irritates dental pulps when placed next to them. Thick mixes minimize this problem.

d. Setting Reactions. The chemical reaction between the powder and liquid of setting phosphate cement produces heat. The amount of heat produced depends upon the rate of reaction, the size of the mix, and the amount of heat extracted by the mixing slab. The setting time of zinc phosphate cement is normally between 4 and 10 minutes. The manipulative factors used to maintain and prolong the normal setting time are lowering the temperature of the mixing slab between 65° and 75°F (if the slab is not cooled below the temperature at which moisture will condense on it), slow incorporation of the powder, mixing over a large area of the cool slab, and, within optimum limits, using a longer mixing time. The less powder used in ratio to the liquid the longer the cement will take to harden. Good technique minimizes the rise in temperature and acidity of the setting cement which can injure the pulp. The setting reaction consists of dissolving the surface of powder particles by the liquid, resulting in a supersaturated solution which crystallizes and encases the undisclosed powder particle. This condition is typical of a cored structure found in most dental materials of this type. The undisclosed powder particles are called the core, and the crystalline phase encasing them is called the matrix. Generally, for increased strength, decreased shrinkage, and resistance to solubility, it is advisable to incorporate as much powder as possible to reach desired consistencies.

e. Clinical Uses. Zinc phosphate is used as an intermediate base, a cementing medium, and a temporary restoration.

(1) A thick mix of zinc phosphate cement is used as an intermediate base beneath a permanent restoration. The layer of phosphate cement used as a base under metallic restorations protects the pulp from thermal shock. When used under silicate cement restorations, the cement protects the pulp from irritation by the acid of the silicate.

(2) Zinc phosphate cement is used to cement crowns, inlays, and fixed partial dentures permanently into place upon remaining tooth structure. It is also used to hold splints, orthodontic appliances, and other appliances in place upon teeth, to cement facings to bridges, and to cement certain types of artificial teeth to artificial denture bases. A thin mix of cement is used to seat the restoration or appliance completely into place. The cementing medium does not cement two objects together as ordinary glue does. Instead the cement holds the objects

together by mechanical interlocking, filling the space between the irregularities of the tooth preparation and the cemented restoration.

(3) A thick mix of phosphate cement is often used as a temporary restorative material when restorative work cannot be completed at one appointment or when it is inadvisable or impractical to insert a more lasting restorative material. Silver alloy filings are sometimes included in the mix to make the material more resistant to wear if it is to be left in place a long time.

f. Equipment for Manipulation.

g. Proportioning Powder and Liquid. Although desirable, a measuring device is not usually employed for proportioning the powder. The amount of each ingredient will depend on the amount desired and the operation to be performed. Experience gained in manipulation and desired consistencies will enable the dental assistant to estimate accurately the amount of powder to be used according to the number of drops of liquid dispensed. The closely estimated powder is placed on one end of the cool, dry glass slab and divided into six equal segments. An additional small amount of powder is often placed on the corner of the glass slab for use if the estimated powder is insufficient for the desired mix. The liquid is dispensed with the dropper supplied by the manufacturer. Usually 3 drops of liquid are used for a thick mix and, depending on the dentist's needs, 4 or more for the thin mix. The drops are dispensed in the center of the slab or they may be dispensed over a wide area. The close estimation of powder, according to type of mix and number of drops, and the small increments will enhance the slow incorporation of powder which slows the setting reaction, enabling the manipulator to incorporate the maximum amount of powder to attain desired consistencies. This will help obtain cement with optimum physical properties.

h. Mixing. Mixing is done by the slow incorporation of the segments one at a time. This procedure aids in neutralizing the acid and achieving a smooth consistency. A considerable portion of the slab is used. Mixing is done with a moderate circular motion of the spatula blade held flat against the slab. The spatula should be rotated occasionally to incorporate the material that collects on the top of the blade. A good rule is to spatulate for about 20 seconds before adding the next segment. If this is done the mixing time is not critical and completion of the mix will take about 1 1/2 minutes. It is important to reach the desired consistency by using more powder and not to allow a thinner mix to stiffen by crystallization.

i. Characteristics of Completed Mixes. When a thick mix is ready for use it will have a puttylike consistency and a dull, glossless appearance. When a thin mix is ready for use, it will be similar in appearance to thick cream. When material for a thin mix is freshly mixed, if a drop on the end of the spatula is placed on the slab and the spatula is raised, the material left on the slab will peak, hold its form momentarily and gradually spread out.

j. Precautions.

(1) Prevent loss or gain of moisture in liquid cement by keeping bottles tightly stoppered.
(2) Dispense drops only when ready to mix.
(3) Use a cool, dry slab which has not been cooled below the dew point.
(4) Use the same brand of powder and liquid.
(5) Add increments of powder slowly.
(6) Use the maximum amount of powder to obtain the desired consistency. To incorporate the most powder, mix the material in a moderate circular motion over a large area of the slab, turning the spatula often.

20. Copper Phosphate Cements

Two types of phosphate cements containing copper oxides have been used in dentistry. They are the red and black copper cements which derive their color from the presence of red cuprous oxide or black cupric oxide. Basically, the copper cements are zinc phosphate cements with copper salts added to the powder, although occasionally the powder may contain 100 percent cupric oxide. The addition of copper is said to produce cement with a germicidal action in the mouth, but this is doubted by many authorities. Although some cement probably is germicidal when first mixed because of the acid in the liquid, this germicidal factor does not persist for any length of time. Many operators use the copper cements in the posterior deciduous teeth when proper preparation has been difficult because of the age of the patient. Their use is diminishing due to high pulpal toxicity and the doubt cast on the germicidal action.

21. Silicate Cements

a. General. Silicate cement is a nonmetallic, permanent-type restorative material used to restore nonstressbearing parts of carious anterior teeth and other teeth where esthetics (appearance) is important. This is because silicate cement, sometimes incorrectly called synthetic porcelain, appears translucent and may be mixed to produce a variety of shades to match tooth color. Because of its lifelike appearance, silicate cement is one of the most popular dental cements. It is the least permanent of the so-called permanent restorative materials.

b. Instruments and Materials Setup.

c. Chemical Composition.

(1) Silicate cement powder is a complex material made of finely ground ceramic compositions which are essentially acid soluble glasses. Its makeup varies with the manufacturer. The main constituent is silica. Other major ingredients are alumina, lime, and fluoride fluxes. Since the color of silicate cement powder can readily be affected by contamination with dust and dirt, the powder must be protected all the time and the mixing instruments thoroughly clean. A single part of soot to 100,000 parts of powder will cause a detectable change in color.

(2) Silicate cement liquid is similar to the liquid zinc phosphate cement liquid. Both are solutions of phosphoric acid which are partly neutralized by zinc oxide and alumina.

(3) The water content of silicate liquid is carefully established by the manufacturer because it is a critical factor in determining the rate and nature of the setting reaction of mixed silicate cement. The liquid consists of about six parts of phosphoric acid to one part of water. Too little water in the liquid increases setting time. An excess of water decreases setting time.

(4) Bottles containing silicate cement liquid should be kept tightly stoppered when not in use to avoid gain or loss of moisture by exposure to the air. To minimize effects of changes in water content of the liquid, manufacturers supply one-third to one-half more liquid than is needed to mix one bottle of silicate powder. Therefore, when 75 percent of the liquid in any bottle has been used, the remaining portion should be discarded.

(5) Liquid designed for silicate cement should not be mixed with zinc phosphate cement, and phosphate cement liquid should not be mixed with silicate cement. Powders and liquids of different brands are not interchangeable and are not to be mixed.

d. Properties.

(1) The major advantage of silicate cement over metallic restorative materials is its natural appearance. It can be prepared to match very closely the shade of the tooth being restored. Its translucency is similar to that of natural tooth structure. Other advantages are its relative ease and speed of manipulation and low conductivity of heat. Another advantage of silicates is that their thermal dimensional change is almost the same as that of tooth structure. Thus, despite the amount of thermal change, tooth structure and silicate will vary in dimension at about the same rate.

(2) Properties that limit the use of silicate cement are low crushing and edge strength, brittleness, setting contraction, some solubility in mouth fluids, and a comparatively short life expectancy.

(a) The crushing strength of silicate cement is between 23,000 and 24,000 psi. In comparison, the crushing strength of enamel is 100,000 psi, amalgam 45,000 psi, and dentin 30,000 psi.

(b) Silicate cement is more brittle than metals and alloys. This makes the cement unsatisfactory when used on occlusal and incisal surfaces, which is why the dental officer does not bevel the margins of cavities prepared for insertion of silicate cement. Brittleness must always be considered in evaluating a dental restorative material.

(c) Silicate will shrink slightly upon setting. This results in staining around margins. If insufficient powder is added to the mix the degree of shrinkage is much greater.

(d) Silicate cement is soluble in the fluids of the mouth. Excess liquid in the mix increases the solubility of the cement. For this reason, the liquid should be thoroughly incorporated with as much powder as can be wetted. Because of this solubility, it is often necessary to replace "washed out" silicate restorations.

e. Setting Reactions. The setting reaction of silicate cement is one in which the outer surface of powder particles is dissolved in the liquid to form silicic acid and phosphates. The silicic acid molecules unite to form a rigid gel. The final result is an interlocked mixture of phosphate crystals, undisclosed particles of powder, and hardened silica gel. The reaction starts rapidly but gradually slows. The temperature has a decided effect on the rate of reaction which in turn determines the amount of powder that can be incorporated in the mix. The silica gel must not be disturbed while forming. Once broken, the parts will not rejoin. Silicate cement that is worked while it is setting becomes. a crumbly or powdery mass.

f. Proportioning Powder and Liquid. When preparing silicate cement, use a glass slab which is reserved only for the mixing of silicate cements and a plastic spatula. The slab should be marked on one end with an "S" to show it is for use only with silicate. It should be clean and free of nicks, scratches, and breaks. Slabs never should be interchanged. Steel spatulas should not be used because they are affected by acid in the silicate liquid and they will contaminate the mix. Before the materials are measured out, the glass slab should be cooled by being placed in water at 65° to 75°F. This should be followed by thorough drying of slab and spatula.

(1) The first step in preparing the cement is to place the portion of powder near the center of the slab. The dentist may have selected a shade which requires blending of powder from two or more bottles. The proper proportion of each should be placed on the slab. An additional small amount of powder should be placed in the corner of the slab to serve as a reserve. With experience, the dental specialist can closely estimate the proper amount of powder to place on the slab. The powder is then divided in halves, and one half is divided into thirds.

(2) Next, place two or three drops of liquid near the powder on the slab. Hold the dropper in a vertical position so that the drops will be uniform in size and let the drops form slowly before falling onto the slab.

g. Mixing Silicate Cement. Starting with the large segment, the powder is incorporated in the liquid one segment at a time, using the spatula in a rapid folding manner and using light pressure. Each segment is mixed only until wet throughout and the next segment is then immediately added. Since the gel structure is almost completely formed after 1 minute, the total mixing time should not exceed 60 seconds. The normal setting time of silicate cement is between 3 and 8 minutes. The only safe way to maintain and prolong the setting reaction is to lower the temperature of the mixing slab. Slabs are usually cooled between 65° and 76°F for mixing if this is not below the point where moisture condenses on the slab. To avoid disturbing the gel, the mix must be completed in 1 minute so the reaction will occur when the material is confined and conformed in the cavity preparation.

h. Characteristics of a Completed Mix. When the mix is ready for use, it will have a heavy dough-like appearance and consistency. A glossy appearance or stickiness indicates too little powder. Flakiness indicates too much powder or prolonged mixing. Optimum properties are attained only by using the maximum of powder within the limitation that all powder particles are wetted by the liquid and mixing time is not exceeded. Too little or too much powder or prolonged mixing time will lower the physical properties previously discussed.

i. Precautions.

(1) Preserve acid-water ratio.

(a) Keep bottles tightly stoppered.
(b) Discard bottles of liquid when 25 percent remains or if they have been left open.

(c) Use dry equipment which has not been cooled below the dew point.
(d) Dispense drops only when ready to mix.
(e) Use the same brand of powder and liquid.

(2) To maintain the desired shade, you must use clean equipment and clean technique.

(3) Use a slab which is properly cooled and free of nicks and scratches.

(4) Mix rapidly within the limitation of mixing time.

(5) Use the maximum powder to get the desired consistency.

22. Zinc Oxide and Eugenol Cement

This cement, composed of a powder that is basically zinc oxide and a liquid known as eugenol, is used for many dental purposes ranging from temporary restorative materials to surgical dressings and impression pastes.

a. Chemical Composition. Zinc oxide is dispensed as a powder, eugenol as a liquid. They are mixed together the same way as zinc phosphate cement. By National Bureau of Standards specifications, the powder must contain between 70 and 100 percent zinc oxide. The manufacturer may add hydrogenated resins to increase strength and zinc acetate to hasten the set. Eugenol is usually derived from oil of cloves because it contains more eugenol (82 percent) than do the oils of cinnamon, orange, or bay. Eugenol is an obtundent (pain-relieving agent). It is a clear liquid which gradually changes to amber when exposed to light.

b. Physical Properties. This cement soothes pain, makes tissue less sensitive to pain, is slightly antiseptic, and is low in thermal conductivity. It is protective because it provides a good marginal seal when placed in tooth cavities. The crushing strength of pure zinc oxide and eugenol cement is about 2,000 psi, which is low in comparison to that of other cements. The crushing strength can be increased to 5,000 psi by the addition of hydrogenated resin.

c. Uses.

(1) The most frequent use of zinc oxide-eugenol cement is as a treatment restoration. When placed for treatment of fractured teeth, lost restorations, advanced caries, and pulpitis it helps prevent pulpal irritation and exerts a palliative effect on the pulp.

(2) It is used as a temporary cementing medium for crowns; inlays, and fixed partial dentures that may later be cemented more permanently with zinc phosphate cement.

(3) It is used as an intermediate base to provide insulation between metallic restorations and vital tooth structure. Because of the cement's low crushing strength, its use for this purpose is sometimes contraindicated where the base is expected to support a permanent restoration. Usually, when the base is to support a permanent restoration, the dentist will require a zinc phosphate cement base to place over the zinc oxide and eugenol cement.

(4) It is used in pulp capping for near and direct exposures of the pulp but this use is declining. Calcium hydroxide is usually used for pulp capping.

(5) It is used as a surgical packing or dressing after certain oral surgery procedures. An example of this is the surgical dressing applied and adapted over the gingival area after a gingivectomy. This dressing protects the area and makes the tissue less sensitive.

Section IV. DENTAL WAXES

23. General

Many different waxes are used in dentistry. The composition, form, and color of each wax are designed to facilitate its use and to produce the best possible results. The discussion in this section is limited to clinical aspects.

24. Inlay Wax

Inlay wax is used to prepare patterns which are to be reproduced in gold or some other material in the fabrication of inlays, crowns, and fixed and removable partial dentures.

a. For success in these procedures, the wax must have properties which enable very close adaptation to the prepared portions of the tooth to be restored; must provide freedom from distortion; must permit detailed carving without flaking or chipping; and must not leave excessive residue when it is removed from a mold by burning. The wax should harden at body temperature but soften at a temperature low enough to permit it to be manipulated in a plastic state in the mouth without injury to pulp or oral tissues. Its color should contrast with the colors of teeth and oral tissues to facilitate carving, except that ivory wax is used to avoid risk of color contamination when porcelain or acrylic resin restorations are constructed. Because of the importance of certain qualities of these waxes, the American Dental Association has developed certain specifications with which an inlay wax must comply to be acceptable.

b. Inlay wax is available in blue, green, ivory or deep purple sticks, preformed shapes for partial dentures, and solidly packed cans. Inlay wax is hard at room temperatures and breaks if bent sharply. This wax remains hard at mouth temperature and may be carved either in or out of the mouth. It is softened with dry heat until plastic or by immersion in warm water.

25. Baseplate Wax

Baseplate wax is used mainly for making occlusion rims and for holding artificial teeth to baseplates during the fabrication of dentures.

a. The wax is composed mainly of beeswax, paraffin, and coloring matter, which is mixed together, cast into blocks, and rolled into sheets. The sheets are red or pink, 3 inches wide and 6 inches long. Baseplate wax is relatively hard and slightly brittle at room temperature but becomes soft and pliable when heated.

b. Baseplate wax must be capable of holding porcelain or acrylic teeth in position at normal room temperature but it should not be brittle. It should maintain uniform consistency at room temperature and at mouth temperature.

c. Two types of baseplate wax, hard and medium, are listed in the Federal supply catalog. The hard type is suitable for use in warm climates but tends to crack and flake at low temperatures. The medium type is suitable for use at low temperatures but flows excessively at high temperatures.

26. Sticky Wax

Sticky wax becomes sticky when melted and has the property of adhering to the surfaces of various materials. Sticky wax is composed of beeswax, paraffin, and resins. It is usually supplied as hexagonal sticks of various colors, often orange or purple. It is brittle at room temperature and assumes a thick liquid consistency when heated. The wax has many uses in a dental clinic or laboratory. For example, it is used to hold together broken pieces of a denture being repaired and to assemble and hold together components of fixed partial dentures and wrought partial dentures in preparation for soldering.

27. Utility Wax

Utility wax is a pliable wax issued in stick form. Its most common uses are: providing rim locks and otherwise adapting impression trays for individual impressions, building up post-dam areas on impressions, and forming a bead or border on preliminary and final impressions. Utility wax is plastic and tacky at room temperature and so it may be used without heating. It is usually red in color.

28. Disclosing Wax

Disclosing wax is used to determine points of unequal pressure in a denture. These points, which may be causing discomfort to the patient, are located by painting the wax on the tissue side of the denture base and holding the denture in place under pressure in the mouth. The wax flows away from the pressure points, revealing the points needing relief.

29. Boxing Wax

Boxing wax is used to form a box around impressions of the mouth when making a cast (model). This boxing limits the flow of gypsum material, either plaster or stone. Boxing wax is usually issued in red strips, measuring about 1 1/2 inches wide, 12 inches long, and 1/8 inch thick. The wax is soft and pliable at room temperature, making it easy to form. For further softening a strip of wax can be passed through an open flame.

30. Impression Wax

Impression wax is discussed with impression materials in paragraph 44.

Section V. GOLD AND GOLD ALLOYS

31. General

For most dental purposes, pure gold cannot be used alone because it is too soft; however, it can be combined with other metals to produce alloys which can be used to fabricate every type of dental restoration or prosthesis where metal is indicated. The basic types of gold alloys used in dentistry are casting gold, gold solder, wrought gold, and gold plate. The principal metals used to combine with gold for dental gold alloys are silver, copper, platinum, palladium, and zinc. The following discussion of dental gold and gold alloys is limited to aspects of clinical interest.

32. Fineness, Carat, and Weighing

The amount of gold in a gold alloy may be rated in terms of fineness or carat. Fineness is determined by the parts per thousand of pure gold contained in the alloy. In terms of fineness, pure gold is 1,000 fine, and an alloy with three-fourths pure gold is 750 fine. In the carat system of rating, the carat refers to the parts of gold determined by dividing the substance into 24 units and then counting the number of units of gold. Thus, a 24-carat substance would be pure gold and a 12-carat alloy would be one-half gold. In weighing precious metals like gold and platinum the troy system of weight is used. In this system, the basic units of measurement of alloy quantity are grains, pennyweights, and ounces. Gold alloys are recorded and issued by the troy system as indicated below.

24 grains (grs)	=1 pennyweight (dwt)
20 pennyweights (dwt)	=1 ounce (oz)
12 ounces (oz)	= 1 pound (lb)

33. Casting Gold Alloy

Casting gold alloy is used in the fabrication of various restorations. It is alloyed and made into ingots suitable for melting and casting into molds for the restorations. Casting gold alloy may be classed into four types: soft, which is used for inlays not subjected to stress; medium, which is used for ordinary inlay work; hard, which is used for full crowns, three-quarter crowns, and retainers; and extra hard, which is used for saddles, clasps, and one-piece cast partial dentures. Alloyed casting gold can be whitened (white gold) by adding palladium, platinum, or silver and used for crowns and abutments requiring great strength and hardness.

34. Annealing and Tempering Gold Alloys

Through the use of controlled heat and rate of cooling, gold alloys can be annealed (softened) or tempered (hardened). Gold alloys are hardened by slow cooling. This is the opposite of steel which is softened by slow cooling. Rapid cooling from a high temperature will soften a gold alloy but harden steel. Rapid cooling is done by quenching the heated gold alloy in tap water.

35. Gold Alloy Solder

Gold alloy solder is used for joining the parts of fixed partial dentures, for building up or forming restorations, and for gold repairs. Soldering is the process of joining metals by means of a solder or a lower fusing metal.

36. Wrought Gold Alloy

Wrought gold alloy is used in dentistry for the construction of clasps and orthodontic appliances.

37. Gold Foil

Gold foil is a restorative material in which the metal is used in a pure state. It is an excellent material for permanently restoring tooth structure and is used most often for restorations on facial surfaces, proximal surfaces on anterior teeth. and occlusal surfaces of posterior teeth Its chief disadvantages are color high thermal conductivity, and difficulty in manipulation. Gold foil is available in either an adhesive or a nonadhesive form. To prevent pellets of adhesive foil from sticking together before use, their surfaces are treated with moisture or gas residues. When ready for use, the moisture and gas residues are vaporized by heating.

38. Gold Plate

Gold plate is used less often than are casting gold alloys, wrought gold alloy, or gold alloy solder. It is used in the fabrication of some types of crowns and often used in repair procedures, such as repairing a hole in a gold crown with solder.

Section VI. DENTAL IMPRESSION MATERIALS

39. General

a. An essential preliminary step in constructing prosthetic restorations is obtaining an accurate cast (model) of the patient's mouth (maxillary or mandibular arch or both). This is done by making an impression, which is a mold or negative reproduction, of the teeth and their surrounding tissues or of edentulous (without teeth) areas, using one of the impression materials described below. The cast then is formed by pouring artificial stone or other suitable material in the mold.

b. One method of classifying impression materials is the way in which they harden. Plaster of paris and metallic oxide impression pastes, for instance, harden by chemical action. Modeling plastic (impression compound), however, softens when heated and hardens when cooled, without a chemical change. These materials which soften under heat and solidify when cooled, without chemical change, are classed as thermoplastic substances.

c. Impression materials also may be classified according to rigidity, plasticity, elasticity, and use. Perhaps the better way to classify them is according to their rigidity when set. Impression materials that are inelastic when set include modeling plastic, impression plaster, and metallic oxide impression paste. Elastic impression materials include the hydrocolloids and polysulfide and silicone base impression materials. The uses, properties, and manipulation of these materials are discussed below. The manufacturers' instructions should be followed in all cases. Variables in specific information stated below apply in most cases.

d. A good impression material has the following desirable qualities:

(1) It is plastic at a temperature which is comfortable to the patient.

(2) It does not irritate the mouth.

(3) It sets completely at or slightly above mouth temperature.

(4) It sets uniformly and without distortion during setting.

(5) It is cohesive but not adhesive.

(6) After it solidifies, the material does not flake when trimmed with a sharp knife at room temperature.

(7) It does not change shape or dimensions at normal room temperature and humidity.

40. Modeling Plastic Materials

a. Modeling plastic materials, which are moldable thermoplastic substances, are used extensively to make impressions for complete dentures, inlays, and fixed partial dentures. They are used alone or with other impression materials to form trays and for post-seal and border molding of impressions. These materials become grainy and brittle with insufficient heat, and sticky and adhesive with excessive heat.

b. Modeling plastic materials are supplied in colors indicative of their softening or working temperatures. The types most often used are cake form (red cake and black cake) and stick form (red stick and green stick). Black cake is harder and softens at a higher temperature than red cake. For this reason it is considered more a tray material and less a true impression material than the red cake. Green stick type is a low-heat material used for impressions for crowns, fixed partial dentures, post-dam (seal at the posterior border of maxillary edentulous impressions), and establishing peripheral borders of edentulous impressions.

c. A typical formula for modeling plastic material is 45 percent shellac, 30 percent talc, 2.5 percent glycerin, and 22.5 percent wax, palm oil, tallow, and coloring matter.

d. Red cake modeling plastic softens in a water bath between 130° and 140°F. Black modeling plastic material must be heated between 140° and 150°F before its working temperature is reached. Green modeling plastic material softens between 120° and 130°F. In each case, the manufacturer prescribes the correct temperature of the water. The water must cover the material completely to assure uniform softening. Gauze is placed over the tray in the water bath to keep the modeling plastic material from sticking to the metal. This also facilitates cleaning the water bath later. Red and green stick types have the same compositions and working temperatures as the corresponding cakes.

e. When soft and smooth, the modeling plastic material is adapted to the tray previously selected by the dental officer. For complete maxillary edentulous impressions, the material is rolled into a ball and pressed down into the tray as desired. For complete mandibular impressions, the material is rolled into a cylinder-shaped mass for insertion into the tray. After it is adapted to the tray, the material is brushed with a flame to remove fissures and fingerprints. All that remains to be done before making the impression is the tempering (moistening and returning to proper temperature) of the material by dipping the tray containing the material momentarily into the water bath.

41. Metallic Oxide Impression Paste

a. General. Metallic oxide impression paste is used as a corrective impression material in denture fabrication. It is also used to make impressions for rebasing or relining dentures. Metallic oxide impression paste is usually supplied in separate tubes as a base and a hardener, which are mixed together. When mixed, the ingredients will harden in the mouth, allowing enough time for the molding of the border of the impression by the dentist to accommodate muscle attachments. The base ingredient usually is zinc oxide, which is premixed with inert oil (linseed) to form one of the pastes. The liquid or hardener ingredient (eugenol) is premixed with inert powder to form the other paste. The two constituents of metallic oxide impression paste (base and hardener) are usually of different colors.

b. Manipulation. The two pastes are usually mixed on a parchment pad with a stainless steel spatula or a tongue blade. The correct proportion is obtained by squeezing equal lengths of material from the tubes onto the mixing pad. Both sides of the spatula are wiped in the brown paste. Then the brown paste is mixed into the pink paste and is spatulated until a uniform color without streaks is obtained. Mixing time is generally 1 minute. Before the selected tray is loaded, the mix should be spread over the mixing area to express any air bubbles. Then the entire mix is picked up and the tray is loaded. If the material sets too rapidly a drop of oleic acid or petrolatum may be added during mixing to retard the set. If it sets too slowly, a drop of water is added. Before mixing the paste, the dental assistant should spread petrolatum around the lips, cheeks, and chin of the patient to prevent the paste from sticking to the patient's face.

42. Hydrocolloids

a. General. Hydrocolloids are elastic impression materials with which accurate impressions of oral tissues, including undercuts and other interferences, can be obtained readily and accurately. An undercut (fig. 9) is a hard or soft tissue area so located that it mechanically resists or prevents insertion or removal of restorations, impressions, or other material. Hydrocolloids are used for making impressions for fabricating complete dentures, fixed and removable partial dentures, crowns, and inlays and for duplicating casts. Hydrocolloid materials will deform momentarily, thus allowing the impression to be withdrawn, but will regain its original shape which accurately reproduces tissues as they exist in the oral cavity.

b. Types. The two basic types of hydrocolloids are reversible (agar), which can be softened by heat and hardened by cooling and can be used repeatedly, and irreversible (alginate), which hardens when mixed with water and cannot be softened again. Irreversible hydrocolloid is obtained in a large can or a small individual pack. The manufacturer's mixing instructions are always followed. Both materials are composed mostly of water. After the impression is made, the gel consists of fibrils of gelled material suspended in water. If water is lost by evaporation or synerisis (exudation of water from inside the material) the impression will shrink. If the hydrocolloid is placed in water, it is subject to imbibitions (uptake of water) and it will swell. There is no effective way to store the hydrocolloid impression, and the cast must be poured at once.

c. Manipulation.

(1) Reversible (agar) hydrocolloid. Special conditioners are used for manipulating reversible hydrocolloid. Various types are available with a compartment for boiling, storing, and conditioning the material. Syringes are used to inject the material onto critical areas and a water-cooled tray is used for gelation of the impression. The first step is to reduce the hydrocolloid gel to a fluid sol by placing the filled syringes and tubes in boiling water for 10 minutes. If a material is reliquefied after a previous gelling, at least 3 minutes should be added to the boiling time, since each time this material is reduced to a sol and the gel allowed to reform, it is harder to break down. Insufficient boiling results in a grainy, stiff mass that will not produce the fine detail required. After the material is liquefied, it may be stored in the storage compartment until needed. A storage bath temperature of 150°F is usually ideal. A lower temperature may result in partial gelation and inaccurate reproduction of fine detail. Before the dentist can make the impression, the material must be cooled or tempered in the conditioning bath. This conditioning will increase the viscosity of the material so it will not flow out of the tray or cause discomfort to the patient. The hydrocolloid is expressed from the tube into the preselected tray and placed in the conditioning bath for 10 minutes at 115°F. Then the dental assistant passes the filled syringe to the dentist. While the dentist is covering the critical areas in the mouth, the assistant should remove the tray from the bath and scrape the water-soaked outer layer from the material in the tray. This step is necessary for a complete bonding between the hydrocolloid in the tray and the injected hydrocolloid. The tray is passed to the dentist who makes the impression. Gelation of the hydrocolloid is accomplished by the circulation through the tray of cool water (60° to 70°F) for at least 5 minutes.

(2) Irreversible (alginate) hydrocolloid. Special equipment is not required to manipulate irreversible hydrocolloid but the manufacturer's directions for mixing it must be followed strictly. Directions for the temperature of the water, proportions of powder to water, and mixing time are most important in preserving the gel strength. Maximum gel strength is required to prevent fracture and assure elastic recovery. Mixing time is especially important; 1 minute is usually specified. Too little spatulation may reduce gel strength as much as 50 percent. Too much spatulation will break the gel as it forms and reduce gel strength. The required measurement of powder is sifted into the measured amount of water in a rubber mixing bowl to minimize the trapping of air bubbles. The mix is stirred vigorously for the specified time, monitored by a time clock. Then the dental specialist loads the material in a preselected tray in such a way as to avoid trapping air bubbles. Excess material in the bowl is usually given to the dentist to cover certain areas in the mouth. Then the dental specialist passes the filled tray to the dentist who makes the impression.

43. Polysulfide Base Impression Material

a. General.

(1) This material is used to make impressions for crowns, inlays, fixed and removable partial dentures, and complete dentures, especially in areas containing undercuts. It is composed of synthetic polysulfide base material and accelerator. It is supplied as pastes which, when mixed properly, solidify to an elastic condition. The material comes in two tubes, one tube

containing polysulfide base material (white paste), and the other containing accelerator (brown paste).

(2) Several polysulfide base impression materials are available. Most of them can be obtained in light (injectible), heavy, and regular types. The light type is used with the heavy type for gold restorations and removable partial dentures. The regular type is used mostly for complete dentures.

b. Manipulation.

(1) When using polysulfide base impression material, the dental specialist will need the following items: a customized tray, a syringe, light and medium or heavy-bodied polysulfide base impression material, and an adhesive. The customized tray is usually made of acrylic resin and constructed on a cast obtained from a preliminary impression of irreversible hydrocolloid material.

(2) Normally, a multiple mix technique is employed. The tray material (heavy or medium bodied) is mixed first. Equal lengths of the two pastes (brown accelerator and white polysulfide base) are expressed on a parchment pad and spatulated until the color of the mix is uniform without streaks. Then the material is placed in the tray, whose inner surface has been painted with an adhesive, and set aside. Next the syringe material is mixed the same way as the tray material. The syringe is filled and passed to the dentist who injects the material into the prepared area of the mouth. The filled tray then is passed to the dentist.

(3) The work of the dentist and the dental assistant must be timed so that neither the tray nor the syringe material has cured to the extent that they do not bond when brought together. If the material sets too rapidly the set may be retarded by adding a drop of oleic acid during mixing or by cooling the tubes in a refrigerator before mixing. If the material sets too slowly, a drop of water is added to hasten the set.

44. Impression Wax (Iowa Wax)

Impression wax may be used to make corrective linings for complete and partial denture impressions. It may be used also for corrective lining impressions for rebasing dentures. The patient's original denture teeth are used and a new acrylic base is processed.

Section VII. CAST MATERIALS

45. Gypsum Products

A number of gypsum products are used in dentistry. Plaster of paris and artificial stone powder are the ones used most as cast materials.

46. Chemistry of Gypsum Products

A general understanding of the chemistry of gypsum products will enable the dental specialist to use them wisely and increase his knowledge of why they react as they do. Gypsum is composed mainly of calcium sulphate dihydrate. A dihydrate is a material consisting of two parts of water to one part of the compound. Calcium sulphate dihydrate therefore is one part calcium dihydrate and two parts water.

a. In the manufacturing process gypsum is converted to plaster of paris and artificial stone by a process called calcining. Methods of calcining differ for plaster of paris, type I artificial stone, and type II artificial stone (die stone) except that in all processes the gypsum is first ground to a fine powder of particle size. Plaster of paris is derived when the gypsum is subjected to heat in an open vat. Type I artificial stone is produced when the gypsum is processed by steam heat under pressure. Type II artificial stone (die stone) is made by boiling the gypsum in a 30 percent solution of calcium chloride. The chloride then is washed away and the stone is dried and ground to the desired fineness.

b. Essentially, in all products, the reaction converts calcium sulphate dehydrate in to calcium sulphate hemihydrates by the removal of 1 ½ of the 2 molecules of water ($2C_aSO_4 \bullet 2H_2O + heat \rightarrow (C_aSO_4)_2 \bullet H_2O + 3H_2O$). The properties of the different products are due to the particle size and structure of the resulting powder that determine the amount of water necessary to float the powder during manipulation. Chemically the plaster and artificial stone are identical but the plaster particles are rough, irregular, and porous. The artificial stone particles are prismatic, more regular in size and dense. When the plaster or artificial stone is mixed with water, a hard substance is formed and the process described above is reversed ($3H_2O + (C_aSO_4)_2 \bullet H_2O \rightarrow 2CaSO_4\,2 \bullet H_2O + heat$). In the setting reaction, crystals of gypsum will form in clusters after the hemihydrates dissolves in the water. These nuclei of crystallization intermesh and become entangled with one another, giving the set material its strength and rigidity. During manipulation enough water must be added so that the reaction will take place. Additional water is needed to float the powder particles so they can be stirred and poured into the impression to form the cast. The more water that must be used for this purpose the weaker the material will be upon set.

47. Uses and Manipulation of Gypsum Products

a. Plaster of Paris.

(1) *Uses.* Plaster of paris is used for pouring casts, making matrices for prosthodontic restorations, attaching casts to articulators, and general use in the dental laboratory where strength is not important. Its crushing strength is 2,600 psi.

(2) *Manipulation.* Water-powder ratios are used as stated by the manufacturer. Before manipulation, the can containing the material should be agitated to disperse evenly all elements in the powder. A clean, dry, rubber bowl and plaster spatula are used to manipulate the material. First, the water is measured and poured into the rubber bowl. The powder is weighed and sifted into the water to avoid trapping air bubbles. Then the mix is spatulated 30 to 60 seconds with a knifing or stirring motion including all powder from the sides of the bowl. Whipping the mix will trap air and so should be avoided. Before the material is poured, the mix is vibrated to remove any air bubbles unintentionally trapped.

(3) *Setting time.* The initial setting time for plaster of paris is 5 to 10 minutes. The initial set is the stage at which the plaster loses its glossy appearance and is hard enough to hold for carving. The final set for plaster of paris is about 45 minutes and is the stage at which the plaster achieves a dry, hard condition. The setting of plaster of paris can be hastened by using less water, by mixing longer, by using chemical accelerators, or by using warm water (up to 85°F). Reversing these processes or using chemical retarders will lengthen the setting time. The most satisfactory results are obtained by following the manufacturer's directions.

b. Artificial Stone.

(1) *Uses.* Artificial stone is used in making master casts and dies and for general laboratory use when a very hard, strong product is needed. Since artificial stone particles are

nonporous, the finished product is hard and dense. This provides an excellent cast for the fabrication of prosthetic restorations. The crushing strength of artificial stone is 7,500 psi.

(2) *Manipulation.* Artificial stone is mixed much like plaster of paris. The average mixing ratio is 30 cc of water to 100 grams of stone powder. This ratio may vary somewhat with different manufacturers. The required amount of water is placed in a rubber bowl and the stone powder added slowly. All powder should be smoothed below the water before spatulating. Spatulation should be thorough without whipping the mixture; whipping can trap air bubbles which weaken the cast. The bowl should be vibrated during the mixing to make air bubbles rise to the surface. Spatulation should be completed in 30 to 60 seconds; after that the bowl should be vibrated again. The use of mechanical spatulation helps to reduce air bubbles.

(3) *Setting time.* The initial setting time for artificial stone is usually 8 to 10 minutes, the final setting time 25 to 45 minutes depending upon the. type of stone mixed. The surface hardness can be increased by soaking the cast several hours in a solution of borax.

Section VIII. MISCELLANEOUS DENTAL MATERIALS

48. Calcium Hydroxide

Calcium hydroxide is a fine white powder used in operative procedures primarily for pulp capping (protection for an exposed or nearly exposed pulp) since this material accelerates the formation of secondary dentin. Calcium hydroxide is available as powder, paste, and liquid. The powder must be mixed with sterile water or xylocaine to form a paste. The paste and liquids are premixed commercial preparations ready for immediate use. Because of its low crushing strength, calcium hydroxide alone is not used as an intermediate base. When applied, it is usually covered with zinc phosphate cement or a zinc oxide and eugenol cement.

49. Root Canal Filling Materials

These materials are used to fill previously prepared root canals. This treatment is part of root canal or endodontic therapy. Root canal filling materials consist of tapered gutta-percha or silver points in various standard sizes and root canal sealers or cements. Root canal cements often consist of a zinc oxide and eugenol preparation. A good root canal filling material is insoluble in tissue fluids, opaque to (not allowing) the passage of x-rays, reasonably easy to remove, nonirritating to periapical (around the apex or root tip) tissues, nonabsorbent to moisture, and dimensionally stable after insertion into a root canal.

a. *Gutta-Percha.* Gutta-percha is used for a temporary filling (supplied as a stick) and as a root canal filling material supplied as points. Gutta-percha is the refined coagulated milky exudate of trees in the Malay Peninsula. It is pink or gray in color. It softens when heated and is easily molded. When cool, it maintains shape fairly well. Gutta-percha points long have been a root canal filling material of choice because of the material's advantages. It has a high thermal expansion. It does not shrink unless used with solvent. It is radiopaque, conducts heat poorly, and is easy to remove from the root canal. It may be kept sterile in antiseptic solution, is impervious to moisture, and is bacterioostatic (prevents the growth or multiplication of bacteria). Disadvantages of gutta-percha are that it shrieks when used with a solvent and is not always easy to introduce into the root canal.

b. Silver Root Canal Points. The dentist may use silver root canal points in filling the root canal. Silver points have the advantages of gutta-percha but are easier to insert. Sight selection of silver points is easy because they come in the same sizes and tapers as standard root canal broaches and reamers. The main disadvantages of silver points are that they are hard to remove from the root canal and are more expensive than gutta-percha.

50. Temporary Stopping Material

Temporary stopping material is used primarily as a temporary filling material. It usually consists of gutta-percha, waxes, zinc oxide, fatty acids, and possibly powdered feldspar or silex. This material dissolves to some extent in fluids of the mouth. It is easier to handle than gutta-percha but does not wear as well. It can be made plastic by heat or by solution in chloroform or eucalyptol.

51. Cavity Lining Varnish

Cavity lining varnish is used as a seal under otherwise unbased restoration. It is composed of resins dissolved in a volative thinner. Cavity lining varnish is used extensively to seal dentin tubules (small tubes in the dentin that contain dentinal fibers) and thus isolate the pulp of the tooth from the acidity of silicate or zinc phosphate cement and in some cases, to help prevent marginal leakage around restorations. Cavity lining varnish is issued premixed, usually with a bottle of thinner. The bottle of varnish should be kept tightly sealed when not in use. If the varnish gets too thick, thinner should be added to restore its original consistency.

52. Dental Resins for Restorative Dentistry

a. General. Resins are used as restorative and denture base materials. (A denture base is that part of a denture which contacts the soft tissues and supports the artificial teeth.) A synthetic resin, methyl methacrylate (acrylic resin), is the most widely used resin for these purposes. Two forms of this material are used: an auto polymerizing type, which sets or cures to form a satisfactory result at room temperatures, and a heat-polymerizing type, which is processed by application of heat under pressure.

b. Composition. Acrylic resins are made as a liquid and a powder which are mixed when ready for use. The liquid, called monomer, is composed of a derivative of methyl acrylic acid, an inhibitor (usually hydroquinone), and a tertiary amine (usually dimethyl-p-toluidine). The autopolymerizing acrylic monomer includes an accelerator. Monomer vaporizes readily in air with characteristic ether-like odor. It must be kept tightly stoppered to prevent evaporation when not in use. Monomer is readily contaminated by other materials and should not be allowed to contact the rubber bulb of the dropper or be stored in the same compartment with eugenol or other essential oils. For this reason, zinc oxide and eugenol cannot be used as a base for resin restorations. The powder, called polymer, is available in a variety of shades which can be mixed to closely match most teeth. Since contaminants can affect the cure and the color of the material, contamination of both polymer and monomer should be avoided.

c. Uses.

(1) Autopolymerizing acrylic resin is used in operative dentistry as a direct restorative material, in the construction of acrylic resin facings for some full crowns, and in the construction of temporary crowns, fixed partial dentures, and space maintainers. It is used in prosthetic dentistry to repair complete and partial dentures, to fabricate individualized impression trays, to fabricate oral surgical and periodontal splints, and as a baseplate material.

(2) Heat-polymerizing acrylic resin is used in restorative dentistry to fabricate crowns and parts of pontics. It is used in prosthetic dentistry to fabricate bases and saddles for dentures, to fabricate individualized impression trays, to fabricate oral surgical and periodontal splints, to repair dentures, and for other purposes.

d. Manipulation. Manufacturer's directions must be followed strictly.

53. Dental Porcelain

Dental porcelain is manufactured as a powder. When it is heated to a very high temperature in a special oven it fuses into a homogeneous mass. The heating process is called baking. Upon cooling, the mass is hard and dense. The material is made in a variety of shades to match closely most tooth colors. Baked porcelain has a translucency similar to that of dental enamel, so that porcelain crowns, pontics, and inlays of highly pleasing appearance can be made. Ingredients of porcelain include feldspar, kaolin, silica in the form of quartz, materials which act as fluxes to lower the fusion point, metallic oxide and binders. Porcelains are classified into high-, medium-, or low-fusing groups, depending upon the temperature at which fusion takes place.

a. High-fusing porcelains fuse at 2,400°F or over. They are used for the fabrication of full porcelain crowns (jacket crowns).

b. Medium-fusing porcelains fuse between 2,000° and 2,300°F. They are used in the fabrication of inlays, crowns, facings, and pontics. A pontic is the portion of a fixed partial denture which replaces a missing tooth.

c. Low-fusing porcelains fuse between 1,600° and 1,950°F. They are used primarily to correct or modify the contours of previously baked high- or medium fusing porcelain restorations.

54. Baseplate Material

Baseplate materials are used in complete and partial denture fabrication, in making the occlusion-rim foundation, and in the fabrication of impression trays. Baseplates are usually softened over an open flame, then molded over a cast and trimmed. They are composed of shellac resins and wax modifiers.

55. Polishing Materials

a. Tin Oxide. Tin oxide is used to polish teeth and restorations. A fine white powder, it is used in paste with water or glycerin.

b. Pumice. Pumice is used as an abrasive and polishing agent for acrylic resins, amalgams, and gold. It consists mainly of complex silicates of aluminum, potassium, and sodium. Two grades of it are listed in the Federal supply catalog: flour of pumice and coarse pumice.

c. Chalk (Whiting). Chalk is used for polishing acrylic resins and metals. It is composed primarily of calcium carbonate.

d. Tripoli. Tripoli is a polishing agent usually used for gold and other metals. It is made from certain porous rocks.

e. Rouge (Jeweler's). Rouge is used for polishing gold and is composed of iron oxide. It is usually in cake or stick form.

f. Zirconium Silicate. Zirconium silicate is used for cleaning and polishing teeth. It may be mixed with water or stannous fluoride solution for caries prevention treatment. Instructions must be followed exactly to obtain the proper powder-liquid proportions for full effectiveness.

56. Intermediate Restorative Material

Intermediate restorative material consists of a powder, that is 80 percent zinc oxide and 20 percent polymethyl methacrylate, which is mixed with a liquid containing 99 percent eugenol and 1 percent acetic acid. Although this a temporary restorative material, its compressive strength is twice that of zinc oxide and eugenol cement and only slightly less than zinc phosphate cement. Its tensile and sheer strengths are greater than zinc phosphate cement. Supplied in three colors, the material is used as follows. Ivory is used in anterior teeth where affected dentin is left in the cavity preparation. Red or pink is used in posterior teeth where affected dentin is left in depth of the cavity preparation. Blue is used in posterior teeth where both affected and infected dentin are removed.

GLOSSARY OF DENTAL SCIENCE

CONTENTS

GLOSSARY OF DENTAL SCIENCE

Abrasion—The mechanical wearing away of tooth structure through mastication, sharp particles, incorrect toothbrushing, or friction of clasps.

Abrasive—A substance containing sharp particles used for smoothing and grinding; for example, pumice.

Abutment—A tooth used to retain, support, and stabilize a fixed partial denture or removable partial denture by a clasp, inlay, or crown.

Acidogenic bacteria—Bacteria which can produce acid.

Aciduric—Ability of microorganisms to grow in an acid environment.

Aerobe—A type of microorganism (bacteria) that requires free atmospheric oxygen to live.

Aerodontalgia—Toothache associated with a decrease in atmospheric pressure such as is experienced at high altitude.

Agar-agar—A gelatinous material obtained from certain seaweeds used in the reversible hydrocolloid impression materials.

Alginate—An irreversible hydrocolloid impression material which cannot be used more than once.

Allergy (hypersensitivity)—Exaggerated specific sensitivity to a substance harmless in similar amounts to most people.

Alveolar osteitis—A painful condition caused by infection and disintegration of the blood clot following tooth extraction (dry socket).

Alveolar process—The cancellous and cortical bone which surrounds and supports the teeth in the maxilla or mandible.

Alveolar ridge—The ridge formed by the alveolar process of the maxilla or mandible. Also called an alveolar arch.

Alveolectomy—The trimming of the alveolar process.

Alveolus—1. Cavity, pit, recess. 2. Air cell of the lungs. 3. Tooth socket.

Amalgamator—A mechanical device for mixing dental amalgam.

Ameloblast—Enamel-forming cell.

Ampere (amp)—A unit for measuring the strength of an electric current. Represents the amount of current.

Anabolism—The building up phase of metabolism.

Anaerobic—Cannot live in the presence of oxygen.

Analgesia—Loss of pain sensation without the loss of consciousness as a result of the administration of a drug.

Anastomosis—A joining; a connection between blood vessels.

Anatomic teeth—Denture teeth designed to conform in general with the anatomy of the natural teeth.

Anatomical articulator—An instrument which can be adjusted to copy closely the movements of the patient's mandible.

Anesthesia—Complete elimination of the sensation of pain. The tactile (touch) and temperature sense also may be absent.

Anneal—Softening a metal or alloy by controlled heating and cooling. Annealing facilitates working a metal and minimizes brittleness.

Anode—The positive pole of an electric source. In dental radiography, the positive side of the tube holding the tungsten target which emits radiation.

Anodontia—Failure of tooth formation; congenital absence of teeth.

Anodyne—Any agent or drug which relieves pain.

Anterior palatine foramen (greater palatine foramen)—A foramen located in the palatal curvature lingual to the roots of the second molar. It forms the opening of the pterygopalatine canal and transmits the greater palatine nerve and blood vessels.

Anteroposterior—Extending from the front backward.

Antiseptic—A substance which will inhibit bacterial growth.

Antrum of Highmore—*See* Maxillary sinus.

Apex—The pointed end of any conical structure; the tip of the root of a tooth.

Aphthous stomatitis—Lesions of the oral mucous membrane which start as small vesicles and later break, leaving ulcers. Also called canker sores.

Apical foramen—The opening at the end of the root of a tooth through which the tooth receives its nerve and blood supply.

Apicoectomy—Removal of the apex of the root of the tooth.

Apothecaries' weight—A system of weights used in dispensing drugs.

Approach arm—The metal which extends from the major connector out to the retentive tips of a bar-type clasp.

Arkansas stone—An especially hard, smooth stone used to sharpen dental instruments.

Arthritis—Inflammation of a joint.

Articular—Pertaining to a joint.

Articulate—To join, fit, or interrelate by mechanical means (articulate the teeth).

Articulation—Anatomically, a joint or place of union between two or more bones. In dentistry, the contact relationship between the occlusal surfaces of teeth while in action.

Articulator—A device used to hold casts of the maxillary and mandibular teeth and dental arches in the proper positional relationships and to permit duplication of certain jaw movements.

Asepsis—A condition of being free of infection, or absence of infectious material.

Asphyxia—Loss of consciousness as a result of too little oxygen and too much carbon monoxide in the blood. Suffocation causes asphyxia.

Aspirator—An appliance for removing fluid from the mouth or any cavity of the body by suction.

Astringent—A drug which shrinks the tissue cells, thus inhibiting secretion or flow of body fluids.

Attrition—The wearing away of tooth substance (enamel, dentin, or cementum) under the stress of chewing (mastication).

Autogenous soldering—Joining two metals by heat alone.

Axial surface—Any surface of a tooth which is parallel to the long axis, such as the facial surface.

Back action clasp—A circumferential-type clasp modified so that the connection to the denture is attached at the terminal end of the lingual arm rather than at the occlusal rest.

Backing—The metal support which attaches a facing to a prosthesis.

Bactericide—A substance which kills bacteria.

Bacteriostatic—An antiseptic or substance which prevents the growth or multiplication of bacteria.

Balance (in occlusion)—The simultaneous contacts of tooth surfaces in different parts of the mouth which prevent tipping of the denture.

Bar—A connector used in partial denture design to join different parts of the denture.

Bar clasp (Roach clasp)—vertical projection—A type of partial denture clasp, such as the T-clasp, which approaches the survey line of the tooth from the cervical area. Named for Doctor Roach, an American dentist.

Base metal—A metal other than a noble metal. Examples of noble metals are gold, platinum, and palladium.

Baseplate—A temporary foundation representing the base of a denture which is used for making jaw relationship records and for the arrangement of teeth.

Bell-crowned—The crown of a tooth which is largest at the occlusal surface and constricted or tapered toward the cervix. Decidous molars, permanent incisors, and bicuspids are good examples.

Bennet movement—The lateral shift of the condyle first described by a British dentist.

Bifurcated—Divided in two parts or branches.

Bilateral—Having two sides. Any partial denture having a major connector is said to be bilateral.

Biscuit bake—That stage in baking porcelaine which just precedes fusion into a glasslike substance.

Blockout tool—Cylindrical rod used in the surveyor spindle to remove excess wax between the height of contour and the gingival border of abutment teeth on master casts and paralleling the undercuts approximately the edentulous areas. (Also called wax trimmers.)

Body (of a clasp)—The rigid part of the clasp formed by the junction of the occlusal rest, the shoulders, and the connector.

Boley gage—A caliper-like instrument calibrated in millimeters and used for fine measurements in the laboratory.

Bonwill triangle—An equilateral triangle with the base corners in the center of each condyle of the mandible and the apex at the mesial incisal edge of the lower centrals or midline of the edentulous ridge. Doctor Bonwill believed each side of the triangle averaged about 4 inches.

Borax (sodium tetraborate)—A white crystalline substance used as a flux in soldering or as a retarder in the setting of plaster of paris and hyrdocal.

Border molding (muscle trimming)—The shaping of an impression material by the movement of the tissues adjacent to the borders of an impression.

Boxing—Preparing a form, usually in wax, around an impression to give proper form and thickness to the base of the cast and to the tissue borders of the cast when it is poured.

Bracing—Resistance to displacement in a horizontal direction.

Braze—To join with hard solder.

Brinell hardness—An index number denoting relative surface hardness of a material abbreviated B.H.N. Used in testing soft metals and nonbrittle materials such as gold, copper, and silver.

Bruxism—Habitual grinding of the teeth. Often limited to the sleeping period or during mental or physical concentration or strain.

Buccal frenum—The string-like tissue which attaches the cheeks to the alveolar ridge in the bicuspid region.

Buccal notch—The V-shaped notch in the impression or denture formed by, or for, the buccal frenum.

Burlew discs—Rubber wheels impregnated with pumice and used for polishing and smoothing dental restorations.

Burnish—The drawing or flattening out of a malleable metal through pressure.

Burnout—The process of eliminating the wax pattern from the mold by means of heat.

Butterfly partial (stay plate) "flipper"—A horseshoe-shaped maxillary acrylic partial denture usually supplying one or two teeth and often retained with clasps. A preferable term is "temporary removable partial denture."

Cancellous—A lattice-like bony structure.

Carborundum—An abrasive used in many dental stones and points.

Cast—Reproduction of the mouth or teeth in plaster or similar material upon which a dental prosthetic restoration is fabricated. Casts may also be used as diagnostic aids.

Cast base—A complete or removable partial denture having most of the tissue area cast in metal with the remainder made of acrylic.

Casting—The process of pouring molten metal into a mold.

Cathode—A negative terminal of the roentgen ray tube.

Cathode ray—An electron emitted from the surface of the cathode.

Caustic—A substance, such as phenol, capable of chemically burning and destroying tissue.

Central ray—The roentgen ray that is at the geometric center of the central beam.

Centric occlusion—Natural contact relation of the maxillary and mandibular teeth when the mandible is moved from rest position to a closed position.

Centric relation—The furthermost retruded position of the mandible from which lateral movements can be made at a given degree of jaw opening. It is the position from which all jaw movements start.

Cervical—Pertaining to the neck of a tooth.

Cervical line (cementoenamel junction)—That line where the cementum and the enamel join.

Cervix—A neck or constriction.

Chalk—Calcium carbonate. A powder used for final polishing and as a separating media when adapting baseplates.

Characterization, denture—Modification of the form and color of the denture teeth and base to produce a more natural appearance.

Chayes attachment—A type of precision attachment used in removable partial denture prosthesis. Named for the designer, Doctor Herman Chayes.

Cheek retractor—An instrument used to hold the lips and cheeks out of the operator's way.

Chemotherapy—Treatment of a bacterial disease with a chemical agent which has a specific harmful effect upon the causative bacteria but is relatively harmless to human tissues.

Chisel—A sharp, beveled instrument used for cutting tooth structure as an aid in cavity preparations.

Chisel (bone)—A sharp, beveled, cutting instrument used to cut bone.

Chrome-cobalt alloy—One of the group of alloys used in dentistry as a material for partial denture frameworks.

Clasp—The metal part of a partial denture which partly encircles or contacts the abutment tooth or teeth and helps to retain, support, and stabilize the appliance.

Clasp arm—The portion of the clasp which extends from the body of the clasp out to the end of the clasp.

Clasp tip—This refers to the terminal one-third of the clasp arm. Sometimes called the "finger."

Cleft palate—Congenital fissure of the palate and roof of the mouth. It is caused by failure of the maxillary bones to unite at the midline.

Cocoa butter—A fatty oil made from the seeds of the chocolate plant. It is used as a protective coating for newly placed silicate restorations.

Cohesion—The sticking together of molecules of the same material.

Compensating curve—A curvature developed in the occlusal arrangement of denture teeth for the purpose of obtaining balanced occlusal contacts.

Condensation—The process of making a substance more compact as with dental amalgam.

Condylar inclination—The amount of inclination from the horizontal of the condylar path as recorded in degrees on the articulator.

Condyle path—The path followed by the mandibular condyle in the temporomandibular joint during movements of the mandible.

Connector—In partial dentures, a part of the appliance which serves to connect two or more parts such as one saddle with another. The lingual bar is a connector.

Contact area—The area of a tooth that normally touches an adjacent tooth.

Coronal—Pertaining to the crown of a tooth.

Cortical bone—Very hard, dense bone; the outer protective cover.

Counter die—The reverse image of a die.

Crest of the ridge—The high point of the alveolar ridge.

Cross-bite—A condition in which the mandible lies so far outside the maxillae, that normal arrangement of the teeth is not feasible. In this case, the mandibular teeth in the bicuspid and molar regions may be set to overjet the maxillary teeth.

Crown, anatomic—That part of the tooth covered by enamel.

Crown, artificial—A fixed restoration of the major part or of the entire coronal part of a natural tooth with an artificial substance.

Crown, clinical—That part of the tooth visible in the mouth.

Crucible—That part of a casting machine in which the metal or alloy is melted before casting. Also a porcelaine container used to hold acid for pickling.

Crystabolite—A form of quartz or sand (silicon dioxide) highly resistant to heat. Often used as a component of investment material.

Curve of Spee—A curve formed by the occlusal alignment of the posterior mandibular teeth, beginning at the tip of the cuspid and continuing distally to the anterior border of the mandibular ramus, as first described by the German anatomist, von Spee.

Cuspid line—The vertical line which the dental officer scribes on the occlusion rims to indicate the position that the cuspid tooth is to occupy in the setup. It may indicate the center or the distal surface of the cuspid, depending upon the technique followed by the dental officer.

Dappen dish—Trade name for a glass medicine dish commonly used in dentistry (medicament dish).

Debubblizer—A wetting agent used to lower the surface tension of the investment and the water repellency of the wax pattern before investing.

Dental arch—The arch formed by the alignment of the teeth in a jaw or artificial denture.

Dental fluorosis—The effects of excessive fluoride on ameloblasts during the formation of enamel, causing an enamel defect.

Dentalgia (odontalgia)—Toothache.

Dental papilla—That portion of a developing tooth bud which will form the pulp and dentin of the tooth.

Dentifrice substances (toothpastes and powders)—Substances used to aid the brush in removing debris.

Dentimeter—An instrument used to obtain an accurate measurement of the perimeter (circumference) of a tooth or crown. The measurement may be used to construct a crown or ferrule.

Dentulous—Having natural teeth present in the mouth.

Denture base (saddle)—That part of a partial denture which fits on the alveolar ridge and holds the teeth. It may be metal, acrylic resin, or vulcanite, but is usually made of acrylic resin.

Denture border (periphery)—The circumferences or outer border of a denture.

Detergent—A wetting agent. Used in denture fabrication to help remove wax from the denture mold.

Developing solution—A chemical solution used for developing dental radiographic films.

Dewpoint—The temperature of the atmosphere at which the moisture begins to be deposited as dew (droplets of water).

Diamond point—A rotary cutting instrument which incorporates diamond particles.

Diastema—A space between the teeth. Most commonly a space between the maxillary central incisors in adults.

Diatoric recess—The hollow opening or slot found in denture teeth for holding them in the denture base material.

Die—An exact, positive reproduction of an object. Used especially for crowns, inlays, and fixed partial dentures.

Dilaceration—A sharp bend in the long axis of a tooth resulting from an injury during development.

Direct retainer—A clasp or attachment applied to an abutment tooth to hold a removable partial denture in position.

Distal—Away from the midline of the face following the curvature of the dental arch.

Disto-occlusion—The class of occlusion in which the mandible is in distal relation to the maxillae.

Dry foil—An adhesive tinfoil used to protect an area in the mouth from moisture.

Ductility—The property of a metal which permits it to be drawn into a wire without breaking. Gold is very ductile.

Duplicating (cast)—The process of producing an exact, positive copy of a cast by means of a mold.

Duplicating (denture)—A procedure by which an entire denture base is replaced with new material.

Edentulous—Without teeth.

Electrode—Either pole or terminal of an electric source.

Electrolyte—The solution used in electroplating.

Embrasure—The occlusal, facial, or lingual sloping space formed by the contacting proximal surfaces of adjacent teeth.

Enamel rod—Microscopic rods which form the bulk of the enamel and are held together by an intercementing substance.

Epulis—A fibrous tumor located on the gingiva.

Equilibration (of occlusion)—To equalize. To remove high spots and areas of interference. To adjust the contact areas between the maxillary and mandibular teeth so that each tooth carries its equal share of the occlusal load.

Erosion—The chemical wearing away of the tooth structure.

Erythema dose—The amount of radiation producing only temporary redness of the skin, like sunburn.

Exfoliation—Falling off in scales or layers. The loss or shedding of deciduous teeth is called exfoliation.

Exostosis—A bony growth projecting outward from the surface of a bone or tooth.

Extraoral tracer—A device used for registering centric jaw relation. The tracing device itself extends outside the mouth.

Face bow—A device used to record the relationship between the maxillary and mandibular arch and to transfer this relationship to the articulator.

Face bow fork (bite fork)—The device used to attach the face bow to the maxillary occlusal rim for a face bow transfer.

Facial—Pertaining to the face. The surface of the tooth or restoration nearest the lips or cheeks. Used synonymously with the words buccal and labial.

Facing—The thin veneer of porcelain or acrylic which closely fits a metal backing; used in fixed and removable partial dentures.

Festoon—Carving in the base material of a denture to resemble the contours of the replaced natural tissues.

Fineness—The proportion of pure gold in an alloy. A fineness of 1,000 is 100 percent pure gold.

Finishing—The process of smoothing and trimming before the final polish.

Finishing knife—Instrument used for trimming off excess restorative materials.

Fistule—An abnormal passage connecting two body cavities, running between a body cavity and the surface, or connecting an abscess with a cavity on the surface.

Fixed partial denture—A prosthodontic restoration replacing one or more teeth which is cemented into place and cannot be removed by the patient.

Fixing solution—A chemical solution used for fixing dental radiographic films.

Flange—The part of the denture or saddle which extends facially or lingually from the ridge crest to the periphery.

Flap—The section of tissue (mucosa, underlying connective tissue and periosteum) raised from the alveolar bone to secure surgical access to underlying structures.

Flash—The overflow of excess denture base material resulting from overpacking the denture mold.

Flask—A metal frame constructed in sections in which a mold is formed in plaster of paris or in artificial stone for the packing and curing of a denture.

Flasking—The act of investing in a flask; the process of investing the cast and a wax denture in a flask preparatory to molding the denture base material into the form of a denture.

Floss—In dentistry, a thin silk or nylon yarn which may be waxed or unwaxed used as part of the prophylaxis treatment to clean the proximal surfaces of the teeth. It may be used as a ligature placed below the cingulums and around the necks of anterior teeth to secure rubber dam material to the teeth.

Flow— The ability of a material to flow or deform in shape under a given load without increasing the magnitude of the applied force.

Flux—A substance used to prevent or remove an oxide film from the surface of a heated metal. In porcelain work, an agent which lowers the fusion temperature of the porcelain.

Focal infection—An infection in a circumscribed area of the body which constitutes a possible source of infection in some other part of the body or in the body in general.

Foil—An exceedingly thin sheet of metal. Tin, gold, and platinum foils are used in dentistry.

Forceps—Metallic instruments used to grasp and manipulate an object. Many types of forceps are used in dentistry.

Foreshortening of image—The term used in dental radiology denoting the abnormal shortening of a tooth or teeth on a dental radiographic film.

Fossa (dental)—A cavity, pit, or small hollow.

Free-end saddle—Refers to a saddle extension of a partial denture which has no posterior abutment.

Free-way space—The space between the occlusal surfaces of the teeth when the mouth is at rest.

Frenectomy—Removal of either of the folds of mucous membrane on the middle of each lip, connecting the lips with the gums.

Frenum or frenulum—The small band or fold of connective tissue covered with mucous membrane which attaches the tongue, lips, and cheeks to adjacent structures.

Frequency—The number of times per second an alternating current changes direction.

Fulcrum—The support upon which a lever rests when a force is applied. In partial dentures, an abutment tooth may act as a fulcrum for the prosthesis.

Fusible metal—An alloy which melts and solidifies at a relatively low temperature.

Fusion (of teeth)—Result of union of two tooth germs so that the resulting teeth are united by dentin and either cementum or enamel.

Gage (gauge)—A measurement such as is used with wrought wire or hypodermic needles. The act of measuring. An instrument used to measure.

Galvanic current—A current of electricity produced by chemical action between two dissimilar metals suspended in a solution.

Galvanism—A current of electricity produced by chemical action. A galvanic shock is sometimes produced when a gold crown or prosthetic restoration from one dental arch occludes with an amalgam restoration of the opposing arch.

Gelation—Solidification of a liquid substance in which a gel forms and acts as a matrix between the undissolved particles.

Gemination of teeth—A condition in which a single tooth germ divides and produces two crowns on a single root.

Gingival recession—The shrinking away or pulling back of the gingiva from its normal position around the tooth.

Gingival sulcus—The space between the tooth and the free margin of the gingiva.

Glaze—The final firing of porcelain which imports a high gloss to the material.

Glenoid—Resembling a shallow cavity. Glenoid fossa: the fossa of the temporal bone which the condyle of the mandible approximates, thus forming the temporomandibular joint.

Gothic arch tracer, needlepoint tracer—A mechanical device with a marking point attached to one jaw and a graph plate or tracing plate attached to the other jaw. It is used to trace and record the pattern and extent of movements of the mandible. The point of a properly made tracing indicates centric relation of the patient's jaws.

Grain growth—The merging of smaller grains into larger grains of metal under high heat. This produces a brittle metal.

Gram—A unit of weight in the metric system equal to the weight of 1 cubic centimeter of water.

Greenstick fracture—A condition in which one side of the bone is broken; the other side is bent.

Groove—A line depression in a tooth surface.

Hamular—A hooklike process distal to the tuberosity. Hamular notch: an indentation formed at the junction of the hamular process with the posterior border of the maxillary tuberosity.

Hard palate—Bone covered by mucous membrane which forms the roof of the oral cavity.

Heat soaking—The process of allowing an invested inlay or partial denture to remain in the oven at the burnout temperature for a predetermined length of time to remove all carbon from the mold before casting.

Heat treatment—The controlled heating and cooling of metals and metallic alloys to produce desirable physical properties.

Height of contour—A line encircling a tooth designating its greatest circumference or points or greatest radius or prominence.

High lip line—The horizontal line which the dental officer marks on the occlusal rim to indicate the approximate level of the upper lip when the patient smiles.

High tension current—Current which has high voltage or electrical pressure.

Hinge joint—A joint which moves in only one phase, as the finger joints.

Hoe—A dental hand instrument shaped like a hoe used in cavity preparation.

Horizontal overlap (overject)—The horizontal overlap of the maxillary teeth over the mandibular teeth.

Hydrocolloid—Elastic colloidal materials which are mixed with water to make dental impressions.

Hygroscopic expansion—Expansion resulting from absorption of moisture.

Hyoid bone—A movable horseshoe-shaped bone located above the thyroid cartilage at the base of the tongue: Some muscles which make up the floor of the mouth are attached to this bone.

Hyperemia—An increased amount of blood in a locality.

Hyperplasia—Overgrowth of a part due to a multiplication of its elements. Increase in number of cells.

Hypertrophy—Abnormal enlargement in the size of a tissue or organ. Increased size of individual cells.

Hypoplasia—Defective formation of an organ or tissue charactized by decreased or arrested growth or development. A retarded or defective development of a part of a tooth.

Immediate denture—A complete or partial removable denture which is made before the teeth to be replaced are extracted and is inserted when the last teeth are extracted.

Impaction—A tooth which is either partially or wholly unerupted long after the normal eruption time.

Impactor—An engine-driven instrument used to remove bone or split teeth with mallet and chisel-like action.

Impression—A negative reproduction of a given tissue area made to reproduce a positive form or cast of the area.

Impression paste—A material, usually supplied as a base and a hardener, which is mixed and used as a corrective impression material.

Impression plaster—Plaster of paris with a high starch content. Used to make complete denture impressions.

Impression tray—A receptacle or device used to carry,

confine, and control and impression material for making an impression.

Inclination—The deviation of the long axis of a tooth from the perpendicular line.

Indirect inlay technique—An inlay technique in which the wax pattern is prepared on a die rather than in the prepared tooth.

Indirect retainer—A part of a partial denture which holds the denture in place by resisting tipping forces.

Induration—Abnormal hardness or firmness of tissue.

Infra—Prefix meaning below.

Initial set—The first hardening of a material.

Inlay—A restoration formed to fit a tooth cavity and then cemented to place (usually a gold alloy restoration).

Insertion—The area of attachment of a muscle, organ, or part. Also the process of placing a restoration or denture.

Interdigitation—Interlocking or fitting together of opposing parts, as with the maxillary and mandibular teeth.

Interocclusal record (checkbite)—An index of the teeth in a certain jaw position, usually made of soft wax or plaster, whose purpose is to enable the specialist to relate the casts in this same position on the articulator.

Interproximal—Between the adjacent surfaces of two teeth.

Invest—To surround, envelop, or embed in an investment material.

Investment cast—A cast poured in investment material. Cast metal dentures are made on investment casts.

Jacket crown—A complete veneer restoration usually made of acrylic, resin, or porcelain.

Jaw relation—Any relation of the mandible to the maxillae.

Kennedy bar (continuous lingual clasp)—The auxiliary bar sometimes used in lingual bar partial dentures.

Kilovoltage (abbreviation kV or kVp for peak kilovoltage)—The unit of electrical pressure which forces the current through a circuit. A kilovolt equals 1,000 volts.

Knoop hardness—A measurement of the relative hardness of brittle materials such as glass, porcelain, and tooth enamel or hard metal clasps such as chrome-cobalt.

Labial bar—A metal bar contoured to the labial aspect of the mandibular tissues used to connect two parts of a mandibular partial denture.

Labial frenum—A frenum which attaches the upper or lower lip to the alveolar ridge at, or near, the midline.

Labial notch—The V-shaped opening in an impression or denture which is formed by, or for, the labial frenum.

Lamina dura—The cortical bone lining the tooth socket.

Leukoplakia—White, diffuse patches on the mucous membrane of lips, tongue, cheeks, and floor of mouth.

Lichen planus—Oral lesions which consist of small or grayish-white papules, slightly elevated and arranged in net-like formation.

Ligament—A tough, fibrous band which connects bones.

Line-angle—Angle made by two surfaces of a tooth uniting along a line.

Lingual bar—A metal bar contoured to the lingual aspect of mandibular tissues used to connect two parts of a mandibular partial denture.

Lingual flange—The part of a denture or impression which extends from about the crest of the ridge to the periphery on the lingual surface.

Lingual frenum—The fold of tissue which connects part of the freely movable portion of the tongue with the floor of the mouth.

Lingual plate—The plate of bone forming the lingual wall of the tooth socket (alveolus) or a solid plate of metal which is continuous with the lingual bar of a partial denture and rests against the lingual surfaces of the anterior teeth. It functions as a connector, an indirect retainer, and sometimes as a periodontal splint for loose teeth.

Lingual rest—A rest on the lingual aspect, usually of an anterior tooth, which provides support to a prosthesis.

Lobe—A part of an organ or gland demarcated by fissures or cleavages. That part of a tooth which has formed from a single developmental center.

Malar process—The bony extensions of the temporal and maxillary bones which unite with the zygomatic bone to form the zygomatic arch. Sometimes called cheekbone.

Malignant—Dangerous to life; virulent or invasive. A neoplasm that metastasizes.

Malleability—The property of a metal which permits it to be extended in all directions without breaking.

Mallet—A small, light hammer used to manipulate metal or as a tapping instrument.

Malocclusion—Abnormal interdigitation of the maxillary and mandibular teeth.

Mamelon—One of three tubercles sometimes present on the cutting edge of an incisor tooth, particularly a recently erupted one.

Mandrel—A spindle or shank upon which abrasive, cutting, or polishing wheels, stones, or disks are mounted for use in a dental handpiece or a dental lathe.

Marginal ridges—The elevations of enamel which form the mesial and distal margins of the occlusal surfaces of the bicuspids and molars and the mesial and distal margins of the lingual surfaces of incisors and cuspids.

Master cast—A cast made from the final impression.

Master impression—An exact, detailed impression of the hard and soft structures of a mouth.

Materia alba—The whitish deposits on the necks of teeth composed mainly of mucous material from saliva, shed epithelial cells, and micro-organisms which collect in the absence of good oral hygiene.

Matrix—A strip of material placed around a tooth to assist in the placement of a restoration.

Matrix retainer—A device designed to hold the matrix in proper position on a tooth.

Maxillofacial—Pertaining to the jaw and the face.

Median—Designating the plane which divides a part lengthwise into symmetrical halves.

Melting range—The range of temperature from that at which a substance begins to melt (solidus) to the temperature at which it is completely molten (liquidus).

Meniscus—A crescent-shaped body such as the interarticular cartilage in the temporomandibular joint. In liquid measures, it is the crescent-shaped surface of the liquid drawn so by surface tension.

Mesial surface—Surface of a tooth closest to the midline.

Metastasis—Transmission of disease from one organ or part to another by way of the blood vessels or lymph channels.

Methyl methacrylate—Acrylic resin. A synthetic resin which is used as the denture base material for dentures, and to a limited extent, as a restorative material.

Midline—An imaginary vertical line drawn between the central incisors.

Milliampere (abbreviation ma, mas = milliampere seconds)—One thousandth part of an ampere.

Mill-in (milling)—Refinement of the occlusion by removing interferences with an abrasive paste.

Modeling plastic—A thermoplastic material used for making impressions.

Modulus of elasticity—A measure of the elasticity of a substance in relation to the stress to which it is subjected.

Monomer—The acrylic resin liquid which is mixed with the acrylic resin powder (polymer).

Mottled enamel—Enamel with white flecks or blotches due to excessive fluoride; they may turn brown later.

Mounting—The attachment of dental casts to a mechanical articulator.

Mounting ring—Removable metal piece which attaches to either the upper or lower member of an articulator and to which the dental casts are fixed in mounting.

Mucobuccal fold—The area of folding of mucous membrane lining the vestibule, from lips and cheeks onto the alveolar bone. It forms the superior and inferior boundaries of the vestibule.

Mucous membrane—Moist, mucus secreting tissue which lines the oral cavity.

Mucus—The viscid secretion that covers mucous membranes. Mucin, a protein, is a constituent of mucus.

Mulling—The manual working of freshly mixed amalgam in a squeeze cloth or rubber dam to produce a smooth plastic mass.

Muscle tone—Slight state of contraction found in all healthy muscle.

Noble metal—A metal not readily oxidized at ordinary temperatures or on heating; for example, gold.

Nonanatomic teeth—Denture teeth which are designed in a manner which does not conform to the anatomy of natural teeth.

Oblique ridge—The diagonal ridge of enamel found only on the maxillary molars. It connects the mesiolingual cusp with the distofacial cusp.

Obtundant—A substance which deadens pain.

Occlusal—The biting, grinding, or chewing surfaces of molars and bicuspid teeth.

Occlusal balance—A relationship between opposing arches in occlusion in which there is contact between occluding units on both sides of the opposing arches.

Occlusal plane—The plane established by the incisal edges of the incisors and the occlusal surfaces of the bicuspid and molar teeth of the maxillae and mandible.

Occlusal surface—The chewing or grinding surface of a posterior tooth. Anterior teeth do not have occlusal surfaces.

Occlusion—The natural fitting together of the maxillary teeth with the mandibular teeth.

Occlusion rim former—A manufactured device used to form the wax into the usual shape for a complete denture occlusion rim.

Occlusion rims—Occluding surfaces built on temporary or permanent bases for making maxillomandibular relation records and for arranging teeth.

Odontalgia (dentalgia)—Toothache.

Ondontoma—A tumor derived from one or more parts of the tooth germ. It may be soft, calcified, or a mixture of both.

Ohm—A unit of electrical resistance.

Opacity—Inability to transmit light.

Overlay—A inlay or splint which fits over the biting or grinding surface of a tooth.

Palatal bar—The metal piece used to connect the right and the left side of maxillary partial denture. It is contoured to the palatal tissue.

Palatine—Adjective: referring to the roof of the mouth. Noun: the posterior bone which gives support to the palate.

Palpation—Using the fingers to feel the external surfaces of the body and structures beneath.

Papilla—A mound of tissue.

Papillae of tongue—Fingerlike elevations seen on mucous membrane of the tongue.

Papilloma—Stalked, wartlike tumor growth projecting from the surface of the skin or mucous membrane.

Papule—A small, circumscribed, solid elevation of the skin.

Path of insertion—The direction in which a removable partial denture is inserted upon and removed from the abutment teeth.

Pennyweight (DWT)—One twentieth part of a troy ounce; 24 grains equal 1 DWT.

Percussion—A method of diagnosis employing tapping over parts of the body or teeth.

Periapical—Around the apex or root tip.

Periapical radiography—The making of radiographic images of individual teeth so as to portray the root and surrounding area as well as the crowns of the teeth.

Pericoronitis—Inflammation of soft tissue around the crown of a partially erupted tooth. Usually around the crown of the mandibular third molar.

Pickling—Removal of surface oxidation of a gold alloy by heating in an acid or other pickling agent.

Pinledge—A thin cast inlay which depends, in part, for its retention on small parallel pins. The pins are cast into the inlay and fit into small holes prepared in the tooth.

Pit—A pointed depression in the surface of a tooth. Pits occur most often at points where several developmental lines meet as on the occlusal surface of molars. Pits are also found at the end of the facial (buccal) grooves of molars.

Plaster of paris—A white powder, calcium sulfate, formed by clacining gypsum which, when mixed with water, hardens on drying.

Plexus—A cluster or network of vessels or nerves.

Point angle—Angle made on a tooth by the convergence of three walls at a point.

Polymer—The powder of acrylic resin which is mixed with the acrylic resin liquid (monomer).

Polymerization—The reaction which takes place between the powder and liquid during the curing of acrylic resin.

Pontic—That part of a fixed partial denture which is suspended between the abutments and replaces a missing tooth or teeth.

Porcelain—A tooth-colored material consisting mainly of kaolin, feldspar, and flux. It is used in dentistry for inlays, jacket crowns, denture teeth, and in fixed partial dentures.

Posterior palatal seal (post dam)—The seal at the posterior border of a maxillary denture.

Precision attachment—Specially machined male and female parts used in partial dentures for attaching a prosthesis to an abutment tooth.

Pre-extraction record—Any record or records made for planning treatment before extraction of teeth.

Preliminary impression (snap impression)—An initial impression used to pour a cast upon which a tray is fabricated for making the final, more accurate impression.

Process—Any marked prominence; a projection or outgrowth from a larger structure, usually a bone.

Profile record—A registration or record of a patient's profile.

Prominence—An elevation or projection such as on the surface of a bone.

Proportional limit—The amount of stress a metal will stand before it is permanently stretched or bent. Proportional limit, elastic limit, yield strength, and yield point are terms which can be used interchangeably.

Prosthesis—Replacement of a part by artificial means.

Protrude—To project forward.

Protrusive occlusion (bite)—Contact relation of the maxillary and mandibular teeth when the mandible is brought forward as in biting a thread.

Proximal—That tooth or other surface, nearest to another tooth or surface, in the same arch or body.

Proximal surface—The surface of a tooth which lies next to another tooth. Nearly always the mesial or distal surface unless the tooth is rotated or the proximal teeth are missing.

Pulpotomy—The partial removal of the pulp of a tooth (usually the pulp chamber contents).

Pulp stones—Calcified bodies sometimes found in the pulp chamber and canals.

Pumice—Spongy, volcanic lava used as a polishing material in powder form.

Purulent—Consisting of, or containing pus; associated with the formation of, or caused by, pus.

Pustule—Small elevation of the outer skin layer filled with pus or lymph.

Radiation—The emission and spread of energy through space in the form of waves.

Radicular—Pertaining to the root of a tooth.

Radiograph—An image of tissues produced upon film by the passage of X-rays.

Radiographic image—The image seen on a dental radiograph.

Radiolucent—An area that appears dark on film indicating that the X-rays have passed through it easily. Examples are soft tissue, pulp, or an abscess.

Radiopaque—An area that appears light on a film; indicates that X-rays have not passed through it easily. Gold, enamel, metal, or bone produce radiopaque areas.

Rebasing—Refitting a denture by replacement of the denture base material without changing the occlusal relations of the teeth.

Reciprocal arm (bracing arm)—The ridge arm of a clasp so located on the tooth as to oppose any pressure exerted by the retentive arm. It acts to stabilize the prosthesis and resist lateral displacement.

Rectifier—A device by which alternating current can be changed to direct current.

Reducing flame—The part of the blow pipe flame which is least apt to cause oxidation of the metal when melting or soldering.

Refractory model or cast—A cast made from a heat-resistant material.

Registration—A record of desired jaw relations used to transfer the relations to an articulator.

Relief—Material added to a cast or scraped from an impression to relieve pressure over certain areas in the mouth.

Reline—Resurfacing of the tissue surface of a denture to improve its fit.

Removable partial denture—A removable prosthesis which replaces less than the full complement of teeth in one arch; can be removed by the patient.

Reservoir—A small bulb of wax attached to a sprue for the purpose of providing additional molten metal when a casting begins to soldify and shrink.

Resin—A group of organic substances, either natural plant products or artificially produced, used as a denture base material. In prosthetics, methyl methacrylate, referred to as acrylic resin.

Resorption—The gradual destruction or loss of tissue or other material by dissolution.

Rest—A metallic lug or projection of a removable partial denture which lies on the occlusal, incisal, or lingual surface of a tooth and resists vertical displacement of the prosthesis.

Restoration—Any artificial replacement of missing tooth structure, teeth, or other tissues.

Retainer—Any type of attachment applied directly to an abutment tooth to hold a prosthetic restoration in place.

Retention—Mechanical security against dislodgement or change of position.

Retrusion—Setting or pulling back.

Reversible hydrocolloid—An impression material made ready for use by heating and cooled within the mouth to set the material and gain the impression. Technically, this procedure may be repeated with the same batch of material by subsequent reheating, but sanitary considerations prohibit its reuse in the oral cavity.

Ridge—A linear elevation of enamel on the surface of a tooth; the area of the maxillae and mandible formerly occupied by the natural teeth.

Ridge lap—The part of an artificial tooth which normally overlaps the alveolar ridge.

Ring (casting ring)—A metal cylinder used to contain the pattern and confine the investment in cast gold work.

Rongeurs—Forceps used to remove bone.

Rouge (jeweler's rouge)—A red powder, usually prepared in cake form, used on a buff or chamois wheel to impart a high luster to metal or resin.

Rubber polishing cups—Small rubber cups used to polish teeth and restorations by rotary application of pumice or other polishing material.

Rugae—The elevated folds or wrinkles of soft tissue situated in the roof of the mouth just behind the maxillary anterior teeth.

Safeside disc—An abrasive disc having one smooth side to prevent damaging adjacent surfaces or structures.

Sagittal plane—Any vertical plane passing through the body parallel with the sagittal structure.

Saliva ejector—A mouthpiece used to remove saliva from the mouth by suction.

Sandpaper discs—Various-sized discs with different grits of sandpaper on their surface, used for smoothing and polishing teeth and finishing restorations.

Scale—To remove calculus from the teeth with special instruments.

Scalers—Instruments designed to remove calculus from the teeth.

Scratch brush—A wire brush or wheel used to remove debris from burs or files.

Semirigid broken-stress fixed partial denture—A fixed partial denture in which one of the connections between the units is composed of a male and a female joint which allows some movement instead of the usual rigid, immovable solder joint.

Separating medium—A coating applied to a surface to prevent another surface from adhering to it.

Septum—The bone between the roots of multrirooted teeth. A portion of hard or soft tissue.

Serious—Resembling, producing, or containing serum.

Serrated—Indented with many shallow crosscuts; toothed like a saw blade.

Setting expansion—The increase in dimension which takes place concurrently with the setting or hardening of certain materials such as plaster of paris.

Setting time—The time necessary to harden or solidify.

Setup—A broad term usually denoting a full maxillary and mandibular arrangement of denture teeth in wax.

Shank—That part of a dental instrument which connects the handle to the working part.

Shell crown—A metal cap designed to fit a prepared tooth (may reproduce the crown, and may be made of gold plate).

Soft palate—Flexible mass of soft tissue, posterior to the hard palate.

Solder—A fusible alloy used to unite two metallic edges or surfaces; the act of uniting two metals by the use of a fusible alloy.

Spatula—One of several flat, blunt, knifelike instruments used for spreading and mixing plaster, cement, silicate cement; mixing ointments and masses; or manipulating wax.

Splint—A prosthesis used for the fixation or support of displaced, fractured, or movable parts. In dentistry, splints are used to support loose teeth and to hold fractured jaw fragments in correct alignment during healing.

Spot grinding—The process of perfecting the occlusion of a restoration by marking premature contacts with carbon paper or other agent and removing the interferences with small stones.

Sprue—A cylinder of metal or wax which is attached to the wax pattern of an inlay, crown, or partial denture to form a passage into the mold after the pattern has been invested.

Sprue former—The base to which a sprue is attached while the wax pattern is being invested preparatory to casting.

Stone (abrasive)—Rotating cutting instruments in which diamond particles, carborundum, or other abrasive particles are incorporated.

Stone (dental)—Artificial stone. A nonporous form of calcined gypsum which is used to pour casts. Stone set more slowly and is denser and harder than plaster of paris.

Stress breaker (checker)—A device incorporated into a fixed or removable partial denture to reduce the stress on an abutment tooth.

Study cast—A plaster or stone duplication of oral tissues used for study and treatment planning.

Succedaneous teeth—Permanent teeth which replace deciduous teeth in the dental arch.

Sulcus (in a tooth)—A linear depression in the surface of a tooth, the slopes of which meet at an angle. A sulcus is always found along the surface of a developmental line.

Supernumerary tooth—An extra tooth; one more than the normal number.

Supplemental—An additional cusp, groove, or tooth.

Support—Resistance to vertical components of masticating (chewing) force.

Surgical template—A translucent acrylic resin base formed to duplicate the tissue-contacting portion of an immediate denture and used as a guide in surgically trimming the alveolar process to fit the immediate denture.

Surgical tray—*See* Surgical template.

Surveying—Establishing the path of insertion of a dental prosthesis by using a dental surveying instrument.

Surveyor—An instrument used to locate and mark the greatest circumference of one or several abutment teeth at a given tilt of the cast.

Swage (verb)—To shape a piece of metal between a die and a counterdie.

Syncope—Fainting caused by a marked decrease in blood supply to the brain.

Talc (soapstone)—French chalk. A mineral of fine particle size sometimes used as a separating medium in adapting baseplates on stone casts.

Tang—The connector between clasp body and the frame of a partial denture.

Tartar—Calculus.

T-clasp—A vertical projection-type removable partial denture clasp which is formed approximately in the shape of a T.

Tempering—The procedure of imparting a desired degree of hardness to a metal, also called heat hardening.

Tensile strength—A measure of resistance to breakage. The terms "ultimate strength," "ultimate tensile strength," or "strength" have practically the same meaning and may be used interchangeably.

Tetanus (lockjaw)—An acute infectious disease in which some of the voluntary muscles of mastication are in a constant state of contraction.

Thermal expansion—Increase in size following, and resulting from, an increase in temperature.

Thermoplastic—A material which can be made soft by the application of heat and which hardens upon cooling.

Thermosetting—Becoming set and unmoldable upon being subjected to heat.

Thrush (moniliasis)—A fungus infection of the oral mucosa occurring most in children and attended with the formation of white spots or patches.

Tissue-borne—A term used to describe a dental prosthesis which depends entirely upon the soft tissues and alveolar ridges for support.

Tooth-borne—A term used to describe a dental prosthesis or part of a prosthesis which depends entirely upon the abutment teeth for support.

Topical—To the surface or to a particular spot.

Torque—A twisting force.

Tragacanth—A gelatinous gum; in powder form sometimes used in dentistry to secure a baseplate in the mouth during try-in.

Transformer—A device by which low voltage can be stepped up to high voltage or high voltage stepped down to low voltage. Known as either a step-up or stepdown transformer.

Transillumination—Transmission of a strong light through anterior teeth and interproximal areas to facilitate oral diagnosis.

Translucent—Transmitting light, partially transparent.

Transverse ridge—Ridge formed by junction of two triangular ridges.

Traumatic occlusion—An abnormal biting force.

Trial packing—A series of closures and adjustments in the quantity of acrylic resin dough packed in a flask preliminary to final closure for curing.

Triangular ridge—The ridge of enamel which descends from the tip of a cusp to the central part of the occlusal surface of a bicuspid or molar.

Trifurcated–Having three roots.

Troy weight–The system of weights used for weighing gold.

Try-in–A preliminary insertion of a complete denture wax-up (trial denture) of a partial denture casting, or of a finished restoration.

Tubercle–A small eminence.

Tuberosity–A rounded swelling or projection. The maxillary tuberosity is the characteristically prominent area located at the distal end of the maxillary ridge.

U-Clasp–Roach-type clasp shaped like the letter U.

Undercut–In dentistry, an undercut is a tissue area so located or so angled in relation to surrounding tissue that it mechanically resists or prevents insertion or removal of restorations, impressions, or other material.

Undercut gage–A gage used with a surveyor to determine the amount of undercut present on a tooth for the correct positioning of clasp arm tips in the undercut.

Unilateral partial denture–A partial denture which is confined solely to one side of the mouth.

Unit–Each abutment restoration or pontic is considered a unit of a fixed partial denture. A fixed partial denture from first bicuspid to first molar supplying the second bicuspid would consist of three units.

Vault–The palate or roof of the mouth.

Vertical dimension–A vertical measurement of the face between any two conveniently located points, one above and one below the mouth, usually in the midline. These measurements are made with the teeth or occluding rims in centric occlusion or with the jaws in rest relation.

Vertical overbite (overbite)–A vertical overlap of the maxillary teeth over the mandibular teeth. Usually confined to anterior teeth.

Vestibule–That part of the oral cavity which lies between the teeth and gingivae, or residual ridges, and the lips and cheeks.

Vibrating line–An imaginary line marking the division between the movable and immovable tissues of the palate.

Vibrator–A mechanical device used to transmit vibrations and thus exclude air bubbles from a mix of plaster or stone during the pouring of investment material.

Vulcanite–A denture base material made of rubber cured or hardened by pressure and heat. Not widely used.

Wash–A corrective lining used in obtaining a final impression.

Waxing up–The contouring of a pattern in wax, usually referring to the shaping in wax of the contours of a trial denture.

Wax pattern–Wax which has been formed into the size and shape desired in a finished restoration, and which, when invested and burned out, produces a mold in which the casting is made.

Welding–Joining of metals by heat and pressure.

Whiting–Purified calcium carbonate used in polishing and as an antiflux.

Working model–A cast upon which laboratory work is accomplished.

Wrought wire–In dentistry, a gold alloy in wire form which is shaped by bending to the desired form.

Yield point, yield strength–The amount of stress a metal will stand before it is permanently stretched or bent. Proportional limit, elastic limit, yield strength, and yield point are terms which can be used interchangeably.

www.ingramcontent.com/pod-product-compliance
Lightning Source LLC
LaVergne TN
LVHW080015210926
848481LV00011B/3032